RECENT ADVANCES IN
ANÆSTHESIA AND ANALGESIA

RECENT ADVANCES IN ANÆSTHESIA AND ANALGESIA

NINTH EDITION

Edited by

C. LANGTON HEWER

M.B., B.S.(Lond.), M.R.C.P.(Lond.), F.F.A.R.C.S.

*Consulting Anæsthetist to St. Bartholomew's
Hospital and to the Hospital for Tropical Diseases,
London, etc.*

With 48 Illustrations

J. & A. CHURCHILL Ltd

104 GLOUCESTER PLACE, LONDON, W.1

1963

First Edition (C. L. H.)	.	.	1932
Second Edition	.	.	1937
Third Edition	.	.	1939
Fourth Edition	.	.	1943
Fifth Edition	.	.	1944
		Reprinted	1946
Sixth Edition	.	.	1948
Seventh Edition	.	.	1953
Eighth Edition (C. L. H. and A. Lee)			1957
		Reprinted	1958
Ninth Edition	.	.	1963

Printed in Great Britain

PREFACE TO NINTH EDITION

ADVANCES in anæsthesia and analgesia have become so rapid in recent years that the specialty is tending to become a group of sub-specialties. There are now two ways of presenting these advances in book form. The first is for the author to summarize all the new work which he considers sound and then to write a series of review articles giving the references of the papers which he has consulted. In my opinion, there are already too many books of this nature. They cannot be authoritative because one writer cannot possibly have sufficient knowledge of the whole field to give proper emphasis to all the various developments.

The alternative plan is for an editor to decide what aspects of the subject should be covered and then to ask anæsthetists who are actually working in the various sub-specialties to contribute articles embodying their own personal experience and opinions. This plan has been followed in this edition and I am most indebted to the ten contributors for their willing, and indeed enthusiastic, response. Dr. R. J. Hamer-Hodges unfortunately died before completing his chapter on Anæsthesia for Obstetrics, but Dr. M. E. Tunstall has very kindly finished and revised this section.

It should be clearly understood that no attempt has been made to cover the whole range of anæsthesia and analgesia. This is out of the question for a relatively small book and preference has been given to practical rather than theoretical advances. Contributors have been given a completely free hand and this has resulted in a little over-lapping; for example, cardiac resuscitation has been described twice, but from slightly different angles.

Although Dr. J. Alfred Lee has not taken part in the actual production of this edition, he has given me much helpful advice for which I am most grateful. The publishers have, as usual, solved the many difficult problems with speed and efficiency and for this I thank them.

C. LANGTON HEWER

LONDON

CONTENTS

CHAPTER 1

INHALATION ANÆSTHESIA

JAMES PARKHOUSE

General considerations — Apparatus — Drugs — Some Special Problems. (Emergency Procedures—Dental Anæsthesia—Anæsthesia and the Elderly Patient.)

GENERAL CONSIDERATIONS

ALTHOUGH it has been suggested[1] that the future of anæsthesia does not lie with the volatile agents, it is true at present that the introduction of drugs into the body by way of the respiratory passages has certain advantages.

Continuous administration can be achieved, using concentrations nicely adjusted to the requirements of the moment, without fear of the prolonged or unusual effects which are always possible when drugs metabolised in the body are given continuously by other routes. The anæsthetist cannot squeeze his patient's liver or kidneys to hasten the elimination of a drug, but he can do something like this to the lungs.

The uptake, distribution and elimination of inhalation anæsthetic agents have been studied both theoretically and experimentally for many years, and much early work is available for reference[2] concerning chloroform,[3-7] ether,[8-10] cyclopropane[11] and ethylene.[12] In particular, the classical work of Haggard on ether,[10] first published in 1924, has recently been reprinted.[13]

From the practical point of view, the development of a new method of estimating anæsthetic agents in a gas mixture or a biological fluid such as blood often gives the necessary impetus for clinical investigation. An example of this was the use of the mass spectrometer[14] for the study of the composition of anæsthetic gas mixtures,[15] and the measurement of blood concentrations of ether[16] and nitrous oxide.[17] Similarly the present success, in many fields, of gas chromatography has coincided with a revival of interest in the pharmacokinetics of general anæsthesia.[18, 19] Gas chromatography is a technique which may ultimately enable "on the spot" analysis to be made during anæsthesia, thus putting many theoretical calculations and clinical impressions to the test.

Three techniques may be used to study the pharmacokinetics of anæsthesia: (a) Samples may be taken from various parts of the venous system, or from an artery of the patient for analysis.[20] (b) Since the uptake and distribution of an inhalation agent obey physical laws relating to solubility, concentration gradient etc., simple or elaborate mathematical expressions may be derived from which the blood and tissue concentrations at any given time can be predicted. Studies of this kind date from the end of the last century,[10, 21-24] (c) The taking up of an agent by the body can be mimicked either by a large digital computer or a simple analogue computer in terms of electrical current, capacitance etc.[25-26]

Often, in the past, clinical studies were of limited value since the conditions of the "experiment" were not well standardized. Now that muscle relaxants are in use and quantitative apparatus is available, this difficulty need not arise. A "precision system",[27] incorporating a quantitative vaporizer, a respiration pump and a non-rebreathing valve, has been used for studying the metabolic effects of halothane,[28] the halothane-ether azeotrope[29] and chloroform,[30, 31] the general conclusion being that with adequate ventilation acid-base balance is not seriously disturbed by any anæsthetic agent. A similar system has been applied to the study of blood trichloroethylene concentrations during anæsthesia,[32] the findings showing a fair measure of agreement with calculated predictions.[33]

Consciousness. Since the traditional purpose of the inhalation agents is to secure a reversible state of unconsciousness, a few remarks concerning consciousness and unconsciousness may not be out of place. The importance of the brain stem reticular system in maintaining the alertness of the waking brain is now accepted.[34] In the absence of an intact reticular system the experimental animal, or the human patient, lapses into a coma from which he cannot be roused; the pertinence of the neurophysiological suggestion (long suspected by many laymen!) that sleep is the normal state of the organism thus becomes clear. The reticular system has a rich blood supply, and abounds in synapses, which are known to be preternaturally sensitive to the effects of anæsthetic agents,[35] so that whatever detailed theory of narcosis may ultimately prevail it is clear that depression of the reticular system must be an early and essential factor in the production of anæsthesia.

It is possible, however, not only to be asleep or awake, but half asleep and half awake. In like manner most attempts to define precisely when a patient is "conscious" and when he "becomes unconscious" are destined to failure; as the induction of anæsthesia proceeds, the probability that the patient will respond to a given stimulus or recall it later decreases. At some stage, for practical purposes, amnesia becomes complete—and what happens thereafter we cannot find out without the application of special psychological techniques, since the patient cannot tell us. Even during deep anæsthesia impulses continue to arrive at the sensory cortex;[36] the fact that they are not "consciously" perceived does not necessarily guarantee their psychological innocuity. Attempts have been made to uncover subconscious memories by hypnosis and other abreaction techniques, and it has even been suggested that by this means extensive recollection of events during anæsthesia is possible.[37] "Awareness" during surgery[38] has attracted more attention since use of the muscle relaxants has made very light anæsthesia practicable. It is probably more common at present than many anæsthetists would like to admit.[39]

Oxygen. When hypoxia occurs during the administration of ether or chloroform with air it results from respiratory obstruction or depression rather than from the reduced oxygen content of the inspired mixture.[45] Except with high concentrations of ether under an open mask,[41] this latter reduction is insignificant.

With endotracheal intubation and controlled respiration it should always be possible to maintain normal arterial oxygen saturation without resort to additional oxygen. Even during thoracic surgery Poppelbaum[42] experienced no difficulty unless respiration was interrupted. With ether, patients breathing spontaneously also maintain a good colour unless abdominal distension or position on the operating table interferes with respiratory movements.[40] Merrifield[43] concluded that under normal conditions oxygenation was usually satisfactory during spontaneous breathing with azeotrope/air anæsthesia, but he noted that assisted respiration was occasionally required. The findings of Ikezono[44] et al. were substantially the same for ether-air administration.

The rate at which arterial oxygen saturation falls during a period of apnœa was studied by Weitzner et al.[45] During apnœa after air breathing arterial oxygen saturation fell to undesirable levels after about one minute and "dangerous" levels after one and a half minutes; this contrasted with the period of at least two minutes of full saturation which could be relied upon after filling the lungs with oxygen. This is immediately obvious, during the use of ether-air anæsthesia with a muscle relaxant, to the anæsthetist who works single-handed and who is in the habit of leaving the bag unsqueezed while setting up a drip; to most clinicians cyanosis is apparent when arterial oxygen saturation has fallen to between 75 and 85%,[46] and at this stage P_{CO_2} will be approximately twice the normal.[47] Thus, if ventilation is resumed at this stage no serious harm is likely to result; happily we have become unused to seeing cyanosis in the anæsthetized patient and it is easy to exaggerate the dangers of *very brief* periods of hypoxia. In circumstances in which repeated interruptions of ventilation are necessary, e.g. for suction, the disadvantages of using air unenriched with oxygen are sufficiently obvious to require no further comment.

Carbon Dioxide. Several new methods of measurement have facilitated the study of carbon dioxide metabolism during inhalation anæsthesia. The CO_2 content of gas samples may be measured instantaneously by means of an infra-red analyser;[48] the tension of CO_2 in the blood may be measured either directly by means of an electrode,[49] or indirectly.[50, 51] The potentialities and limitations of these methods cannot be discussed here,[52, 53] but there is no doubt that they have enabled a wealth of data to be obtained with regard to anæsthesia and controlled respiration.

For some years anæsthetists have been obsessed by the danger of unsuspected carbon dioxide accumulation during anæsthesia, and in the curarized patient hyperventilation has become the rule. Recently, however, it has been suggested that, except with faulty technique or during thoracic surgery, CO_2 retention is seldom a serious hazard to the fit patient.[54] Remarkably few E.C.G. changes have been noted during the inhalation of 30 % CO_2 in man.[55]

It is well known that if the lungs of an experimental animal are filled with oxygen and connected to a source of pure oxygen full arterial saturation is maintained for 30–60 minutes in the complete absence of breathing.[56, 57] During this state of apnœic diffusion oxygenation CO_2 retention is a limiting factor. A similar state of affairs has been demonstrated during anæsthesia for bronchography.[58] An organic compound, T.H.A.M.,[59] has been described which buffers the effects of accumulated CO_2 and improves the survival of animals during apnœic diffusion respiration; the potential value of this in the anæsthetized patient remains to be seen.

Respiration. In contrast to the above mentioned view, even more vigorous hyperventilation has been advocated during nitrous oxide-oxygen anæsthesia;[60] very low P_{CO_2} levels have been reported and it has been claimed that electroencephalographic patterns resembling those of deep anæsthesia can be produced. This slow wave activity is probably similar in nature to that of sleep; the respiratory centre is part of the reticular system and it has been demonstrated that low blood CO_2 levels may remove some of the "drive" to the mid-brain reticular system just as they similarly affect the respiratory centre.[61] Hyperventilation should thus produce a deeper level of narcosis with any given concentration of nitrous oxide. It should be remembered, however, that CO_2 is itself a narcotic in high concentrations, and one recent study suggests that *more* nitrous oxide is required during hypocapnia.[62]

Extreme hyperventilation raises once more the question of whether the undoubted effects on conscious state are perhaps the result of cerebral hypoxia[63, 64] consequent upon the decreased blood flow known to occur.[65] Advocates of vigorous hyperventilation are at some pains to attempt a refutation of this suggestion,[66] but it is doubtful whether an E.E.G. pattern of large slow wave activity is anything more to be proud of than a constriction of the cerebral vessels; if anæsthesia requires to be deepened the reticular system must be depressed in some way, and if the patient comes to no harm the mechanism of this depression is mainly of academic interest.

The effect of *posture* on ventilation, during halothane anæsthesia, has been studied,[67] thus supplementing the work of Case and Stiles on the vital capacity of conscious subjects.[68] The lithotomy and prone positions appear to cause no significant change in ventilation; Trendelenburg, kidney and prone "jack knife" positions tend to reduce ventilation more than the lateral or reverse Trendelenburg. Raising the gall bladder rest reduces ventilation by 5–15%.

Actual respiration must always be related to respiratory requirement; Radford's nomogram[69] may be used to estimate this requirement according to body weight. During anæsthesia other factors must be taken into consideration, including the effect on dead space of face masks, endotracheal tubes and drugs which may alter bronchial calibre.[70] Nunn[71] has suggested a modification of the Radford nomogram for use during anæsthesia, and has shown that approximately 15% may be deducted from the requirement because of the lowering of metabolism, while approximately 15% should be added to allow for increased physiological dead space: the two factors thus conveniently cancel out. In the case of controlled ventilation physiological dead space may reach 50% of tidal volume with some forms of very rapid inflation.[72]

As far as the clinical anæsthetist is concerned one of the most important advances in connection with respiration is the development of compact measuring instruments such as the Wright respirometer[73] which make it possible to measure rather than guess the minute volume at any time.

Electroencephalography. Information relating to the E.E.G. during anæsthesia has been collected in a recent book.[74] Here may be found a description of the patterns characteristic of various depths of anæsthesia with all the commonly used inhalation agents. In practice the distinction between the several deeper planes is now of little value. As a means of guiding the curarized patient through the less well signposted region of light anæsthesia the E.E.G. has proved disappointing. Although Artusio has claimed to distinguish three E.E.G. "levels" during analgesia (the classical Stage 1 of Guedel) with ether,[75] it seems that expert interpretation is required, and the same changes are certainly not evident with analgesic concentrations of nitrous oxide.[76] Even during *anæsthesia* with nitrous oxide and muscle relaxants E.E.G.'s very similar to those of the conscious patient have been observed; there are, however, changes in response to photic stimulation which may prove applicable to clinical anæsthesia.[77]

Hypotension. Numerous techniques are now available for lowering the blood pressure; methonium compounds, trimetaphan and trophenium, halothane and "total" spinal block have all found advocates. The initial wave of enthusiasm for "controlled hypotension" has nevertheless paled, and there is at present fairly general agreement that many of the indications for a "bloodless field" are more imaginary than real.

In a survey of hypotensive anæsthesia in Great Britain, Hampton and Little[78] found a mortality of one in 500 cases and a morbidity of one in 38. As Gray[79] remarked, this represents an indictment which cannot be ignored. More recently, over 9,000 hypotensive anæsthetics have been reported from East Grinstead.[80] In this series there were four cases of cardiac arrest and several other complications possibly attributable to the technique, although most of these were avoidable. Linacre[81] reported 1,000 gynæcological operations performed with hypotensive anæsthesia without apparent increase in mortality or morbidity, and Rollason and Hough[82] found the same in the case of prostatectomy, although their series included only 40 hypotensive anæsthetics. Although it has been claimed that the flicker-fusion test often reveals transient impairment of cerebral function after induced hypotension[83] interpretation of this test requires caution.

It has been said that the young patient with a healthy cardiovascular system will withstand hypotension well, but it is by no means proven that old age constitutes a specific contraindication,[82] and even apparently healthy young patients may have coronary artery disease.[84, 85] Gray[79] suggested that when hypotension is essential to safeguard the life of the patient or make the operation possible, it should be combined with moderate hypothermia; many anæsthetists would regard this view as unnecessarily extreme. All are agreed that regardless of indications or technique full oxygenation and scrupulous avoidance of head-up tilt are essential.

Reflex Disturbances. There can be little doubt that reflexes have been "overplayed" in the past as a cause of mishaps for which an error on the part of the anæsthetist was responsible.[86] None the less it would be unreasonable to suppose that the multifarious autonomic disturbances to which the waking man is liable should magically disappear under the influence of a whiff of gas. During upper abdominal surgery, in particular, sweating, pallor, bradycardia and hypotension are commonly seen when the viscera are manipulated during very light anæsthesia. Loder again drew the attention of anæsthetists to this fact,[87] and advocated splanchnic block, combined with infiltration of the vagus for gastric surgery, in addition to light general anæsthesia and a muscle relaxant. Geddes and Gray[60] thought that vigorous hyperventilation might be responsible for a lower incidence of reflex disturbances in their cases, but this may have represented no more than the effect of something equivalent to the deepening of anæsthesia.

In support of Crile's[88] "anoci-association" theory, it would certainly seem to be true that the only way to ensure that operative stimuli do not reach the central nervous system is to block them peripherally. Argument centres chiefly around the belief that when such stimuli do reach the central nervous system the patient is less well if his ability to react is undepressed, than if he has no option but to lie mute and unresponsive.

APPARATUS

For various reasons it seems that the desirability of quantitative administration of anæsthetic agents, and indeed the whole problem of knowing exactly what the patient is breathing at any time during the anæsthetic, is at last assuming its full importance in the minds of anæsthetists. The breathing systems with which we have grown up, "closed" and "semi-closed", open drop and the various modifications of Ayre's T-piece, were not designed with this requirement in mind. The very terminology is confusing; the Magill attachment, when properly used, approximates to an open or non-rebreathing system, and is therefore most appropriately termed "semi-open".[89] "Semi-closed" should be used to refer to an absorption system with a gas flow in excess of the basal requirement and some spillage through a partly or intermittently opened expiratory valve.

As with the study of pharmacokinetics, there are three possible lines of investigation: (a) Gas samples may be taken during an actual anæsthetic.[90–94] (b) Theoretical expressions may be derived to explain the behaviour of the apparatus, so that it becomes possible to predict what should occur in clinical practice.[90, 91, 95–98] (c) Models may be constructed to simulate the performance of a live patient.[92, 93, 99, 100] Elucidation of the behaviour of apparatus in these three ways represents one of the main trends of thought during the last few years.

In contrast to this is the concept that knowledge of what the patient is breathing is best obtained not through the application of more and more complex mathematical formulæ and instruments of research to our traditional arrangements of apparatus, but through the revision of everyday methods in such a way as to eliminate as many causes of uncertainty as possible.[101] For practical purposes it is always possible to know the composition of the inspired mixture if known concentrations of the anæsthetic drug are admitted into a system in which there is no rebreathing. When suitable inhalers or vaporizers and valves are available this presents no difficulty, and thus there is much interest in quantitative apparatus and non-rebreathing valves: this may be regarded as the second main trend of thought concerning apparatus for inhalation anæsthesia at the present time.

Theoretical Work

Mapleson[95–97] derived mathematical expressions from which certain practical recommendations can be made for several anæsthetic systems. With the Magill attachment he calculated that a fresh gas flow equal to the patient's minute volume should ensure that no significant amount of rebreathing takes place. Molyneux and Pask[90] as a result of both calculations and measurements in the operating theatre, were not prepared to commit themselves to any such simple relationship. Sykes[93] showed that the Magill attachment is very inefficient when used for controlled ventilation, the apparatus dead space being as much as 400 ml at tidal volumes commonly used for adult patients.

For the T-piece arrangement Mapleson concluded that a fresh gas flow equal to twice the minute volume would prevent rebreathing regardless of the length of the reservoir tube. A more searching mathematical treatment of the T-piece from Japan[98] reached the conclusion that a higher fresh gas flow would be necessary. Woolmer and Lind,[99] and Inkster[100] had previously studied the performance of the T-piece in models in which a mechanical pump imitated the breathing of a patient; their findings showed a fair measure of agreement with Mapleson's calculations.

In all these studies a great deal of over-simplification is required in order to achieve a reasonable basis for calculation; many assumptions are made[96] and the anæsthetist should hesitate before regarding the conclusions as being directly applicable to the anæsthetized patient. One point to be observed is that nearly all the recommendations that are made assume that the anæsthetist knows his patient's minute volume—a practical difficulty noted by Molyneux and Pask.[90] Even if the respiration is measurable and fairly constant, and even now that high flow oxygen rotameters are commonly available, it is not always possible to meter enough gas to supply a hyperventilating patient with twice his minute volume.

Foldes et al.[91] made simple calculations from which they were able to produce tables relating fresh gas flow to inspired nitrous oxide concentration using a circle system. For the same type of system Gray[94] stressed the importance of using high gas flows and adequate nitrous oxide concentrations initially to achieve effective levels of nitrous oxide in the blood without undue delay. Mapleson and his colleagues have also studied circle systems,[92, 97, 102] but they were principally interested in the behaviour of vaporizers placed either inside the circuit (V.I.C.) or in the fresh gas supply line leading to the circuit (V.O.C.). This is of importance with regard to the use of halothane, the cost of which makes a non-rebreathing system impracticable in most circumstances unless very low concentrations are used with muscle relaxants. Mapleson and his colleagues dispelled some bizarre notions about the build-up in concentration of halothane, or its disappearance, when such arrangements are used.

With both V.I.C. and V.O.C. arrangements, increase in the vaporizer concentration control setting leads to a rise in concentration of the volatile agent in the circuit. If the fresh gas flow is increased, the concentration setting remaining constant, vapour concentration falls with the V.I.C. arrangement and rises with the V.O.C. arrangement. With the V.I.C. arrangement an increase in the patient's ventilation leads to an increase in the inspired vapour concentration; with the V.O.C. system inspired concentration may fall but the more efficient alveolar ventilation resulting from increased tidal volume may cause the alveolar vapour concentration, and thus the depth of anæsthesia, to increase.[92] The effect of changes in pulmonary ventilation constitutes one of the main distinctions between the V.I.C. and V.O.C. arrangements, since if the vaporizer is inside the circuit movement of gases over the surface of the liquid agent, and hence vapour concentration, is dependent on respiratory activity. This has been said to constitute a built in safety factor if respiration becomes depressed, but it is also a potentially dangerous feature if the anæsthetist begins to assist respiration without altering the vaporizer control setting. There can be no doubt that use of a calibrated vaporizer *outside* the circuit is less liable to lead the anæsthetist into difficulties.[102] In practice, a clear distinction must always be made between the concentration control setting of a vaporizer and the vapour concentration actually inhaled by the patient.

Quantitative Apparatus

The E.M.O. inhaler, since its introduction in 1956,[103] has come to be used in all parts of the world; together with the Oxford Inflating Bellows,[104] by means of which the patient's lungs can be ventilated at any time, it enables a high standard of anæsthesia to be provided for any kind of surgical procedure in complete independence of gas cylinders and supplies of expensive drugs.[105, 106] There are still a great many countries in which nitrous oxide is expensive or even unobtainable, soda-lime is scarce and poor in quality and even cylinders of oxygen are obtained from overseas. To bring the advantages of modern anæsthesia to practitioners in these countries is surely one of the most important "Recent Advances" in the specialty.[107] From the United States, Hingson,[108] after visiting many countries, lends support to this view.

The E.M.O. apparatus is essentially an *inhaler*, rather than a vaporizer—although it will deliver quite accurate concentrations of ether when a constant flow of gases passes through it, its real purpose is as a draw-over apparatus for administering ether-air mixtures. With this in mind the E.M.O. is designed to offer a very low resistance to breathing, and internal compensation mechanisms ensure a constant concentration of ether despite considerable variations in flowrate pattern. A less accurate ether-air apparatus is marketed by Drager, and the E.M.O. has also been copied in the U.S.S.R. Nandrup[109] has described a mechanically driven vaporizer for delivering ether-air mixtures. E.M.O. inhalers are also made for halothane and other liquid agents.

As an alternative to the standard Oxford Inflating Bellows, Poppelbaum[42] uses an ingenious "double bellows": when the bellows is expanded air is drawn from the atmosphere into an outer compartment while simultaneously expired gas is sucked from the patient's lungs into a separate inner compartment. When the bellows is compressed the patient's lungs are inflated with fresh air from the outer compartment while the contents of the inner compartment are discharged to the atmosphere. This apparatus is of considerable interest as a *manual* method of applying a negative phase during expiration. The Ambu bag[110] may also be used with the E.M.O. as an alternative to the Oxford Inflating Bellows.[111]

For the quantitative administration of halothane the Fluotec vaporizer is also available.[112] This is not intended as a draw-over apparatus—resistance to breathing is rather high and performance is best with a constant stream of gas passing through. These limitations, however, permit a great saving in bulk and weight and the Fluotec has become justifiably popular as an addition to the Boyle apparatus. When low flows of gas are used to vaporize halothane from a Fluotec —less than 2 L/min—a calibration chart should be consulted; with the mark II apparatus the concentrations delivered are considerably *higher* than the dial setting in these circumstances. Similar vaporizers are available for other agents—the Azeotec, Chlorotec and Tritec.

An alternative approach to the problem of "quantitative" administration has gained considerable popularity in the United States since the original descripton by Lucien Morris of the "Copper Kettle".[113] This is a vaporizer made of copper, the very high thermal conductivity of which provides considerable temperature stability during vaporization, particularly if the table top of the anæsthetic machine is also made of copper. In the case of ether, the gases leaving the "kettle" are 50–60% saturated with vapour.[114]

In Germany a compact halothane analyser has been devised which can be incorporated in a circle system;[115] the concentration of halothane in the circuit is thus "monitored" constantly, and the introduction of more halothane is automatically regulated by the "Narkostat" to maintain the concentration within the circuit at the vaporizer control setting. If this apparatus were to prove reliable in practice and sufficiently rapid in response, it would have a wide appeal.

Circuit Arrangements

Few basic changes have been made in recent years in the general design of circle absorber systems. In the United States there has been a tendency to adopt much larger soda-lime canisters, sometimes with several compartments, so that fresh soda-lime can be brought into use by simply rotating the container. Transparent canisters are available for use with coloured soda-lime. These are misleading, however, since channelling of gases may cause the central core of soda-lime to become exhausted while the visible outer layer remains coloured. In a to-and-fro system the size of the soda-lime canister is important in relation to the tidal volume of the patient; in a circle system this is less important from the point of view of efficiency, but some large canisters offer considerable resistance to breathing, especially with poor quality soda-lime. Miniature circle systems are in use in the United States for pædiatric anæsthesia.

The high cost of halothane has tempted many anæsthetists to use this agent in a "closed" system, or at least with a relatively small flowrate of fresh gases. The introduction of a calibrated vaporizer into the fresh gas line has been advocated by some workers,[116] while others use a vaporizing bottle within the circuit.[117] The behaviour of these two arrangements, V.O.C. and V.I.C., has been discussed above.

Portable Apparatus

Apart from the E.M.O. inhaler, portable apparatus has been designed with several purposes in mind, and along several lines.

In 1954 Hingson[118] suggested the use of a simple portable apparatus utilizing "Sparklet" cylinders to deliver mixtures of oxygen and cyclopropane, oxygen, cyclopropane and nitrogen, or nitrous oxide and oxygen. From this was developed the Western Reserve Midget machine which delivers a non-flammable mixture of oxygen, cyclopropane and helium into a 6 l bag. A miniature soda-lime canister is provided and also a nipple for attaching an oxygen supply, if available, for more prolonged anæsthesia. A similar apparatus designed in this country[119] was advocated as an alternative to nitrous oxide-oxygen anæsthesia for dental work. A third version of the same principle has now appeared in the form of the C.O.N. (cyclopropane-oxygen-nitrogen) apparatus.[120] This has been developed for the handling of large numbers of casualties by the armed forces; a double-ended sparklet discharges (simultaneously) oxygen and nitrogen from one end and nitrogen and cyclopropane from the other into a reservoir bag. The final mixture consists of oxygen 30%, nitrogen 30% and cyclopropane 40%. A miniature soda-lime canister is again provided, to fit between the bag and the face mask, and it is claimed that in an adult anæsthesia may be maintained for three minutes before the patient's oxygen consumption reduces the inspired oxygen concentration below 20%. The mask can then be removed, and satisfactory operating conditions may be expected for a further two minutes. Should longer anæsthesia be required the bag must be re-charged from a fresh sparklet. There are no controls to be adjusted and the administrator need do nothing other than maintain a clear airway and hold the mask on the patient's face; induction is extremely rapid and serious trouble is unlikely to be encountered even by an inexperienced administrator. Attractive as this apparatus may be in theory, it is clear that in the desperate conditions envisaged a high mortality would have to be accepted—and one is tempted to wonder how much worse off one would be with a bottle of chloroform and an open mask.

A portable, quantitative chloroform apparatus—the E.S.O.[121]—was made available for paratroops during the last war. Recently, halothane has been exploited in the same way, originally with the intention of equipping antarctic expeditions.[122] Induction is rapid and smooth and with known concentrations (from a Fluotec vaporizer) serious complications are unlikely. Respiratory depression may necessitate either assisted breathing or enrichment of the atmosphere with oxygen; Nunn takes the view that the latter alternative is preferable for the novice, and his apparatus incorporates a supply of oxygen which entrains air so that the patient breathes an oxygen concentration of 30%.

Non-rebreathing Valves[123, 124]

Although a number of non-rebreathing valves have been available in the United States for some years, especially for pædiatric use,[125-128] these were intended for the spontaneously breathing patient. The Oxford vaporizer incorporated a valve for the same purpose;[129] with a draw-over arrangement such a valve is essential to prevent rebreathing. With a "plenum" system rebreathing can be prevented, or reduced to negligible proportions, by appropriate adjustment of the fresh gas flow and use of an expiratory valve. In practice, the advantages of children's non-rebreathing valves are more than outweighed by the large dead space between the functioning part of the valve and the little patient.

In contemporary anæsthetic practice emphasis has shifted towards controlled respiration, and for this a different type of non-rebreathing valve is required—more appropriately described as an inflating valve.[130] Such a valve offers obvious advantages: soda-lime can be dispensed with and quantitative administration of volatile agents becomes possible without elaborate monitoring equipment or difficult calculations.

The Ruben valve[131] is representative of the dual purpose type of valve which may be used to ensure non-rebreathing during spontaneous or controlled respiration. Originally devised for use with the Ambu bag, in conditions in which either resuscitation or anæsthesia is required without other equipment being at hand, the Ruben valve has now found favour in many parts of the world. It is expensive, difficult to sterilize, and less robust than an all-metal valve, but despite these disadvantages it is one of the most satisfactory dual-purpose valves available at the moment. Alternative designs have been described by Sykes.[132]

It must always be remembered that a Ruben valve may stick during spontaneous breathing without giving audible evidence of this fault. When substituted for an expiratory valve with the Magill attachment, the total fresh gas flow must be adjusted to equal the

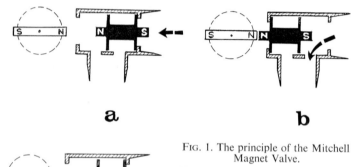

a   **b**

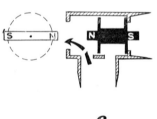

Fig. 1. The principle of the Mitchell Magnet Valve.

(a) The shuttle is repelled by the like pole of the magnet.

(b) Inflation pressure pushes the shuttle across, closing the expiratory port and allowing gas to flow into the lungs.

(c) When inflation ceases the shuttle is again repelled so that rebreathing is prevented and expired gases pass into the atmosphere.

c

patient's minute volume. This, incidentally, affords a convenient index of the adequacy of spontaneous respiration. If the patient's minute volume exceeds the gas supply the reservoir bag empties; if the gas supply is excessive the reservoir bag distends, and this predisposes to "sticking" of the valve, especially if it contains condensation from the expired air. "Sticking" is less likely with a draw-over arrangement than when a stream of gas provides a *vis a tergo*. Another danger is that free movement of the expiratory pin of the Ruben valve may be prevented by the pressure of a towel or a surgeon's hand. For these reasons the valve should not be covered by surgical towels, especially when the patient is breathing spontaneously.

A simple, sturdy and reliable inflating valve has been designed by

Mitchell.[133] This is an all-metal valve which may be boiled or auto-claved; it is actuated by a magnet (Fig. 1).

Apparatus for Pædiatric Anæsthesia

There is still no really suitable valve for babies and small children; elimination of carbon dioxide is still best achieved by the open method or the T-piece during spontaneous breathing, and by a modification of the T-piece or by intermittent occlusion of an endotracheal connector during controlled respiration.[134, 135]

Although small size circle systems enjoy a certain vogue in the United States they have not found favour in this country. Similarly, infant and child size Waters' canisters are less used than formerly. A small size Oxford Inflating Bellows for children has been described.[135]

During the last few years the influence of Rees and his colleagues [134, 136] has spread widely, and for controlled respiration in small children and babies some version of his modified T-piece is now usually employed. It has the great merits of simplicity and reliability; its component parts can be found in almost any anæsthetic room and it can be used with any gas machine. Its behaviour has no more been worked out in scientific terms than that of the original T-piece itself, but in practice it works admirably.

DRUGS

Even among simple organic compounds of a few types, for example ethers and halogenated hydrocarbons, large numbers of potential anæsthetic agents are to be found. A great many of these compounds have now been investigated; Krantz[137, 138] and his colleagues, for example, have studied various ethers systematically during the last two decades, including several compounds which subsequently came to be used clinically—methyl-n-propyl ether,[139] ethyl vinyl ether[140] and trifluoroethyl vinyl ether (Fluoromar).[141, 142]

Since the establishment of a Medical Research Council Committee, interest has centred on non-explosive agents; in particular a number of fluorinated compounds have been studied. Many such compounds have been prepared by Stacey who as long ago as 1948 referred to the chemical inertness and non-flammability of fluorinated organic compounds.[143] Robbins[144] studied the anæsthetic activity of a series of fluorinated hydrocarbons in 1946, without using them in man. Halothane was introduced in 1956[145, 146] and methoxyflurane in 1960.[147]

Artusio and Van Poznak[148] tested several fluorinated hydrocarbons and ethers in dogs, and Burns and his colleagues have published a series of reports on their current investigations of a group of halogenated hydrocarbons,[143] of hexafluorobenzene,[149] difluorotrichloroethane and four fluorinated ethers.[150] Of these difluorotrichloroethane is regarded as worthy of further study. The very similar compound trifluoro-dichloroethane (substance C) was reported on more fully by Burn, Epstein and Goodford;[151] it is a satisfactory anæsthetic in animals with circulatory effects rather similar to those of halothane. It has not been used in man.

Halothane

Halothane (trifluoro, chloro-bromo ethane) has been in clinical use since 1956[152, 153] and so much information is now available concerning its properties and effects[154] that a comprehensive review of the literature cannot be attempted here. Generally speaking it is a highly potent volatile agent capable of producing respiratory and circulatory depression but apparently without serious effect on the liver or other organs;[155] non-flammable, non-irritant, stable in the presence of soda-lime and not appreciably metabolized in the body.[156] It is the most expensive general anæsthetic agent in use.

Halothane anæsthesia is characterised by smooth induction, bronchodilatation, absence of salivation and laryngeal irritability, vasodilatation and hypotension proportional to the concentration administered. Recovery is rapid by the standards usually applied to a volatile liquid agent, but analgesia is poor and awakening is often marked by a period of characteristic shivering.[157] Cardiac arryhthmias are less common than with chloroform[158] but adrenaline should be used with great care.

Dispute continues as to the exact mechanism of hypotension during halothane anæsthesia—a dispute not helped by the margin of error that must be accepted for all methods of measuring cardiac output during anæsthesia. Vasodilatation and myocardial depression no doubt both play a part in the production of hypotension.

Some clinical reports extol the virtues of halothane as the sole agent for practically all types of surgical procedure,[159] even claiming that muscle relaxants are not necessary. Probably fewer anæsthetists see halothane as the herald of a new era than in the humbler role of a useful supplement to nitrous oxide, particularly for minor procedures. There is no doubt that for out-patient and dental work[160] halothane, carefully given, has much to offer. For the anæsthetist who has not been uniformly successful with the use of muscle relaxants in infants, halothane provides a very successful, non-flammable alternative to ether, especially for intrathoracic work.

Halothane offers certain advantages which must be weighed against its cost. It is a good drug but not a magical one; no doubt it will prove as successful in the hands of those who learn to use it skilfully as other drugs have done in the past.

Halothane-ether Azeotrope

Sometimes when two liquids are mixed together in a certain proportion, the resulting mixture is found to have a boiling-point, at constant pressure, which does not alter during vaporization. Thus, the composition of the mixture remains constant. The boiling-point of such a mixture, which is called an azeotrope, is either lower or higher than that of either component. In the latter case, as with the halothane-ether azeotrope, the mixture is "self-correcting"—when the components are mixed in a proportion not exactly equal to that of the azeotrope, evaporation alters the composition of the mixture so that it approaches, from either direction, the azeotropic mixture. The halothane di-ethyl ether azeotrope contains approximately two thirds halothane; the *exact* proportions in which the agents are mixed is unimportant.

The first clinical reports of the use of the azeotropic mixture appeared in 1958.[161] It has many of the characteristics of halothane, but analgesia is better, shivering is not seen, and for a given depth of anæsthesia circulatory[29] and respiratory depression are somewhat lessened. Under conditions of clinical use the limits of flammability of the mixture are not reached.[162]

Theoretical criticism has been levelled at the mixture[163] on the ground that ether depends for its safety upon the effects of sympathetic stimulation,[164] which should be rendered impossible by the autonomic effects of halothane. In practice the azeotrope has proved capable of providing excellent anæsthesia for a wide variety of poor risk cases.[165]

Methoxyflurane (Penthrane)

This is a halogenated ether, 2,2-dichloro-1, 1-difluoroethyl methyl ether. It is an interesting compound for several reasons: although its boiling point (105°C) is above that of water, so that the vapour pressure at room temperature is unusually low, its potency is such that open drop anæsthesia can be achieved. Again, although an ether, the compound can probably be regarded as non-flammable, for practical purposes, at room temperature.[166] The drug is stable in the presence of soda-lime; it is stored in dark bottles and dibenzylamine is added to prevent the formation of acid breakdown products.

Artusio et al.[167] reported a series of 100 patients anæsthetized with methoxyflurane, using circle, semi-closed and open drop methods. They described smooth induction and maintenance, with no increase in mucous or salivary secretion. The agent was stated to provide good muscular relaxation during deeper levels of anæsthesia and even then hypotension was not significant although some respiratory depression occured. Alternatively, during light anæsthesia, muscle relaxants could be used with impunity. With overdosage the blood pressure fell to 80–90 mm Hg systolic, and this was taken as an indication for immediate reduction of the inspired concentration. Cardiac rhythm remained stable, and in the dog adrenaline was injected without mishap. In a subsequent study, Bamforth et al.[168] have shown in dogs that the dose of adrenaline needed to induce ventricular tachycardia during methoxyflurane anæsthesia is similar to that needed during chloroform anæsthesia and more than is needed under cyclopropane.

Dobkin and Fedoruk[169] compared 1.0% methoxyflurane with 2.0% halothane in dogs, and noted that the halothane caused less respiratory depression but greater depression of blood pressure and cardiac output. The metabolic effects of the two drugs were similar.

All workers have noted relatively slow recovery after methoxyflurane anæsthesia, with a tendency to prolonged postoperative amnesia and analgesia. "Hangover", in the form of dizziness, may persist for 48 hours, and this may well limit the appeal of an otherwise promising agent. The slow recovery has been attributed to the high fat solubility of the drug, although the very same property has been invoked as an explanation of the rapid recovery observed after halothane anæsthesia.

New Work on Old Drugs

A few years ago Dundee remarked that it may seem strange to include nitrous oxide in a text devoted to "recent advances."[170] The same might be said of diethyl ether. These, the first two agents to be used for general anæsthesia, have stood the test of time for well over a hundred years and have a secure place in present day practice. Regardless of what current or future laboratory researches may reveal, it is unlikely that the clinical anæsthetist will be much impressed by any alleged dangerous properties of either drug.

There is no question that nitrous oxide has come into its own since the introduction of the muscle relaxants. Too weak to be toxic, this agent is as near to being harmless as anything can be when used with adequate oxygen. Its only disadvantages are the need for cylinders and flowmeters, and the danger of "awareness" on the part of the patient if more than about 35% of oxygen is used.

Ether has been used by Artusio[171] to provide analgesia for major thoracic surgery. Slightly higher concentrations, 3–4%, may be used in conjunction with curare to provide a level of anæsthesia comparable to that of 65% nitrous oxide.[105] Ether-air mixtures will burn, but not explode,[172] and it is worth recalling that there is no instance on record of an ether-air mixture causing serious harm to a patient on account of an explosion.[173]

Work an analgesia, similar to that of Artusio, has been reported with nitrous oxide,[174] and with cyclopropane.[175]

Trichlorethylene, despite continued use in clinical anæsthesia, remains a little studied agent. It has been known for years that this drug is metabolized in the body to some extent; the German chemist Liebreich suggested in 1869[176] that both chloral hydrate and the salts of trichloracetic acid form chloroform in the body, although there has never been the slightest evidence for this belief. It is possible, however, that some of the prolonged drowsiness occasioned by exposure to trichlorethylene may be attributable to production of chloral hydrate, a circumstance to which further reference will be made.

Trichloracetic acid is a known metabolite of trichlorethylene, and this substance was shown by Liebreich to cause narcosis. Joan Powell, in 1945, administered sodium trichloracetate to human subjects and noted no toxic effects,[177] although marked drowsiness occured.[178]

Some recent work from Czechoslovakia[179] throws possible new light on this problem. This work is relevant to the problem of industrial trichlorethylene poisoning, and concerns exposure to considerably lower concentrations than are used clinically. In these circumstances 50–70% of the inhaled trichlorethylene was retained (i.e., metabolized) in the body. In addition to trichloracetic acid two other metabolites were identified:—monochloracetic acid, a toxic substance which occurred only in small amounts, and trichloroethanol which was found in large amounts. This last substance was also found by Butler[180] in the urine of dogs anæsthetised with trichlorethylene. Trichlorethanol closely resembles "Avertin"—tribromoethanol—so that yet another possible reason for prolonged drowsiness is revealed.

Finally, reference should be made to the interesting observation that Disulfiram, which is known to inhibit the metabolism of alcohol

at the aldehyde stage, can also inhibit the breakdown of trichlorethylene, perhaps at a comparable stage, resulting in the accummu-
lation of chloral in the body. Administration of glucose and insulin,
on the other hand, increases the quantity of excreted metabolites.[181]

SOME SPECIAL PROBLEMS

Emergency Procedures

The dangers associated with vomiting and regurgitation continue
to dominate all discussions on the management of these cases.
Vomiting, long known to occur in the second stage, has been regarded by may anæsthetists as a complication of anæsthesia in which
the patient breathes spontaneously, while regurgitation has often
been thought of as a complication peculiar to cases in which muscle
relaxants are used. That regurgitation may occur when these drugs
are administered has been recognized since Gray and Halton's report
in 1948.[182] However, until the mechanism of œsophageal reflux is
further elucidated it would be unwise to assume that this distinction
is so clear cut, and the possibility of regurgitation should always be
borne in mind even in the patient who is breathing spontaneously.

Dinnick[183] has performed a valuable service by drawing the
attention of anæsthetists to the implications of some recent work on
hiatus hernia. Allison[184] distinguished between the "sliding" and
"rolling" types of hiatus hernia, pointing out that in the former the
normal angulation between the œsophagus and stomach disappears
so that regurgitation is likely to occur. Routine use of the head-down
position during barium swallow radiography has disclosed a hitherto
unsuspectedly high incidence of such reflux, especially during the
later months of pregnancy, and subsequent work has shown, not
unexpectedly, that artificial raising of the intra-abdominal pressure
increases the incidence of regurgitation.[185] The significance of this
in acute intestinal obstruction and obstetrical anæsthesia should be
sufficiently obvious.

The importance of the normal angle between the œsophagus and
the stomach was further demonstrated during laparotomy under
general anæsthesia by Greenan,[186] who showed that when the
stomach was pushed upwards and to the left much greater intra-
gastric pressures were needed to cause reflux that when it was pulled
downwards, in which position the cardio-œsophageal angle is reduced.

Probably at least four factors contribute to the normal prevention
of reflux:[187]

(1) A smooth muscle sphincter.[188]

(2) A pinch-cock action of the sling formed by the right crus of the diaphragm.[189]

(3) The cardio-œsophageal angle.[190]

(4) A plug-like action of the mucosal folds in the region of the cardia.[191]

Recently, interest has been aroused by the suggestion of Creamer et al.[192] that the œsophagus behaves as a flaccid tube running from a region of low pressure (i.e. the thorax) to a region of higher pressure (i.e. the abdomen). The pressure on the wall of the intra-abdominal œsophagus causes it to collapse as a "flap valve"; any increase in the difference between the pressures within the abdominal and thoracic cavities, as for example during deep inspiration, would accentuate this closing effect. Although this explanation is attractive, it has aptly been said that "the mystery of the anti-reflux mechanism has been seemingly solved so many times that new hypotheses may reasonably be regarded with scepticism."[193]

With regard to the prevention of complications due to aspiration, there are still several schools of thought, ranging from rapid inhalation induction in the left lateral or head down position (much used for such cases as the "bleeding tonsil") to rapid intubation under suxamethonium in the steep head up position.[194, 195] Enthusiasm for the latter technique depends on the belief that there will not be sufficient positive pressure in the stomach to force its contents steeply uphill if the cardiac "sphincter" relaxes. Even with a steep head-up tilt, however, there is much to be said for passing a stomach tube if not to empty the stomach at least to take off the head of pressure. The fact that such a tube is more likely to render the cardia incompetent should be of no consequence if the principle of the method is sound. Also, the possibility of sudden vomiting after thiopentone, before even suxamethonium has had time to act,[196] should be remembered; administration of a minimal amount of an inhalation agent, to ensure that there will be no memory of the intubation, followed by the rapid injection of a full dose of suxamethonium, is the most logical method of induction if the head up tilt is to be used. The mask should be removed from the patient's face as soon as the relaxant begins to take effect—any attempt to inflate the lungs may raise the intra-gastric pressure sufficiently to cause disaster and the continued presence of the mask will conceal the appearance of gastric contents.

The above remarks should not be interpreted as representing unqualified enthusiasm for the head up position. They are intended as an indication of the most sensible way in which to apply a potentially dangerous technique. Should the head up position prove to be safe—and the evidence is as yet unconvincing—it would rank as one of the really great advances. A major cause of death and postoperative complications would be removed and it would, logically, become possible to anæsthetise any patient regardless of the time of his last meal.

Gastric and œsphageal balloons have been described,[197] but have apparently gained little popularity. Sellick[198] has recently suggested backward pressure on the cricoid as being a reliable means of preventing regurgitation; this may well be a promising suggestion as long as the pressure is applied by a well-instructed assistant. Intubation under topical analgesia is too little practised; unless the anæsthetist has taken trouble to acquire the necessary technique, as few now do, it can be distressing for the patient. When acute intestinal obstruction occurs in a very poor risk patient, especially with chronic respiratory disease, tracheostomy should be performed unhesitatingly.[199]

In assessing the relative merits of the several possible techniques so many factors of unknown significance are encountered that scientific judgment is impossible. Not all patients with full stomachs either vomit or regurgitate during induction; not all patients with incompetent cardias have symptoms. Accidents have occurred with every technique, and no doubt the advocates of each can always find reason for blaming the anæsthetist rather than the method. If competent help is available and all necessary equipment is assembled and tested in advance it is unlikely that the patient will come to much harm. All too often fatalities occur when a junior anæsthetist is alone in the middle of the night, diffident about causing delay by sending for help, reluctant to complain about the lithotomy position, the non-tilting trolley, the absent suction apparatus or the non-urgent nature of the operation.

It is all to the good that anæsthetists now realize so well that a patient's stomach does not invariably empty in four hours. We should beware, however, of a reactionary tendency to believe that since the stomach *may* still contain food after eight, or even twelve hours, there is no point in waiting at all. A sense of proportion should be preserved; as the hours pass the likelihood of vomiting declines.

Dental Anæsthesia

Klock,[200, 201] in America, and Tom[202, 203] in this country, made a useful contribution by pointing out that nitrous oxide can often be used with more than the traditional low concentration of oxygen for dental anæsthesia in the chair. It nevertheless remains true that much of the dental anæsthesia practised in this country carries at least a risk—and at worst much more than a risk—of anoxia. It may be argued that such episodes are brief, and experienced administrators have laid claim to many thousands of "dental gases" without untoward incident. Indeed, dental "gases "are given in such great numbers that to many anæsthetists it seems quite inconceivable that they should be causing significant harm without this occasioning a public outcry.

Such clinical views may command sympathy, if not respect, but they do not alter the fact that it should be unnecessary, at the present time, to use anoxia as an aid to anæsthesia. Many anæsthetists can recall at least one fatality known to them; perhaps the patient was "unsuitable" on account of ischæmic heart disease; perhaps the administrator was foolish or the dentist insistent, but in any event a life was lost unnecessarily for the sake of the most trivial of operative procedures.

Supplementary agents such as thiopentone, trichloroethylene and halothane, or cyclopropane-oxygen-nitrogen mixtures may be used, but the real answer to the problem of dental anæsthesia lies not in this direction so much as through the inculcation of a fresh attitude to the whole matter. It is still regrettably often true that the qualities of a "good" dental anæsthetist are merely ability to induce anæsthesia at lightning speed, without asking too many questions, and an equal ability to secure "instant" awakening. The provision of proper facilities for pre-operative preparation and postoperative recovery, together with a sufficiency of *time*, would render this kind of anæsthetic "piece work" as obsolete as it deserves to be.

Bourne[204] has pointed out that there is a risk of patients fainting in the dental chair, during general anæsthesia. If the head is not immediately lowered, there is grave danger of cerebral ischæmia. The precise incidence of this complication is not known; it has almost certainly been responsible for some of the disasters attributed to nitrous oxide.

Anæsthesia and the Elderly Patient

Old patients sometimes show mental deterioration in hospital, such incidents often being related to the cerebral anoxia of hæmorrhage or pneumonia, and being rendered more likely by nursing in the head-up position. Mental changes have similarly been reported in old people following surgery under general anæsthesia.[205]

A survey has now been carried out by a team including an anæsthetist and a psychologist, to ascertain whether such mental changes are indeed attributable to anæsthesia.[206] The conclusion that emerges from this work is that no patient should be denied an anæsthetic which is otherwise indicated merely on the score of being old. The psychology of old people is complex, but certain facets of their reaction to surgery are readily comprehensible and often predictable.

If an old person is relieved of symptoms as a result of surgery, as by the excision of a large tumour or the alleviation of pain, subsequent questioning often reveals that his mental performance and zest for life have improved—the anæsthetist cannot directly claim credit for this improvement but he should appreciate that he is contributing to a worth while form of treatment. On the other hand if symptoms or disabilities are created by surgery, as in the case of a colostomy or an amputation, loss of interest in life and deterioration of mental performance are unfortunately, but understandably, common. Statistical analysis fails to reveal any specific effect of general anæsthesia.

CONCLUSION

Theoretical work on the inhalation agents and the apparatus used to administer them, and the clinical application of devices which monitor almost every electrical and mechanical impulse generated within the body, have forced upon the attention of the anæsthetist the relevance to his work of many aspects of science and mathematics. There is thus in some quarters a tendency for clinical anæsthesia to become more and more dominated by the dictates of the research worker: according to Woolmer[207] "The anæsthetist of to-morrow will be of a type very different from his predecessor of the days of Hewitt. He will not be an artist but a medical scientist."

To others this prospect is both unattractive and improbable. Happier is the thought that tomorrow's anæsthetist will not after all be so different from yesterday's, or to-day's; that he will still be a physician concerned with applying his skill to the care of sick people. To draw an analogy, one might say that whatever advances may be made in the motor industry—and no driver objects to having a better car—the first duty of the motorist is to steer his vehicle safely. Similarly, although the anæsthetist should be aware of what science and mathematics can offer him, he cannot depend on this knowledge alone. Clinical anæsthesia is still a long way from being an exact science, and it still takes a good doctor to give a good anæsthetic.

References

1. DAVISON, M. H. A. (1959). *Anæsthesia*, **14**, 127.
2. NICLOUX, M. (1908). *Les Anésthesiques Généraux au Point de Vue Chimico-Physiologique*. Doin, Paris.
3. BERT, P. (1883). *C. R. Soc. Biol., Paris*, **35**, 241, 409.
4. NICLOUX, M. (1906). *C. R. Soc. Biol., Paris*, **60**, 147, 206.
5. TISSOT, J. (1906). *J. Physiol. Path. gén.*, **8**, 417, 442.
6. NICLOUX, M., and YOVANOVITCH, A. (1924). *C. R. Soc. Biol., Paris*, **91**, 1285.
7. MCCOLLUM, J. L. (1930). *J. Pharmacol.*, **40**, 305.
8. BERT. P. (1883). *C. R. Soc. Biol., Paris*, **35**, 522.
9. NICLOUX, M. (1907). *C. R. Soc. Biol., Paris*, **62**, 8, 68.
10. HAGGARD, H. W. (1924). *J. Biol. Chem.*, **59**, 737, 753, 771, 783, 795.
11. ROBBINS, B. H. (1936). *J. Pharmacol.*, **58**, 251.
12. NICLOUX, M., and YOVANOVITCH, A. (1925). *C. R. Soc. Biol., Paris*, **93**, 1653.
13. SURVEY OF ANESTHESIOLOGY (1957). **1**, 561, 629.
14. FAULCONER, A. (1953). *Anesthesiology*, **14**, 405.
15. BUCKLEY, J. J., VAN BERGEN, F. H., HEMINGWAY, A., DEMOREST, H. L., MILLER, F. A., KNIGHT, R. T., and VARCO, R. L. (1952). *Anesthesiology*, **13**, 455.
16. JONES, C. S., SAARI, J. M., DEVLOO, R. A., FAULCONER, A., and BALDES, E. J. (1953). *Anesthesiology*, **14**, 490.
17. HATTOX, J. S., SAARI, J. M., and FAULCONER, A. (1953). *Anesthesiology*, **14**, 584.
18. BUTLER, R. A., and HILL, D. W. (1961). *Nature*, **189**, 488.
19. BUTLER, R. A. (1961). Sir Halley Steward Trust Lecture.
20. SEVERINGHAUS, J. W. (1954). *J. Clin. Invest.*, **33**, 1183.
21. ZUNTZ, N. (1897). *Fortscr. d. Med.*, **15**, 632.
22. WIDMARK, E. M. P. (1919). *Acta. med. Scandinav.*, **52**, 87.
23. TEORELL, T. (1937). *Arch. internat. de Pharmacodyn. et de therap.*, **57**, 205, 226.
24. KETY, S. S. (1951). *Pharmacol. Rev.*, **3**, 1.
25. MAPLESON, W. W. To be published.
26. NUNN, J. F. (1960). *Brit. J. Anæsth.*, **32**, 346.
27. DOBKIN, A. B. (1958). *Brit. J. Anæsth.*, **30**, 568.
28. DOBKIN, A. B. (1959). *Anesthesiology*, **20**, 10.
29. DOBKIN, A. B., DRUMMOND, K., and PURKIN, N. (1959). *Brit. J. Anæsth.*, **31**, 53.
30. DOBKIN, A. B., JOHNSTON, H. J., and SKINNER, L. C. (1960). *Canad. Anæsth. Soc. J.*, **7**, 257.
31. DOBKIN, A. B., SKINNER, L. C., and JOHNSTON, H. J. (1960). *Canad. Anæsth. Soc. J.*, **7**, 379.
32. CLAYTON, J. I., and PARKHOUSE, J. (1962). *Brit. J. Anæsth.*, **34**, 141.
33. MAPLESON, W. W., CLAYTON, J. I., and PARKHOUSE, J. To be published.
34. *Brain Mechanisms and Consciousness* (1954). Blackwell, Oxford.
35. LARRABEE, M. G., and POSTERNAK, J. M. (1952). *J. Neurophysiol.*, **15**, 91.
36. MARSHALL, W. H., WOOLSEY, C. N., and BARD, P. (1941). *J. Neurophysiol.*, **4**, 1.
37. CHEEK, D. B. (1959). *Amer. J. clin. Hypnosis*, **1**, 101.
38. PARKHOUSE, J. (1960). *Postgrad. med. J.*, **36**, 674.
39. HUTCHINSON, RUTH (1961). *Brit. J. Anæsth.*, **33**, 463.
40. COLE, P. V., and PARKHOUSE, J. (1961). *Brit. J. Anæsth.*, **33**, 265.
41. FAULCONER, A., and LATTERELL, K. E. (1949). *Anesthesiology*, **10**, 247.
42. POPPELBAUM, H. F. (1960). *Proc. R. Soc. Med.*, **53**, 289.
43. MERRIFIELD, A. J. (1961). *Brit. J. Anæsth.*, **33**, 289.
44. IKEZONO, E., HARMEL, M. H., and KING, B. D. (1959). *Anesthesiology*, **20**, 597.

45. WEITZNER, S. W., KING, B. D., and IKEZONO, E. (1959). *Anesthesiology*, **20**, 624.
46. COMROE, J. H., FORSTER, R. E., DUBOIS, A. B., BRISCOE, W. A., and CARLSEN, E. (1955). *The Lung: Clinical Physiology and Pulmonary Function Tests*, 1st ed., p. 100. Year Book Publishers, Chicago.
47. SCURR, C. F. (1956). *Brit. J. Anæsth.*, **28**, 23.
48. COLLIER, C. R., AFFELDT, J. E., and FARR, A. F. (1955). *J. Lab. clin. Med.*, **45**, 526.
49. SEVERINGHAUS, J. W. (1959). in *Symposium on pH and Blood Gas Measurement*. ed. Woolmer, R. F., p. 60. Churchill, London.
50. ASTRUP, P. (1956). *Scand. J. clin. Invest.*, **8**, 33.
51. ROBINSON, J. S., and UTTING, J. E. (1961). *Brit. J. Anæsth.*, **33**, 327.
52. NUNN, J. F. (1960). *Proc. R. Soc. Med.*, **53**, 180.
53. COOPER, E. A., and SMITH, H. (1961). *Anæsthesia*, **16**, 445.
54. NUNN, J. F. (1959). *Anæsthesia*, **14**, 77.
55. MCARDLE, L. (1959). *Brit. J. Anæsth.*, **31**, 142.
56. DRAPER, W. B., and WHITEHEAD, R. W. (1944). *Anesthesiology*, **5**, 262.
57. HOLMDAHL, M. H. (1956). *Acta. chir. Scand.*, Suppl. 212.
58. JOOSTE, K. H. (1955). *Anæsthesia*, **10**, 59.
59. NAHAS, G. G. (1959). *Science*, **129**, 782.
60. GEDDES, I. C., and GRAY, T. C. (1959). *Lancet*, **2**, 4.
61. BONVALLET, M., and DELL, P. (1956). *Electroenceph. clin. Neurophysiol.*, **8**, 170.
62. MCALEAVY, J. C., WAY, W. L., ALTSTATT, A. H., GUADAGNI, N. P., and SEVERINGHAUS, J. W. (1961). *Anesthesiology*, **22**, 260.
63. CLUTTON-BROCK, J. (1957). *Brit. J. Anæsth.*, **29**, 111.
64. SUGIOKA, K., and DAVIS, D. A. (1960). *Anesthesiology*, **21**, 135.
65. KETY, S. S., and SCHMIDT, C. F. (1946). *Fed. Proc.*, **5**, 55.
66. ROBINSON, J. S., and GRAY, T. C. (1961). *Brit. J. Anæsth.*, **33**, 62.
67. WOOD-SMITH, F. F., HORNE, G. M., and NUNN, J. F. (1961). *Anæsthesia.*, **16**, 340.
68. CASE, E. H., and STILES, J. A. (1946). *Anesthesiology*, **7**, 29.
69. RADFORD, E. P. (1955). *J. appl. Physiol.*, **7**, 451.
70. DOBKIN, A. B. (1958). In *Modern Trends in Anæsthesia*, ed. Evans, F. T., and Gray, T. C., 1st ed., p. 127. Butterworth, London.
71. NUNN, J. F. (1960). *Anæsthesia*, **15**, 123.
72. WATSON, W. E. (1961). Personal communication.
73. WRIGHT, B. M. (1959). In *Symposium on Pulmonary Ventilation*, ed. Harbord, R. P., and Woolmer, R., p. 87. Sherratt, Altrincham.
74. FAULCONER, A., and BICKFORD, R. G. (1960). *Electroencephalography in Anesthesiology*, 1st ed. Thomas, Springfield.
75. ARTUSIO, J. F. (1954). *J. Pharmacol.*, **111**, 343.
76. HENRIE, JOYCE, R., PARKHOUSE, J., and BICKFORD, R. G. (1961). *Anesthesiology*, **22**, 247.
77. CLUTTON-BROCK, J. (1958). *Atti XI Congresso Societa Italiana di Anestesiologia*, p. 65.
78. HAMPTON, L. J., and LITTLE, D. M. (1953). *A.M.A. Arch. Surg., Chicago*, **67**, 549.
79. GRAY, T. C. (1957). *Lancet*, **2**, 383.
80. ENDERBY, G. E. H. (1961). *Brit. J. Anæsth.*, **33**, 109.
81. LINACRE, J. L. (1961). *Brit. J. Anæsth.*, **33**, 45.
82. ROLLASON, W. N., and HOUGH, J. M. (1960). *Brit. J. Anæsth.*, **32**, 276, 286.
83. BERG, O., NILSSON, E., and VINNARS, E. (1957). *Brit. J. Anæsth.*, **29**, 146.
84. YATER, W. M., TRAUM, A. H., BROWN, W. G., FITZGERALD, R. P., GEISLER, M. A., and WILCOX, B. B. (1948). *Amer. Heart J.*, **36**, 334, 481, 683.
85. HAYWARD, G. W. (1952). *Anæsthesia*, **7**, 67.
86. MACINTOSH, R. R. (1949). *Brit. J. Anæsth.*, **21**, 107.
87. LODER, R. E. (1957). *Lancet*, **2**, 468.

88. CRILE, G. W., and LOWER, W. E. (1914). *Anoci-Accociation*. Saunders, Philadelphia.
89. DRIPPS, R. D., ECKENHOFF, J. E., and VANDAM, L. D. (1961). *Introduction to Anæsthesia*, 2nd ed., p. 92. Saunders, Philadelphia.
90. MOLYNEUX, L., and PASK, E. A. (1951). *Brit. J. Anæsth.*, **23**, 81.
91. FOLDES, F. F., CERAVOLO, A. J., and CARPENTER, S. L. (1952). *Ann. Surg.*, **136**, 978.
92. GALLOON, S. (1960). *Brit. J. Anæsth.*, **32**, 310.
93. SYKES, M. K. (1959). *Brit. J. Anæsth.*, **31**, 247.
94. GRAY, T. C. (1954). *Ann. R. Coll. Surg. Engl.*, **15**, 402.
95. MAPLESON, W. W. (1954). *Brit. J. Anæsth.*, **26**, 323.
96. MAPLESON, W. W. (1958). *Brit. med. Bull.*, **14**, 64.
97. MAPLESON, W. W. (1960). *Brit. J. Anæsth.*, **32**, 298.
98. ONCHI, Y., HOYASHI, T., and UEYAMA, H. (1957). *Far East J. Anæsth.*, **1**, 30.
99. WOOLMER, R., and LIND, B. (1954). *Brit. J. Anæsth.*, **26**, 316.
100. INKSTER, J. S. (1956). *Brit. J. Anæsth.*, **28**, 512.
101. PARKHOUSE, J., and SIMPSON, B. R. (1959). *Brit. J. Anæsth.*, **31**, 464.
102. MUSHIN, W. W., and GALLOON, S. (1960). *Brit. J. Anæsth.*, **32**, 324.
103. EPSTEIN, H. G., and MACINTOSH, R. R. (1956). *Anæsthesia*, **11**, 83.
104. MACINTOSH, R. R. (1953). *Brit. med. J.*, **2**, 202.
105. MACINTOSH, R. R. (1955). *Brit. med. J.*, **2**, 1054.
106. LAMBRECHTS, W., and PARKHOUSE, J. (1959). *S. Afr. med. J.*, **33**, 1003.
107. COLE, P. V., and MCCLELLAND, R. M. A. (1961). Mission Hospital Bulletin, No. 12.
108. HINGSON, R. A. (1961). *Anesth. and Analg.*, **40**, 316.
109. NANDRUP, E. (1958). *Nord. med.*, **60**, 1355.
110. RUBEN, H., KNUDSEN, E. J., WINKEL, E., and HJORTH, A. (1958). *Der Anæsthesist*, **7**, 161.
111. Meddelelser fra Sundhedsstyrelsen. Ugeskrift for Laeger, **106**, 793.
112. BRENNAN, H. J. (1957). *Brit. J. Anæsth.*, **29**, 332.
113. MORRIS, L. E. (1952). *Anesthesiology*, **13**, 587.
114. MORRIS, L. E., and FELDMAN, S. A. (1958). *Anesthesiology*, **19**, 642.
115. VONDERSCHMITT, H., and MOYAT, P. (1961). *Der Anæsthesist*, **10**, 196.
116. JOHNSTONE, M. (1961). *Brit. J. Anæsth.*, **33**, 29.
117. MARRETT, H. R. (1957). *Brit. med. J.*, **2**, 331.
118. HINGSON, R. A. (1954). *J. Amer. med. Ass.*, **156**, 604.
119. BOURNE, J. G. (1958). *Brit. med. J.*, **2**, 47.
120. STEPHENS, K. F., and BOURNE, J. G. (1960). *Lancet*, **2**, 481.
121. EPSTEIN, H. G. (1955). *Oxf. med. Sch. Gaz.*, **7**, 107.
122. NUNN, J. F. (1961). *Brit. med. J.*, **1**, 1139.
123. FOREGGER, R. (1959). *Anesthesiology*, **20**, 296.
124. SYKES, M. K. (1959). *Brit. J. Anæsth.*, **31**, 450.
125. LEIGH, M. D., and KESTER, H. A. (1948). *Anesthesiology*, **9**, 32.
126. STEPHEN, C. R., and SLATER, H. M. (1948). *Anesthesiology*, **9**, 550.
127. LEWIS, G. (1956). *Anesthesiology*, **17**, 618.
128. SLATER, H. M., and STEPHEN, C. R. (1951). *A.M.A. Arch. Surg.*, *Chicago*, **62**, 251.
129. EPSTEIN, H. G., MACINTOSH, R. R., and MENDELSSOHN, K. (1941). *Lancet*, **2**, 62.
130. MUSHIN, W. W., RENDELL-BAKER, L., and THOMPSON, P. W. (1959). *Automatic Ventilation of the Lungs*, *1st ed.*, p. 327. Blackwell, Oxford.
131. RUBEN, H. (1955). *Anesthesiology*, **16**, 643.
132. SYKES, M. K. (1959). *Brit. J. Anæsth*,. **31**, 446.
133. MACINTOSH, R. R., and BANNISTER, F. B. (1960). *Grundlagen der Allgemein-narkose*, p. 316. V. E. B. Verlag Volk und Gesundheit, Berlin.
134. REES, G. J. (1950). *Brit. med. J.*, **2**, 1419.
135. PARKHOUSE, J. (1960). *Brit. med. J.*, **1**, 274.

136. REES, G. J. (1958). In *Modern Trends in Anæsthesia*, ed. Evans, F. T., and Gray, T. C., 1st ed., p. 206. Butterworth, London.

137. KRANTZ, J. C., CARR, C. J., FORMAN, S., and HARNE, W. G. (1941). *J. Pharmacol.*, **71**, 2.

138. KRANTZ, J. C., EVANS, W. E., FORMAN, S., and WOLLENWEBER, H. S. L. (1942). *J. Pharmacol.*, **75**, 30.

139. KRANTZ, J. C., EVANS, W. E., CARR, C. J., and KIBLER, D. V. (1946). *J. Pharmacol.*, **86**, 138.

140. KRANTZ, J. C., CARR, C. J., MUSSER, R. D., and SAUERWALD, J. J. (1947). *J. Pharmacol.*, **89**, 88.

141. LU, G., KING, J. S. L., and KRANTZ, J. C. (1953). *Anesthesiology*, **14**, 466.

142. KRANTZ, J. C., LU, G., and BELL, F. K. (1953). *J. Pharmacol.*, **108**, 488.

143. BURNS, T. H. S., HALL, J. M., BRACKEN, A., GOULDSTONE, G., and NEWLAND, D. S. (1961). *Anæsthesia*, **16**, 3.

144. ROBBINS, B. H. (1946). *J. Pharmacol.*, **86**, 197.

145. RAVENTOS, J. (1956). *Brit. J. Pharmacol.*, **11**, 394.

146. SUCKLING, C. W. (1957). *Brit. J. Anæsth.*, **29**, 466.

147. VAN POZNAK, A., and ARTUSIO, J. F. (1960). *J. Toxicol. appl. Pharmacol.*, **2**, 363, 374.

148. ARTUSIO, J. F., and VAN POZNAK, A. (1960). *Fed. Proc.*, **19**, 273.

149. BURNS, T. H. S., HALL, J. M., BRACKEN, A., and GOULDSTONE, G. (1961). *Anæsthesia*, **16**, 333.

150. BURNS, T. H. S., HALL, J. M., BRACKEN, A., and GOULDSTONE, G. (1961). *Anæsthesia*, **16**, 440.

151. BURN, J. H., EPSTEIN, H. G., and GOODFORD, P. J. (1959). *Brit. J. Anæsth.*, **31**, 518.

152. BRYCE-SMITH, R., and O'BRIEN, H. D. (1956). *Brit. med. J.*, **2**, 969.

153. JOHNSTONE, M. (1956). *Brit. J. Anæsth.*, **28**, 392.

154. JOHNSTONE, M. (1961). *Anesthesiology*, **22**, 591.

155. STEPHEN, C. R., MARGOLIS, G., FABIAN, L. W., and BOURGEOIS-GAVARDIN, M. (1958). *Anesthesiology*, **19**, 770.

156. DUNCAN. W. A. M., and RAVENTOS, J. (1959). *Brit. J. Anæsth.*, **31**, 302.

157. BRENNAN, H. J., HUNTER, A. R., and JOHNSTONE, M. (1957). *Lancet*, **2**, 453.

158. DELANEY, E. J. (1958). *Brit. J. Anæsth.*, **30**, 188.

159. JOHNSTONE, M. (1961). *Brit. J. Anæsth.*, **33**, 29.

160. GOLDMAN, V. (1959). *Anesth. and Analg.*, **38**, 192.

161. HUDON, F., JACQUES, A., and BOIVIN, P. A. (1958). *Canad. Anæs. Soc. J.*, **5**, 403.

162. PARKHOUSE, J., and SIMPSON, B. R. (1959). *Brit. J. Anæsth.*, **31**, 186.

163. JOHNSTONE, M., EVANS, V., and MURPHY, P. V. (1961). *Canad. Anæsth. Soc. J.*, **8**, 53.

164. BREWSTER, W. R., ISAACS, J. P., and ANDERSON, T. W. (1953). *Amer. J. Physiol.*, **175**, 399.

165. ADAMS, A. K., LAMBRECHTS, W., and PARKHOUSE, J. (1959). *Acta anæsth. Scandinav.*, **3**, 189.

166. WASMUTH, C. E., GRIEG, J. H., HOMI, J., MORACA, P., ISIL, N. H., BITTE, E. M., and HALE, D. E. (1960). *Cleveland Clin. Quart.*, **27**, 174.

167. ARTUSIO, J. F., VAN POZNAK, A., HUNT, R. E., TIERS, F. M., and ALEXANDER, M. (1960). *Anesthesiology*, **21**, 512.

168. BAMFORTH, B. J., SIEBECKER, K. L., KRAEMER, R., and ORTH, O. S. (1961). *Anesthesiology*, **22**, 169.

169. DOBKIN, A. B., and FEDORUK, SYLVIA (1961). *Anesthesiology*, **22**, 355.

170. DUNDEE, J. W. (1958). In *Modern Trends in Anæsthesia*, ed. Evans, F. T., and Gray, T. C., 1st ed., p. 29. Butterworth, London.

171. ARTUSIO, J. F. (1955). *J. Amer. med. Ass.*, **157**, 33.

172. MACINTOSH, R. R., MUSHIN, W. W., and EPSTEIN, H. G. (1958). *Physics for the Anæsthetist*, 2nd ed., p. 341. Blackwell, Oxford.

173. M.O.H. (1956). *Report on Anæsthetic Explosions including Safety Code for Equipment and Installations,* H.M.S.O., London.
174. WASMUTH, C. E., and HALE, D. E. (1954). *Cleveland Clin. Quart.,* **21,** 46.
175. MENDELSOHN, D., MACDONALD, D. W., NOGUEIRA, C., and KAY, E. B. (1960). *Anesth. and Analg.,* **39,** 110.
176. LIEBRICH, O. (1869). *Ber. Dtsch. Chem. Ges.,* **2,** 269.
177. POWELL, J. F. (1945). *Brit. J. industr. Med.,* **2,** 142.
178. PAYKOC, Z. V., and POWELL, J. F. (1945). *J. Pharmacol.,* **85,** 289.
179. SOUCEK, B., and VLACHOVA, D. (1960). *Brit. J. industr. Med.,* **17,** 60.
180. BUTLER, T. C. (1949). *Fed. Proc.,* **8,** 278.
181. FORSSMAN, S., OWE-LARSSON, A., and SKOG, E. (1955). *Arch. Gewerbepath. Gewerbehyg.,* **13,** 619.
182. GRAY, T. C., and HALTON, J. (1948). *Brit. med. J.,* **1,** 784.
183. DINNICK, O. P. (1961). *Lancet,* **1,** 470.
184. ALLISON, P. R. (1948). *Thorax,* **3,** 20.
185. MARCHAND, P. (1955). *Brit. J. Surg.,* **42,** 504.
186. GREENAN, J. (1961). *Brit. J. Anæsth.,* **33,** 432.
187. ELLIS, H., and McLARTY, M. (1961). *Anæsthesia,* **16,** 435.
188. FYKE, F. E., CODE, C. F., and SCHLEGEL, J. F. (1956). *Gastroenterologia,* **86,** 135.
189. JACKSON, C. (1922). *Laryngoscope,* **32,** 139.
190. BARRETT, N. R. (1954). *Brit. J. Surg.,* **42,** 231.
191. DORNHORST, A. C., HARRISON, G. K., and PIERCE, J. W. (1954). *Lancet,* **1,** 695.
192. CREAMER, B., HARRISON, G. K., and PIERCE, J. W. (1959). *Thorax,* **14,** 132.
193. Editorial (1961). *Lancet,* **2,** 809.
194. HODGES, R. J. H., BENNETT, J. R., TUNSTALL, M. E., and KNIGHT, R. F. (1959). *Brit. J. Anæsth.,* **31,** 152.
195. SNOW, R. G., and NUNN, J. F. (1959). *Brit. J. Anæsth.,* **31,** 493.
196. O'MULLANE, E. J. (1954). *Lancet,* **1,** 1209.
197. MACINTOSH, R. R. (1951). *Brit. med. J.,* **2,** 545.
198. SELLICK, B. A. (1961). *Lancet,* **2,** 404.
199. PARKHOUSE, J. (1959). *Lancet,* **2,** 53.
200. KLOCK, J. H. (1951). *Anesth. and Analg.,* **30,** 151.
201. KLOCK, J. H. (1955). *Anesth. and Analg.,* **34,** 379.
202. TOM, A. (1956). *Brit. med. J.,* **1,** 1085.
203. TOM, A. (1959). *Anæsthesia,* **14,** 184.
204. BOURNE, J. G. (1957). *Lancet,* **2,** 499.
205. BEDFORD, P. D. (1955). *Lancet,* **2,** 259.
206. SIMPSON, B. R., WILLIAMS, M., SCOTT, J. F., and CRAMPTON SMITH, A. (1961). *Lancet,* **2,** 889.
207. WOOLMER, R. (1957). *Anæsthesia,* **12,** 249.

CHAPTER 2

INTRAVENOUS ANÆSTHESIA

J. D. ROBERTSON

Barbiturates — New Non-Barbiturate Drugs — Pharmacology of Intravenous Anæsthesia—Place of Intravenous Anæsthesia—Use of Intravenous Anæsthesia in Special Circumstances—Analeptics.

SINCE its introduction into clinical practice in 1935 thiopentone has remained the most popular intravenous anæsthetic in this country. It is not, however, the ideal agent and, although it is difficult to envisage any compound which would be entirely satisfactory in all circumstances, some of the new drugs now being subjected to clinical trial may avoid some of its disadvantages and prove superior, for example, in minor out-patient anæsthesia. While the duration of action of thiopentone in single doses is relatively brief, the return of consciousness is not due to rapid detoxication but to redistribution in the body and, as a consequence, cumulative action with delayed recovery is likely to occur if too large an initial dose or further injections of the drug are given within a few hours. The chief aim of recent investigations in the field of intravenous anæsthesia has, therefore, been to find a drug from which recovery is rapid and complete, which is free from undesirable side-effects on the respiration and circulation and which is non-irritant to the intima of veins and other tissues. Some of the many new barbiturate and non-barbiturate compounds which have been used as intravenous anæsthetics in man will now be reviewed and an assessment of their merits in comparison with thiopentone attempted.

Two intravenous barbiturate drugs which were introduced several years ago—*thialbarbitone sodium* (Kemithal) and *thiamylal sodium* (Surital, Thioseconal, Thioquinalbarbitone) are still the subject of occasional reports, although neither agent appears to differ sufficiently from thiopentone to come into widespread use as an alternative. Thialbarbitone is about half as potent as thiopentone and has a similar cumulative effect[1] while thiamylal is equipotent with thiopentone and is less cumulative. A comparison of the respiratory depressant effects of thiopentone, thialbarbitone and thiamylal in equipotent doses was made in sixty patients by Swerdlow.[2] He found that the mean apnœa time after the induction dose was significantly lower with thialbarbitone than with thiamylal while the latter was significantly better than thiopentone. Three minutes after the induction dose the respiratory volume changes were similar with all three, but a supplementary dose caused significantly greater respiratory depression with thiopentone than with the other two drugs. Dundee and Riding[3] formed the impression that with equipotent doses recovery was more rapid with thiamylal than following thiopentone. However, in a comparative clinical study of thiopentone and thiamylal no significant difference was observed between the two agents in respect of potency, incidence of laryngospasm and respiratory depression or recovery time.[4]

Several barbiturates have been introduced on the Continent. One of these *Thionarcex* (JL 1074)—sodium-5-ethyl-5 butylethyl-2-thiobarbiturate—has not been used in this country, but clinical reports suggest that it is slightly more potent than thiopentone and that recovery from it is a little more rapid. Dundee and Riding[5] compared sodium thiopentone with another intravenous barbiturate —*Inactin sodium* 5-ethyl-5-(methyl propyl)-2-thiobarbiturate and found that the potency of Inactin was about two-thirds that of thiopentone while the induction and incidence of complications were similar. They concluded that Inactin was as satisfactory as sodium thiopentone for induction of anæsthesia and that there was no significant difference in the action of equipotent doses. These findings have been confirmed by Dundee, Barron and King.[6] The third compound is *buthalitone sodium* (Transithal, Baytenal, Ulbreval, Thialbutone). Chemically, this compound is sodium-5-allyl-5-isobutyl-2-thiobarbiturate. Several clinical reports seem to confirm the claims of the German workers with regard to the rapid recovery of consciousness following the use of this agent. Many of these concern the use of buthalitone in out-patient anæsthesia for short operations such as orthopædic manipulations, incision of abscesses and minor gynæcological operations,[7-12] in dental chair anæsthesia[13-12] and for electro-convulsive therapy.[12, 16, 17] These workers were all impressed by the smoothness of anæsthesia, the rapidity of recovery and the absence of hang-over following its use. However, several remark on the high incidence of side-effects, such as coughing, hiccupping and sneezing, following administration of buthalitone.[7, 9, 10, 18-20] It has been suggested[8] that these are caused by too rapid injection of the drug and that they can be eliminated if the first 1 to 4 ml is administered rapidly and after an interval of $1\frac{1}{2}$ minutes the remainder is given slowly over 3 to $3\frac{1}{2}$ minutes.

Duffield and Ginsberg[10] observed that in three cases when some of the solution was injected outside the vein it did not cause any inflammatory reaction, but in other reports[9, 12] the perivenous injection of a small quantity of a 10% solution was associated with the complaint of a burning pain at the site and one patient showed marked tissue irritation followed by limitation of movement.[9]

Kane and Stephens[21] studied the rate of passage of buthalitone sodium across the human placenta. They noted that there was a distinct tendency for the cord plasma concentration of buthalitone to be lower than that of the maternal plasma at the time of delivery and that there was no indication that the cord level increased with the time between induction and delivery. These findings were in contrast with those with thiopentone which gave equal maternal and cord levels, the latter decreasing as the time between induction and delivery increased.

Clinical assessment of the duration of action of intravenous anæsthetics is notoriously difficult and many of the reports must be considered as impressions. More objective measurement has been attempted by several workers. Simmonds and Blanshard[18] used the time when the patient could be roused by painful stimuli, when he could appreciate the spoken word and when he was fully conscious and able to sit, as indices, claiming that these simple methods could be applied in all cases and were objective. They concluded that buthalitone did not appear to be an advance for out-patient anæsthesia as the rate of recovery showed no statistical difference from that observed after the use of thiopentone. In an attempt to assess the return to full consciousness Simmonds and Curwen[22] compared standard drawings carried out by the patient at varying times following anæsthesia with buthalitone and thiopentone. Again, no statistically significant difference was found between buthalitone and thiopentone. O'Mullane[23] employed the electro-encephalogram to assess duration of recovery in three volunteers following buthalitone and thiopentone. He concluded that the impression gained in a clinical study, that buthalitone provided a more rapid recovery, was shown to be very misleading. Patients receiving thiopentone were much more deeply anæsthetised than those who were given what was considered to be an equipotent dose of buthalitone. The deep anæsthesia lasted for a longer period with buthalitone and then there was a rapid recovery to pattern (1) followed by a slower recovery of consciousness. These findings suggest that buthalitone may be active for even longer than thiopentone though the difference between the two is slight.

Various assessments of the potency of buthalitone have been

carried out, from which it was concluded that buthalitone was about half as potent as thiopentone.[12, 19, 24−26]

Although buthalitone may be substituted for thiopentone for induction of anæsthesia prior to major surgery, the absence of recent reports with Thionarcex, Inactin and buthalitone suggests that none of these drugs have been found to be an improvement on thiopentone.[8,12]

Methitural (Neraval, Thiogenal, Methothiourate, AM 109)

Methitural sodium (methyl-thioethyl-2-pentyl-thiobarbiturate) is another short-acting thiobarbiturate which was introduced on the Continent and which was the subject of several papers from America a few years ago. It was claimed that by introducing a methylthioethyl group in the side chain the breakdown of the drug would be accelerated and liberation of methionine would protect the liver. The potency of methitural has been variously assessed as between a half and two-thirds that of thiopentone. The usual concentration employed for intravenous anæsthesia has been 2·5 or 5%. In the cat, dog and monkey a significantly quicker recovery was observed with equivalent anæsthetic doses of methitural than with thiopentone.[27] This has been confirmed in man by some observers[20, 28−31] while others concluded that there was no significant difference in the duration of hypnosis produced by methitural or thiopentone when equipotent concentrations and doses were used.[19, 32−37]

Studies of the metabolism of methitural and thiopentone in the dog and the rat showed that methitural, like thiopentone, was rapidly absorbed into the body fat depots and was degraded by the liver, but it was eliminated more rapidly than thiopentone[38] and the cumulative effect of repeated doses of methitural was also much less than that of thiopentone or thiamylal.[27] Fitzpatrick, Clarie and Mersch[29] observed rapid and complete recovery following the administration of 0·5% solution as a continuous drip or after intermittent injections of a 2·5% solution and considered that this was due to the reduced cumulative effects of the drug. Others have found that during the maintenance of anæsthesia repeated doses of methitural were large in comparison with those of thiopentone which, they concluded, was due to the significantly faster detoxication of methitural.[30]

The incidence and severity of hypotension following induction of anæsthesia with methitural does not seem to be greater than that with thiopentone and several workers have claimed that apnœa was shorter.[19, 30, 32] There are, however, numerous reports of an increased incidence of hiccup, cough and laryngospasm following administration of methitural and Dundee[31] found that these may be of such severity as to outweigh the advantages from the short action of the drug. Solutions containing more than $2 \cdot 5\%$ were sometimes irritant causing burning and pain at the site of injection and along the vein during the administration.[29, 30, 32, 34]

The absence of any recent enthusiastic report suggests that the claim that methitural has a shorter duration of action than thiopentone has not been confirmed and that the incidence of side-effects is considerably higher than with thiopentone.

N-Alkyl Thiobarbiturates

The distribution of three N-alkyl thiobarbiturates and the duration of their action has been studied in dogs and in man.[39] Two of these compounds are N-methyl thiobarbiturates (Lilly 14694 and Lilly 16213) and the other is N-allyl thiobarbiturate (Lilly 16192). The more rapid recovery from anæsthesia induced with these compounds in comparison with thiopentone was attributed to the almost complete removal of the drug from the plasma and other tissues as a result of their high affinity for fat, the rate of metabolism and the degree of plasma binding being similar to that with thiopentone. As a result of these investigations it was suggested that these compounds may serve as intravenous anæsthetics for use in operative procedures of long duration in which anæsthesia with thiopentone is associated with prolonged recovery of consciousness. However, in view of the fact that the rapid clinical recovery following the administration of the N-alkyl thiobarbiturates was due to withdrawal and retention by the fat and not to more rapid metabolism, the possibility of the danger of maintaining a large reservoir of an active drug in the body fat may be a liability.

Reports on three other methylated thiobarbiturates have recently been published.[6, 40]

The first of these—*Compound B*.137, which is the normal methylated form of Inactin—was compared with Inactin and thiopentone in a clinical trial. It was found that methylation does not appear to alter the potency of Inactin, which is slightly less than that of thiopentone. The authors were unable to substantiate the claim that normal methylation resulted in a more rapid return of consciousness, but it increased the incidence of excitatory side-effects unless opiate premedication was employed. A striking feature of this study was the close correlation between the incidence and severity of spontaneous abnormal muscle movements and the dosage of B.137

used. Respiratory side-effects were not a feature of B.137 anæsthesia. Post-operative venous thrombosis, nausea and vomiting occurred more frequently with the methylated compound than with the non-methylated thiobarbiturates.

Compound B.82, which is the normal methylated form of buthalitone, possessed the disadvantages of the parent drug with regard to respiratory disturbances and, in addition, caused a high increase in the incidence rate of excitatory phenomenon. Slightly more than half the patients developed a generalized erythematous rash within one minute of the injection of B.82, a complication which was not seen with either buthalitone or thiopentone.

The third—*Compound B.133* is N-methyl-5-ethyl-5-isobityl thiobarbiturate and is not related chemically to any thiobarbituate in clinical use. Following the intravenous administration of B.133 the frequency and severity of side-effects was less than with B.82, but was still significantly higher than with the non-methylated thiobarbiturates. The incidence of respiratory side-effects was similar to that for buthalitone and the appearance of a generalized erythematous rash was also a feature of B.133.

From their experience with these compounds in clinical practice, Dundee and his co-workers concluded that the methylated thiobarbiturates are unlikely to have a place in clinical anæsthetic practice.

Spirobarbiturates and Spirothiobarbiturates

Of the many compounds of this type which have been prepared only a few have come to clinical trial. With the spiro-thiobarbiturates the duration of action is claimed to be shorter than that of thiopentone but hiccupping, laryngospasm and retching following anæsthesia have been a source of concern.[41] No recent report on the use of these compounds in anæsthesia has been found.

Methohexitone Sodium
(Methohexital Brietal, Brevital, Compound 25398)

Over two thousand barbiturates have been synthesized and tested in animals in an attempt to find an ultra-short acting oxygen barbiturate. Compound 22451 is a sterio-isomeric mixture of alpha and beta DL,1-methyl-5-allyl-5-(1-methyl-2-pentynyl) barbiturate acid. The sodium salt was found to be a satisfactory intravenous anæsthetic agent which was three times more potent than thiopentone and from which recovery was more rapid.[42] However, shivering, twitching and hiccups were more frequent with Compound 22451 than with the thiobarbiturates[43, 44] and an investigation of its isomers was carried out. The most desirable configuration was found to be the alpha DL form[45] and this was introduced into clinical practice as Compound 25398 by Stoelting[46] and has now been given the name methohexitone. When compared with thiopentone in rats, mice, rabbits, monkeys and dogs it was found to be three times as potent as thiopentone while its action was half as long and it was less likely to accumulate. In a trial on 285 patients who received methohexitone anæsthesia for a wide variety of surgical procedures the impression that recovery was more rapid after the new compound than after thiopentone or thiamylal was confirmed. A double blind study of thiopentone, methitural and methohexitone administered in 2·5%, 5% and 1% solutions, respectively, showed that the rate of recovery of out-patients in a dental clinic was significantly more rapid from methohexitone than from comparable doses of methitural or thiopentone.[35] In the past few years numerous reports from both sides of the Atlantic comparing the duration of action of methohexitone with thiopentone and other intravenous anæsthetics have confirmed the claim that the recovery time is significantly more rapid with methohexitone.[47, 48] Green and Jolly[49] describe a clinical trial of methohexitone in 500 patients, 94 per cent of whom were fit to return home within half-an-hour and 91 per cent were able to leave the dental chair within 6 minutes of receiving the injection.

In other series in which thiopentone, methitural and methohexitone have been compared for out-patient anæsthesia the potency and rapidity of recovery following methohexitone has been confirmed.[50, 51, 52] However, an increased incidence of tachycardia, hiccup and muscle tremor was frequently reported with methohexitone, but this is not generally considered to outweigh the advantage of more rapid recovery.[47, 48] In a study of methohexitone in a series of over 10,000 patients, both as the sole agent for minor out-patient procedures or for induction of anæsthesia for dental, obstetric and general surgical operations, Coleman and Green[53] found that recovery was notably rapid, complete and free from side-effects. They considered that the rate of recovery in patients was quicker than from any barbiturate previously investigated and considered that, in small doses, the drug has great promise for use in out-patients. In their series the average dose was 70 mg ranging from 50 to 220 mg in 1% solution.

There is considerable lack of agreement concerning the incidence of complications associated with the use of methohexitone. Wyant and Chang[48] noted that hiccup was a frequent complication and, in a series in which 3,340 patients were anæsthetized with metho-hexitone, 86 developed marked skeletal muscle twitchings or tremor[54]. Dundee and Moore[55] found that premedication with an analgesic drug, for example, pethidine, significantly reduced the incidence of spontaneous muscle movements as compared with that following the use of atropine. On the other hand, when promethazine or scopolamine, which increase sensitivity to pain,[56-58] were used for premedication, the incidence of muscle twitchings after the injection of methohexitone was greatly increased.[59] They suggested, therefore, that the phenothiazine derivatives and scopolamine are unsuitable drugs to use before methohexitone anæsthesia.[58, 60]

Transient respiratory and circulatory depression has been reported following the rapid injection of methohexitone.[47, 54] In a series of 500 dental patients in whom anæsthesia was induced by the rapid intravenous injection of methohexitone in a dosage of 5 mg/stone of body weight, a transient fall in systolic blood pressure occurred in 70 per cent.[49] Although this would seem to confirm the danger of administering a drug with the potency of methohexitone to patients in the dental chair, the patients all made a rapid recovery and many were fit to return home within half-an-hour. Most other workers have not found respiratory or circulatory depression to be a serious complication with methohexitone and Dundee and Moore[55] con-cluded that it caused an appreciably lower incidence of hypotension than an equivalent dose of thiopentone. In the large series reported by Coleman and Green[53] blood pressures were taken on a large number of patients during the operation and no profound falls were noted.

There have also been conflicting reports about the risk of local irritation following the injection of methohexitone administered as a 1% solution by intermittent intravenous injection or as a 0·1 to 0·2% solution by continuous infusion. In the early reports no evidence was found of venous thrombosis and only mild and brief local tenderness was noted even after a large amount had been deposited extravenously in one case.[46, 47, 50] On the other hand, in the large series reported by Taylor and Stoelting[54] 60 per cent of the patients complained of pain at the site of injection or along the course of the vein during the injection, although none developed thrombophlebitis subsequently. Dundee and Moore[55] have not encountered this high incidence of pain on injection and consider that methohexitone is less irritant to veins and tissues than thio-pentone. Coleman and Green[53] found that extravenous injection of methohexitone produced only a transient and painless erythema and that intra-arterial injections in calves evoked no undesirable response. However, they observed that about 50 per cent of unpremedicated patients were aware of a sensation along the course of the injected vein which in some instances amounted to pain, although it was not recollected in the post-operative period and there was no associated thrombophlebitis.

From these reports it appears that the claims that the recovery of consciousness following methohexitone is rapid and complete have been substantiated. While the incidence of excitatory side-effects is greater than with the thiobarbiturates it is less than that found with other methylated compounds and may be further reduced by avoiding the use of anti-analgesic drugs in premedication. The overall incidence and severity of respiratory and circulatory depression is also probably less frequent than some reports suggest and will be minimal if it is remembered that methohexitone is a potent agent which should not be given too rapidly or in excessive doses. The exact incidence of local irritant phenomena has not yet been fully evaluated, and, although venous thrombosis in the injected vein is not a frequent complication, there is no doubt that a considerable proportion of patients are aware of a sensation passing up the arm during the injection of methohexitone. Further, despite the evidence to the contrary, the possibility of serious damage following intra-arterial injection cannot be ignored and the usual precautions taken during thiopentone administration should also be applied when methohexitone is used.

Methohexitone sodium would seem to be the most promising of the barbiturate drugs recently introduced for intravenous anæsthesia, particularly for out-patient surgery.[61]

New Non-Barbiturate Drugs

Dolitrone (Thiazanedione) is 5-ethyl-6-phenyl-m-thiazane-2,4-dione. It is generally employed for intravenous injection as a 2.5% solution which has pH of about 11 and, being unstable, must be made up fresh for each case.

Initially Dolitrone was used to produce "controlled amnesia," a state of general analgesia without complete loss of consciousness but marked retrograde amnesia, which was found to be satisfactory for dental extractions and dressing of extensive burns.[62, 63] With larger doses Dolitrone produced general anæsthesia comparable to that obtained with thiopentone, but it was claimed that there was little depression of respiration and blood pressure and no cumulative effect or prolonged anæsthesia following repeated doses. The only complications encountered were thrombophlebitis, though this was uncommon, and transient nausea in the postoperative period. Other investigators[64] administered Dolitrone, as a 2·5% solution by intermittent intravenous injection as the sole anæsthetic to 39 patients and by continuous intravenous infusion in a concentration of 0·2 to 0·6%, to 30 patients for a wide variety of surgical procedures and found that it produced a rapid and smooth induction of anæsthesia but that smooth maintenance was difficult to attain, the drug being primarily a hypnotic with little analgesic potency. They found that its main advantage was for obtunding laryngeal and pharyngeal reflexes in very light planes of anæsthesia and that it was a satisfactory general anæsthetic for short operations. However, they considered that Dolitrone was unsuitable as the sole anæsthetic for prolonged procedures because of its depressant effect on the respiration and circulation when large doses were employed. Laboratory studies in dogs and rabbits[65] showed that Dolitrone had about two-thirds the potency of thiopentone and that in equipotent doses the average recovery time was less with the former, although occasionally in dogs this was associated with a period of intense excitement which was not prevented by premedication with morphine. The intravenous injection of Dolitrone always produced a transient hypotension with a considerable increase in heart rate but no instance of serious respiratory depression was observed in dogs with either drug while both reduced the rate of respiration when they were given to unpremedicated rabbits.

Reports on the administration of Dolitrone, to volunteers and to patients undergoing minor surgical and gynæcological procedures in which it has been compared as an anæsthetic with thiopentone and other barbiturates,[20, 66] show that Dolitrone can be classed as an ultra short-acting anæsthetic with minimal respiratory and circulatory depressant activity. On the other hand entirely smooth anæsthesia was exceptional with Dolitrone and other short-acting agents compared with thiopentone anæsthesia, spontaneous movements, coughing and hiccups being disturbing complications. The most serious feature associated with the use of Dolitrone was the high incidence of post-operative thrombophlebitis in the vein used for injection. Although this was less frequent when a 2% solution was employed instead of the usual 2·5% solution, the anæsthesia was less satisfactory with the former and it was concluded that Dolitrone compared unfavourably with the other intravenous anæsthetics now available. Later observers[67] have conceded many of these objections to Dolitrone but consider that further experience with the compound is required before it can be either accepted or rejected.

Glutethimide (Doriden). This compound is α-ethyl-α-phenyl glutarimide and is a close chemical relation to Bemegride. Glutethimide was introduced as an oral sedative-hypnotic, doses of 250 to 500 mg providing satisfactory sedation without residual action on the next day.[68] It was also found to be a useful substitute for oxybarbiturates or narcotics for premedication.[69] However, a blind trial in which the drug was compared with pentobarbitone showed that in equipotent doses the effects were identical and the incidence of hangover drowsiness was no less with glutethimide than with pentobarbitone.

Glutethimide has the disadvantage of being poorly soluble in water and for intravenous administration polyethyleneglycol has been employed as the solvent. In experimental animals doses up to 10 mg per kg of body weight have been found to cause little or no change in blood pressure[68] and this has been confirmed in adult volunteers.[71] Relapse into sleep commonly occurred after apparent recovery from glutethimide anæsthesia and amnesia and release of inhibitions was a uniform finding with alterations of mood which sometimes persisted for as long as 24 hours. Discomfort in the injected vein was a frequent complaint and in a few subjects this was followed by thrombophlebitis. In a recent report[72] glutethimide was considered to be ineffective when administered orally as a pre-operative sedative, but provided satisfactory induction of anæsthesia when injected intravenously. The advantages claimed were rapid onset of anæsthesia with less depression of respiration and greater depression of pharyngeal and laryngeal reflexes than with thiamylal while waking time was found to be shorter. Pain was noted during the injection of glutethimide in 27 per cent of patients and postoperatively localized areas of thrombosis or thrombophlebitis were present in 60 per cent of the cases. A transient fall in blood pressure occurred in all and in 6 of the 58 patients exceeded 30 mm Hg. Bemegride though closely related chemically to glutethimide did not show specific antagonism towards the hypnotic. These observers concluded that the present preparation of glutethimide does not compare favourably with the thiobarbiturates as an intravenous anæsthetic.

Cyclohexamines. Three aryl-cyclohexylamines have been employed clinically as intravenous anæsthetics. These are CI 395 (phencyclidine, Sernyl), CI 400 (Cyclohexamine) and CI 401.

In animal studies, the first of these compounds was shown to produce a cataleptoid state in which the animal was lightly anæsthetized and did not respond to painful stimulation. Although the compound was shown to have some local anæsthetic action, the site of its potent analgesic effect was considered to be at thalamic or midbrain level. Clinical studies[73] showed that, following the intravenous injection of phencyclidine in doses varying between 0·14 and 1·0 mg/kg, patients appeared to lose consciousness and no longer responded to painful stimuli. In sixty-eight patients undergoing various surgical procedures it was found that phencyclidine produced satisfactory anæsthesia for superficial surgery, but that muscle relaxation was poor and in most cases there was a transient but marked stimulation of blood pressure and respiration. Mild excitation was a problem during the procedure in several cases and appeared to increase when the dosage was more than 0·5 mg/kg. An outstanding feature of phencyclidine anæsthesia was the prolonged amnesia for the operative and immediate pre-operative period and this sometimes persisted for as long as twenty-four hours postoperatively. Several patients exhibited marked excitement during the recovery period and alarming hallucinations made many patients restless and noisy. These findings have been confirmed by other workers with phencyclidine[74] and with Cyclohexamine.[75,76] Although it was suggested that the incidence of side-effects, in particular, disorientation and hallucinations in the postoperative period, might be less with Cyclohexamine the experiences of the present author caused him to abandon the drug after its use in a small number of cases. Recently it has been claimed[77] that phencyclidine is a safe and satisfactory general analgesic of sufficient potency to allow skin grafting and other operations to be performed painlessly and without memory of the procedure in children with severe burns. However, although crying, hallucination or delirium occurred in 50 per cent of the children over five years, it was considerably less frequent in young children and the authors consider that the drug merits further trial. The effects of the three cyclohexylamines were studied in one patient with thalamic pain by Kurtzke.[78] Phencyclidine was found to be the safest of the three compounds and was given for 5 months during which pain was effectively controlled. However, termination of its use was necessitated by acute delirioid reaction with some residual brain damage. The author concluded that these three compounds may provide an effective, though hazardous, treatment for thalamic pain but that its use is warranted in this disorder with appropriate safeguards.

Cyclohexylamines have been shown to be potent general analgesics which can be used effectively to produce an anæsthetic-like state for superficial operations. The high incidence of psychotic side-effects during the postoperative period is, however, a very serious disadvantage and is probably sufficient to preclude the clinical use of the currently available compounds.

SCTZ (Hemineurine, Chlorethiazol) is methyl-(4-β-chloroethyl)-5-thiazole and is a hypnotic derived from thiazole fraction of vitamin B1. In mice, rats and rabbits SCTZ was observed to have a marked sedative action but with little analgesic potency or potentiating effect on general and local analgesics.[79] Tachycardia occurred in animals receiving SCTZ parentally but in those under general anæsthesia there was little effect on the heart and only slight and transitory hypotension was observed. In a clinical study of 80 patients[79] in which SCTZ was given intravenously as a 2% solution in a dosage of 1·2 G in 2 or 3 minutes the onset of sleep was rapid and profound. Following one injection sleep lasted for 10 to 20 minutes but could be maintained by a slow drip of the drug, otherwise the patient awoke, although he usually remained drowsy for several hours. Whatever the depth of the sleep, however, the patient continued to respond to stimulation without recovering consciousness or having any memory of this response. In the dosage employed there was little effect on respiration or circulation except when painful stimulation was applied when the heart rate, blood pressure and respiration were notably increased. When used in association with general anæsthetics it was observed that the dose of the anæsthetic required was not diminished by the previous administration of SCTZ. Despite this lack of potentiating action, however, the authors recommended the use of SCTZ to induce sleep or to suppress apprehension before the administration of the general anæsthetic. Postoperatively, awakening was rapid, but drowsiness prolonged lasting for 3 to 5 hours. Contact could be established with the patient, but he fell asleep again when left undisturbed. Because of its lack of analgesic activity, however, it was of little value in patients with severe pain.

The use of SCTZ in 97 patients undergoing neurosurgical procedures has been described[80] and it was confirmed that the drug was a hypnotic with little or no analgesic potency. It was considered that the action of SCTZ was almost entirely limited to the cortex and that the effect on subcortical layers appeared to be very slight when normal therapeutic doses were used. Unless an analgesic was combined with the hypnotic any form of stimulation resulted in motor discharge. Dundee[81] reported a clinical trial of the drug in 40 patients and concluded that SCTZ was not a satisfactory agent for induction or maintenance of anæsthesia because of the absence of analgesic activity. This drug also seems to have some irritant action on the veins following injection. It therefore seems unlikely that it will prove of value as an intravenous anæsthetic agent.

G.29505 (Detrovel). This compound is 2-methoxy-4-allylphenoxy-acetic acid-N, N-diethylamide and is therefore chemically different from the other agents hitherto used as anæsthetics. Pharmacological studies[82] showed that this compound possessed characteristic anæsthetic properties in various animal species, in all of which it was characterized by a rapid recovery of consciousness. An interesting and unusual feature of the drug was the marked but transient respiratory stimulation followed by moderate depression which regularly followed the intravenous injection. As well as being a potent sedative G.29505 was found to possess analgesic and anti-convulsant properties. In later studies on mice[83] it was observed that the anæsthetic effect of G.29505 could be markedly potentiated by premedication with chlorpromazine or perphenazine. The metabolic fate of G.29505 was studied in the rat by Pulver.[84] He found that, following its intravenous administration, measurable concentrations of G.29505 were present in the blood, but that the level fell rapidly and the anæsthetic was no longer detectable after 1 hour, although readily measurable quantities of the metabolites were present for as long as 7 hours. The concentrations of the anæsthetic in several organs of rabbits which had been killed at various intervals following the administration of G.29505 showed that the drug was rapidly deposited in fatty tissue and in organs with a high lipoid content while the metabolite remained in the aqueous phase. Following deposition, G.29505 was released from the brain and spinal cord with relative rapidity while the fat depots were exhausted more slowly, but due to the rapid breakdown rate to intermediary products no measurable blood concentration of G.29505 could be detected once the initial values had fallen to zero, although the metabolite was detectable for several hours. A meta-bolite of G.29505 has been isolated from the urine of experimental animals and identified as 3-methoxy-4-N, N-diethylcarbamedo-methoxycinnamic acid.[85] This metabolite shows very low toxicity and does not possess anæsthetic activity. Thus, the intermediate breakdown of G.29505 takes place rapidly which explains the short duration of anæsthesia, the rapid postoperative recovery and the absence of after-effects. Both the parent compound and its meta-bolite have been shown to pass through the placenta.[86] However, the concentration of G.29505 in the infant blood was found to be remarkably low due partly to its limited transport through the placenta and partly to the low levels in the maternal blood from rapid decomposition of the drug.

Electroencephalographic studies of the effect of G.29505 and other non-barbiturate anæsthetics in animals indicates that G.29505 produces depression almost equally in the cortex and in the reticular system of the brain.[87] This has been confirmed by the application of electrons to different parts of the cortical and subcortical layers during exploration of the brain by steriotaxic methods during neurosurgical procedures in man.[80]

Several clinical reports from Germany[88, 89, 90] have confirmed the rapid onset of anæsthetic action and the rapid and complete recovery of consciousness following the intravenous injection of G.29505. These authors also comment on the stimulation of respiration and the transient depression which followed each successive injection of G.29505 and on the minimal effect produced by the drug on the cardiovascular system. The principal untoward reaction observed was the relatively common complaint of pain in the arm during or immediately following injection of the drug and the frequent occurrence of postoperative venous thrombosis or thrombophlebitis in the injected vein following its use. These authors employed a 2 to 5% solution in 25% sodium benzoate in a dosage of 3 to 5 mg/kg body weight. As it was felt that the venous damage might be due to the solvent G.29505 has now been prepared as an emulsion in 4% lesivan with 5% glucose. In a series of 50 ambulant patients[91] who received this new preparation, 40 who had a single injection showed no adverse effect on the veins. The other 10 were given repeated injections of G.29505 at intervals of 2 or 3 days for electro convulsion therapy and it was found that, after the second or third, half of the patients showed a slight induration at the point of injection and in two cases the reaction was marked. Swerdlow[92] employed this preparation alone or supplemented by nitrous oxide and oxygen in 250 patients undergoing dental extractions or minor casualty or out-patient surgery. He concluded that G.29505 was a useful agent for procedures of short duration and that the method of induction with G.29505 followed by nitrous oxide and oxygen for multiple dental extractions was pleasant for the patient, provided easy management of anæsthesia and was followed by rapid and complete recovery. Thrombophlebitis was observed in twelve cases in the series and in two it was severe with periphlebitic lymphangitis. In one patient, in whom some extravenous spilling had occurred, a marked inflammatory reaction with œdema resulted. All resolved satisfactorily with conservative treatment.

The analgesic activity of G.29505 has been studied by a method employing the application of graded pressure to the anterior surface of the tibia.[93] In contradistinction to the action of thiopentone subhypnotic doses of G.29505 decreased the sensitivity to somatic pain although the effect was very transient.

Because of its short duration of action and mild analgesic potency, G.29505 would seem to be a promising agent for use as the sole anæsthetic for minor procedures or as an induction agent prior to nitrous oxide and oxygen anæsthesia. The high incidence of venous irritation following injection suggests, however, that further modification of the solvent may be required.

Hydroxydione Sodium Succinate (Viadril, Presuren). This is sodium 21-hydroxypregnane-3 : 20-dione succinate and is a water soluble hormonally inactive derivative of pregnanedione. The early pharmacological studies on hydroxydione showed it to be a marked central nervous system depressant of low toxicity in laboratory animals. It was also claimed that cardiac and respiratory depression was less with hydroxydione than with the ultra short-acting thiobarbiturates and that it produced a pronounced relaxant and antispasmodic effect on tracheal smooth muscle.[94-96] In experiments on cats Lerman and Paton[97] observed two distinct responses of the blood pressure and respiration following hydroxydione injection. The intensity of these effects varied considerably with the type of preparation used being well marked in the chloralosed cat in doses equivalent on a mg/kg basis (5 to 10 mg/kg) with that which produces basal anæsthesia in man. In the intact or decerebrate animal, however, as much as five times the anæsthetic dose of hydroxydione was required to cause an effect on blood pressure or respiration. This respiratory and circulatory depressant activity of hydroxydione in dogs anæsthetized with chloralose has been confirmed by other workers[87] and is an interesting phenomenon which may well extend to other anæsthetics such as nitrous oxide.[98] The peripheral synaptic action of hydroxydione was also studied[97] in cats under chloralose and it was observed that hydroxydione in doses which produced considerable hypotension, left the twitch of the tibialis in response to excitation of its motor nerve completely unaffected while the nictitating membrane response to preganglionic excitation was little altered.

The onset of unconsciousness following hydroxydione, even when this is by rapid injection of a 5 or 10% solution, is much slower than with other intravenous agents and the basal anæsthesia produced corresponds more to bromethol than to the thiobarbiturates. It seems likely, however, that amnesia is complete within a few minutes of completing the injection of hydroxydione and patients subsequently have no recollection if the mask is applied while they are still apparently awake.

Many workers consider that hydroxydione is a non-analgesic hypnotic[99 – 103] while others consider that it potentiates the analgesic effect of nitrous oxide and has a slight analgesic potency of its own.[80, 98, 104 – 106] Employing the spring balance technique of analgesimetry[107, 108] it has been found that hydroxydione does not share the anti-analgesic action of the barbiturates but that there is gradually increasing analgesia following injection of anæsthetic doses which is paralleled by the hypnotic action of the drug. Dundee[108] suggested that the analgesic action of hydroxydione may explain the feeling of comfort and postoperative well-being reported after its use by many observers.

Opinions vary on the severity and frequency of respiratory and circulatory depression in patients following the administration of hydroxydione; this is probably related to the rate and dosage employed. In one series,[99] in which hydroxydione was administered as a 1% solution in 5% dextrose and water or normal saline, it was observed that respiratory depression occurred in 22·3 per cent of the patients with some reduction in blood pressure in 62·8 per cent; in only nine cases was this sufficiently severe to warrant the use of a vasopressor. In another large series of 1,000 patients[109] to whom hydroxydione was administered as the main anæsthetic agent or as an adjunct to various types of regional and general anæsthetics, hypotension, tachycardia and apnœa were observed in many cases. On the other hand, several investigators[102, 110] recorded only slight effects on the respiration and blood pressure and it has been claimed[105] that, because of the minimal degree of respiratory depression observed with hydroxydione, it proved useful for anæsthesia in ear, nose and throat surgery. Attention has also been drawn[11] to the delay between the injection of hydroxydione and the appearance of respiratory or circulatory depression. In my own experiences with hydroxydione respiratory depression has not been a serious feature and the risk of immediate respiratory and circulatory depression which may follow the injection of thiopentone has not been seen even after the rapid injection of doses up to 1 G of a 10% solution of hydroxydione. The slow decline in blood pressure which was often observed was not considered to be a disadvantage and produced a reduction in bleeding comparable to that obtained with moderate controlled hypotension by other methods.

Many authors have commented on the marked degree of laryngeal and pharyngeal reflex depression associated with hydroxydione anæsthesia. Because of this and the way in which the endotracheal tube is tolerated it has been recommended for use in head and neck surgery, thyroid operations and neuro-surgery.[80, 102, 112-115] Most authors have found that the muscle relaxation produced by hydroxydione is inadequate for abdominal operations, but combined with a specific muscle relaxant agent these have been carried out satisfactorily.[104] The drug has been found to be particularly suitable for use in elderly patients in poor general condition in whom the light basal anæsthesia obtained with hydroxydione requires only minimal supplementation with potent and toxic general anæsthetic agents.[114, 116] Absence of metabolic disturbances and especially an insignificant effect on the blood sugar level have been reported[117] suggesting that the drug may be a safe anæsthetic for diabetic patients undergoing operative procedures. The inhibition of adrenaline-induced arrhythmias in cats by hydroxydione has been recorded by Taylor and Watson[118] leading them to suggest that the drug might be a useful anæsthetic agent for cardiac surgery. Dow[119] considered that hydroxydione anæsthesia afforded ideal conditions for cardiac catheterization because of its minimal upset of respiration, pulse and blood pressure and its successful use for this procedure in sixty children has been reported.[120] Hydroxydione either does not cross the placental barrier or crosses it only in small amounts and its use has therefore been recommended in operative obstetrics.[121] Several favourable reports[115, 119, 122] have been published on the use of hydroxydione anæsthesia for cæsarean section in which it was claimed that there was little difficulty with fœtal respiratory depression even in cases of fœtal distress.

Many workers have found evidence of venous irritation with subsequent thrombosis or thrombophlebitis in the injected vein following hydroxydione administration and a few have commented on the complaint of pain in the arm during the injection in some patients. In the early clinical trials in the United States it was felt that, to minimize the incidence of venous complications, the drug should be administered in very dilute solution (0·5 to 1% by fast running drip or 2·5% injected into the drip). The incidence of venous thrombosis following hydroxydione administered in this way varied from 3 in 125 patients[104] up to 77·5 per cent.[99] Because of these venous complications and the use of large volumes of fluid given at a fast rate for its administration, hydroxydione has not achieved general acceptance either in the United States or in this country.

However, Stedtfeld,[123] as a result of trials in dogs and later in surgical patients with a new hydroxydione preparation (Presuren), suggested that, by modifications in the technique of administration and particularly by reducing the time in which the solution of hydroxydione remained in contact with the veins, the incidence of thrombosis could be greatly reduced. Employing a rapid injection method with concentrations between 2·5 and 10%, Stedtfeld observed only 6 cases of phlebitis in 158 patients. His findings were confirmed by others[114, 115, 124] using this technique and it has been claimed[115] that the incidence of postoperative thrombophlebitis was not greatly in excess of that caused by more conventional intravenous anæsthetics, although a non-painful venous thrombosis occurred in 26 of the 104 patients observed. The use of 0·25% procaine solution as solvent has been employed to reduce the incidence of injection pain.[125]

Robertson and Wynn Williams[126] studied the venous complications following the administration of hydroxydione in concentrations of 2·5% to 10% administered by various modifications of the rapid injection technique and compared these with a similar series of patients who received 2·5 to 5% sodium thiopentone. They found that in 5 per cent of 359 patients receiving hydroxydione there was evidence of thrombophlebitis while in 35 per cent painless thrombosis at the site of injection, which had not been noticed by the patient, could be detected on careful examination. This incidence was not altered by changes in the concentration of hydroxydione or minor modifications in technique, although it was less than that previously observed when the drug was administered in dilute solution by intravenous infusion. Of the 200 patients who received 5% thiopentone 11·5 per cent had a painless thrombosis and 2 per cent showed evidence of thrombophlebitis while the corresponding figures for the 200 patients receiving 2·5% thiopentone were 5 per cent and 0 per cent. Pathological studies of human and rabbit veins following hydroxydione injection showed that the thrombus consisted mainly of red blood corpuscles with a small admixture of fibrin and that the endothelial lining of the vein was frequently completely absent, although evidence of necrosis or inflammatory signs in or around the vein wall was strikingly absent in most cases. *In vitro* studies, in which 5 and 10% hydroxydione was added to whole blood, showed that, while this had a more lytic action on platelets than thiopentone, there was no detectable effect on the coagulation mechanism. From these studies it was concluded that the thrombosis following hydroxydione injection is the result of damage to the venous intima at the site of injection and that this is due to the chemical composition of the drug rather than its pH or the solvent used.

The major metabolite of hydroxydione has been identified as 3α, 21-dihydroxy 5β-pregnane-20-one (pregnanediolone).[126, 127] This steroid has anæsthetic properties, but preliminary testing in animals has shown that it is too toxic for use in man. In the search for further steroid compounds with anæsthetic potency 3α-hydroxy pregnane-11, 20-dione-3 disodium phosphate (Compound 146, Glaxo) was shown to produce satisfactory anæsthesia in laboratory animals, to have a higher therapeutic ratio than hydroxydione and to be much less irritant on the vascular endothelium as well as being devoid of hormonal activity. Despite these promising features, however, on clinical trial it was found that patients experienced disturbing paræsthesiæ which made it unsuitable as a substitute for hydroxydione.

It, therefore, seems at the present time that, although hydroxydione has valuable properties as a basal anæsthetic, the high incidence of venous thrombosis in the injected vein makes it unlikely that it will receive general acceptance. While the venous complications have undoubtedly been reduced by the introduction of the rapid method of injection, nevertheless, if the advantages of steroid anæsthesia are to be exploited, a new agent rather than a new method of administration is required.

Pharmacology of Intravenous Anæsthesia

Distribution of Thiobarbiturates in Tissues. After the intravenous administration of thiopentone injected in dogs in a single dose over a period of a few seconds, the brain to plasma concentration ratio is the same in 30 seconds as in 3 hours. At both these times the drug is evenly distributed throughout the various areas of the brain.[128] These results indicate that thiopentone passes into brain with extraordinary rapidity unhindered by the blood brain barrier and explains the rapid response of patients to the drug. It is probable that, as with nitrous oxide and other gases, the rate of cerebral blood flow is the limiting factor in the rate at which thiopentone enters the brain. The rate of passage of barbiturates into the brain seems to be related to their fat solubility. Thus, thiobarbiturates penetrate the brain more readily than do their less fat soluble oxygen analogues.

This rapid uptake and equilibration between the brain and blood thiopentone level has also been observed in humans.[129]

Many authors have confirmed the rapidity with which the plasma level of thiopentone falls after injection and in dogs the disappearance of thiopentone from the plasma 45 minutes after the injection and later seemed to proceed exponentially.[130] This rapid early disappearance was previously considered to be the result of the uptake of the drug in the body fat and, once a steady state had been reached in the distribution of the drug between the fat and other tissues, the rate of disappearance from the plasma represented the

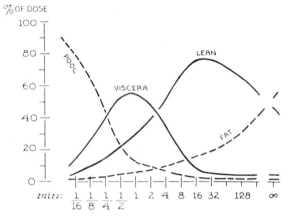

FIG. 2. Distribution of thiopental in different body tissues at various times after its intravenous injection. Time scale (in minutes) progresses geometrically. Final values at infinity (∞). (Price, H. L. *et al.*, 1960. *Clin. Pharmacol. Therap.*).

rate of metabolism since only insignificant amounts appeared in the urine.[131] However, it has been found that thiopentone did not enter fat to a maximum extent in dogs until two to six hours after the injection so that a plasma disappearance rate based on levels as early as 45 minutes after injection must represent more than the metabolism.[130] In man, the uptake of thiopentone into body fat seems to be only slightly more rapid. Price and Conner[132] and Price[133] have come to a similar view by analysis of the kinetics of thiopentone redistribution in the human body, supporting the idea that, contrary to previous beliefs, the role of body fat in determining the duration of anæsthesia is relatively unimportant. Although it appears to be that adipose tissue ultimately contains most of the thiopentone in the body the rate at which fat abstracts the drug from the blood has now been shown to be too slow to make this process clinically important. Saturation of the lean body tissues with thiopentone is probably responsible for the speed with which consciousness is regained after a single intravenous injection of the drug. For this reason the rate at which all these tissues are perfused with blood is important in determining the intensity and duration of narcosis following thiopentone injection. Fig. 2 shows the distribution of thiopentone in different body tissues at various times after its intravenous injection in the humans. Within 1 minute after injection the blood has given up 90% of the dose, principally to the central nervous system, heart, liver and other rapidly perfused viscera and during the ensuing half hour these viscera are in turn depleted of the drug as a result of further redistribution. Of the thiopentone given up by rapidly perfused viscera the other aqueous tissues of the body acquire nearly 80%; the remainder enters fat. The rate at which the central nervous system loses thiopentone therefore depends predominantly on the rate at which the poorly-perfused aqueous tissues of the body gain it. This in turn depends on the rate at which the body is perfused with blood. Fat is so slowly perfused that it cannot begin to concentrate thiopentone to an important degree until after the central nervous system has already lost over 90% of its peak content. Where blood flow to lean tissues is increased, as for example, in apprehension, pregnancy and thyrotoxicosis, a small fraction of the injected drug appears initially in the central nervous system, but where the blood flow to these tissues is reduced, for example in hæmorrhagic shock, the cerebral blood flow is well maintained and the fraction of the dose of thiopentone reaching the central nervous system is abnormally high and its removal slow. Consequently, unconsciousness is prolonged. Thus, the rate of perfusion of indifferent body tissues can have more importance than any other factor in determining the duration of narcosis after thiopentone injection. Further support of the view that, because of its relatively poor blood supply, fatty tissues are of less importance in the rapid removal of thiopentone from blood than the richly perfused lean tissues of the body, is afforded by the finding that weight for weight obese subjects require less thiopentone than lean subjects to attain an anæsthetic of comparable depth and duration.[134, 135] In experiments on rats and rabbits it was found that ingested oil was more efficient than depot fat in reducing sleeping time following thiopentone, probably due to the fact that the effect of the orally ingested fat is due to the chylomicronæmia and hyperlipæmia resulting from fat absorption, since fat dispersed in the blood stream is likely to have a greater surface area and smaller diffusion distance than depot fat.[136] Thus, it appears that, although thiopentone has a great affinity for fat, because of the poor blood supply of the fat depots in the body, uptake of the drug in these tissues is slow and maximum deposition only occurs after about $2\frac{1}{2}$ hours. By this time the fat content of thiopentone greatly exceeds that of other tissues and is a major factor in determining the duration of action of large doses or intermittent repeated doses of thiopentone. After an intravenous infusion lasting more than an hour lean body tissues are saturated with thiopentone and cannot aid in depleting the central nervous system so that recovery, which is delayed, depends on other causes, such as metabolism, excretion and the rapid development of tolerance.

Because of the slow breakdown of thiobarbiturates, when a second dose of the drug is given while the fat depots are already partly filled with the drug, the plasma level will remain high with subsequent prolongation of sleep. A comparison of the cumulative action of four thiobarbiturates in the rat and the dog[137] has confirmed previous observations that the cumulative action of thiopentone can be detected 24 hours after an injection, and that thiamylal is less cumulative than other thiobarbiturates. As the removal of these drugs from the fat depends on detoxication these results suggest that thiamylal is broken down more rapidly than thiopentone, thialbarbitone and thioethamyl.

Detoxication. Frey[138] has carried out a comparative investigation on the breakdown and excretion of short-acting anæsthetics in dogs. He found that the breakdown of thiopentone in dogs appeared to follow two paths—side chain oxidation with the retention of the thiobarbiturate structure and desulphuration to pentobarbitone. The findings of pentobarbitone as a metabolic product of thiopentone is of considerable practical importance and Frey has suggested that the after-effects, particularly with prolonged thiopentone anæsthesia, are primarily attributable to pentobarbitone. After thiopentone anæsthesia, pentobarbitone was demonstrated in the urine and plasma for at least twice as long as after the injection of an equimolar dose of pentobarbitone itself. This finding was explained by the fact that, of the thiopentone stored in the body fat, small amounts are continuously being desulphurated and liberated in the plasma and excreted in the urine. The total excretion time for thiopentone was found to be as long as 6 to 7 days which is only a little less than that of the long-acting barbiturates, barbitone and phenobarbitone.

Acute Tolerance. It has been noted that the blood level of thiopentone is not a reliable guide to the depth of anæsthesia and that there is a wide variation in the blood level at which normal patients awake. Brodie[139] showed that the plasma concentrations at the time of orientation after small total doses of thiopentone were lower than the corresponding levels after larger total doses. It has also been observed that the incremental doses required by patients receiving higher induction doses of thiopentone were greater than those required by patients receiving smaller doses and the suggestion has been made that the peak level reaching in the brain, whether during induction or maintenance, determines the blood level at which the patient will awake.[140] With small total doses relative to the initial dose this peak is more likely to be reached in induction, while with larger total doses the peak may be exceeded by one of the later supplementary injections particularly if these are large.

Plasma Binding. Some factors influencing the distribution, metabolism and action of barbiturates have been reviewed[141] and attention drawn to the fact that thiobarbiturates are more strongly bound to the albumin fraction of the serum protein than their oxygen analogues. Thus with thiopentone about 65% is bound, in contrast with 5% for barbitone. The active concentration of thiopentone in the blood depends on the proportion of the barbiturate that is free in the plasma and this is dependent on the proportion that is rendered pharmacologically inactive by being bound to the plasma proteins. This binding is reversible and varies with the albumin content and pH of the blood as well as with the concentration of thiopentone. The first two factors are unlikely to vary much in normal patients, but when there is an increase in the concentration of barbiturate the percentage bound diminishes although the total amount increases. Consequently patients who have received large amounts of thiopentone will have proportionately more free drug per mg/kg injected than those receiving smaller doses and the level of anæsthesia is correspondingly deeper.

Anti-analgesia. Recent studies [142, 143] have demonstrated that subnarcotic doses of thiopentone antagonize the analgesic action of nitrous oxide, morphine and pethidine and it was suggested that this anti-analgesic action of thiopentone is probably a feature of all barbiturates. With larger doses of thiopentone the pain threshold was shown to rise but when, following redistribution of the drug, the blood level fell the anti-analgesic effect of the drug returned. It has also been shown that promethazine and scopolamine increase the sensitivity to pain[56, 57, 58] and that the use of these drugs as premedication before barbiturate anæsthesia is associated with an increased incidence of postoperative excitement.[59, 144] Although attention has been drawn[145] to the pitfalls of analgesimetry by pain-threshold techniques the findings of Dundee and his associates have considerable support in clinical practice. The recent trend to employ tranquillizing agents, particularly promethazine derivatives, in pre-medication or to potentiate thiopentone anæsthesia[146, 147] may by increasing the anti-analgesic effect of the latter cause an increased incidence of excitatory complications in the recovery period. It would appear that, despite the drawbacks of analgesic drugs, they possess advantages not hitherto fully realized and that their replace-ment in premedication or supplementary anæsthesia by agents which have been shown to possess anti-analgesic activity is likely to cause an increase incidence of skeletal muscle twitching and postoperative restlessness following barbiturate-nitrous oxide-oxygen anæsthesia.

Place of Intravenous Anæsthesia

In recent years general anæsthesia has continued to displace local analgesia in several fields of surgery, such as ophthalmic, ear, nose and throat and out-patient procedures, and, although the use of intravenous anæsthesia alone has generally been unsatisfactory because of the slow recovery of full consciousness following large doses of thiopentone, it seems probable that some of the new agents now becoming available, together with nitrous oxide and suxa-methonium, will produce further encroachment into the domains of local analgesia. In addition, many of the untoward effects encountered in patients suffering from cardiovascular, respiratory and metabolic disturbances following intravenous anæsthesia are now better under-stood and consequently largely avoidable. The place of intravenous anæsthesia, though not of individual agents, will, therefore, now be reviewed in the light of some recent developments.

Cerebral Angiography. Stark[148] has compared general anæsthesia with local analgesia for patients undergoing cerebral angiography and has described a technique of general anæsthesia which has proved satisfactory in 100 consecutive cases. He found that the induc-tion of anæsthesia with an intravenous barbiturate commonly produced a fall in blood pressure of a transitory nature, but considered that the rise in intracranial pressure which was liable to occur during induction of anæsthesia by inhalational methods was a greater risk to the patient. Falls in pressure of 20 mm. Hg or more occurred in 40 per cent of the cases who had a subarachnoid hæmorrhage, but in patients with intracranial tumours only 25 per cent had comparable hypotension during induction of anæsthesia with thiopentone. Although a rise in blood pressure of 20 mm. Hg or more was observed during anæsthesia in several patients with subarachnoid hæmorrhage specific treatment with a hypotensive drug was only required on one occasion. The author attributed this hypertensive response to temporary ischæmia of the vasomotor centre caused by the increased cerebrovascular resistance produced by thiopentone, although other factors may have played a part.

Translumbar Aortography. In translumbar aortography carried out as an aid to urological diagnosis and for investigation of peripheral vascular disease, with thiopentone sodium used as the sole agent for anæsthesia, the absence of adequate respiratory control in the prone position associated with such risks as coughing and laryngospasm as well as the lack of analgesic activity of the drug have been found to be serious disadvantages and extra-aortic extravasation has been a not infrequent complication. Using a technique of general anæsthesia with thiopentone as an induction agent only, followed by intubation and controlled respiration with gas, oxygen and trichlorethylene or pethidine anæsthesia, Stuart[149] claimed that, in his experience of over 1,000 cases, good operative and postoperative conditions were consistently produced.

Cardiac Surgery. Several authors have discussed the use of intravenous anæsthesia in patients undergoing cardiac operations. All are agreed that the effects of thiobarbiturates on the myocardium, central vasomotor mechanism and peripheral vessels tend to cause a fall in blood pressure with consequent reduction in coronary blood flow. These drugs must therefore be given very slowly and in minimal dosage to avoid such undesirable effects.[150, 151] In a series of 420 mitral valvulotomies anæsthetized by Gray and Riding[152] the authors concluded that, because of their circulatory depressant effects, the use of thiobarbiturates should be reduced to a minimum and if possible should be excluded completely. A reduction in the dosage of barbiturates was achieved by the use of pethidine and later by gradually extending the use of nitrous oxide in induction. They point out, however, that they were unable to show objectively that the reduction in the dosage of thiopentone had been justified by their results.

Thoracic Operations. The experiences of Moore[153] on the use of intermittent doses of thiopentone during surgery has confirmed the general opinion that this method has numerous disadvantages. He found difficulty in knowing when further doses of thiopentone were indicated during the course of anæsthesia, and by limiting the use of thiopentone to the induction dose only the recovery period was shortened.

Experiences in the use of balanced anæsthesia with intravenous barbiturates and narcotics together with muscle relaxants and nitrous oxide oxygen inhalation has been described in 200 patients with advanced pulmonary tuberculosis undergoing pneumonectomy, lobectomy or segmental resection.[154] The patients were divided into two groups according to the premedication given, the first group receiving barbiturates with morphine or pethidine and scopolamine or atropine intramuscularly; while the second group received chlorpromazine with atropine or scopolamine. It was found that the type of operation did not influence the amount of thiopentone needed but that patients having chlorpromazine required approximately 20% more thiopentone than those having an analgesic drug in the premedication.

Laryngoscopy and Bronchoscopy. Although local analgesia is still used for endoscopic procedures, general anæsthesia is now widely employed and the combined use of thiopentone and suxamethonium with or without local analgesia provides excellent conditions for these examinations. Various methods of overcoming the problems of ventilation and oxygenation have been described in recent years.

Macintosh[155] suggested that with topical anæsthesia and intermittent injections of thiopentone and suxamethonium the patient can breathe spontaneously and adequately. Kensall[156] employed a similar technique which allows bronchoscopy to be carried out while oxygen is being passed into the sidearm of the bronchoscope and artificial respiration maintained by manual compression of the patient's chest. The use of a cuirass to produce adequate movement of the chest has also been found to offer a satisfactory solution to the problem.[157, 158] In another method described by Cheatle and Chambers,[159] with patients under thiopentone anæsthesia and made apnœic with suxamethonium, a piece of portex tubing 3 mm internal diameter is passed into the trachea as far as the carina and a flow of oxygen of 3 litres a minute delivered through it. Additional doses of suxamethonium are given during bronchoscopy to maintain respiratory paralysis. Determinations of oxygen and carbon dioxide content and of pH of arterial blood of their patients showed that oxygenation was adequately maintained, but that there was a rise in the carbon dioxide content and a consequent fall in arterial blood pH. These changes were not thought to be dangerous because of the short period required for bronchoscopy. Other anæsthetists[160, 161] have combined intravenous barbiturate anæsthesia with nitrous oxide/ oxygen administered via a small bore endotracheal tube and a short-acting muscle relaxant drug for bronchoscopic and laryngoscopic procedures, including biopsies and cord striping for polyps and other lesions. The Magill tubes used varied in size from a No. 4 for the average adult down to a No. 0 tube for children under 4 years of age. In children between 2 and 6 years no barbiturate was given for induction, but light sleep was induced with nitrous oxide/oxygen and in those under 2 years of age ordinarily no premedication or anæsthetic was given, but repeated small doses of suxamethonium only.

The difficulty of maintaining satisfactory gaseous exchange in patients during bronchoscopy due to the competition between surgeon and anæsthetist for the airway is reflected in the numerous anæsthetic techniques which have been described. While it is difficult to say which method is best it seems unlikely that those which rely on spontaneous respiration through a narrow-bore endotracheal tube or those in which gas exchange is dependent on oxygen insufflation will meet with general approval.

Intraocular Surgery. Increasing use is now being made of general anæsthesia in preference to local analgesia for many ophthalmic operations. Cataract extraction under general anæsthesia may be complicated by increases in intraocular pressure with corresponding loss of vitreous. Such changes in tension may be due to straining or coughing, increase in tone in the ocular muscles or rises in venous pressure. Intravenous anæsthesia is frequently chosen in such cases because induction is easy and rapid with no stage of excitement, it produces a consistent fall in intraocular tension and postoperative vomiting is usually slight. Some authors[162, 163] advocate the use of intravenous injection of thiopentone sodium in dilute solution for induction along with small doses of a relaxant to aid in obtaining reduced intraocular tension. They believe that the best results are obtained when an endotracheal tube is avoided and the patient is allowed to breathe spontaneously. Others[164-169] combine the use of an induction dose, sometimes followed by intermittent injections of an intravenous barbiturate along with a relaxant and endotracheal nitrous oxide/oxygen anæsthesia. Condon[165] employed thialbarbitone sodium rather than thiopentone sodium as he found that the former caused less respiratory depression with equivalent depths of anæsthesia and that in many cases of apnœa or respiratory depression thiopentone was responsible rather than any relaxant employed. Sandiford[168] recommends that for intracapsular extractions respiration should be controlled throughout whereas in the extracapsular extractions spontaneous respiration should be retained.

Intravenous Anæsthesia for Obstetrics. Because of the claim[170] that equilibrium between maternal and fœtal blood and thiopentone was not reached until 10 to 12 minutes after injection and that delivery after this time would result in dangerous depression in the infant, several authors[171, 172] have suggested that when thiopentone is used the infant should be extracted as rapidly as possible, i.e. within 4 minutes, if fœtal respiratory depression is to be prevented. Other studies,[173-175] however, have indicated that there is no appreciable placental barrier to thiopentone, the drug reaching the fœtus at a rate which probably depends on the mother's circulation time so that the fœtal level is at a maximum at the onset of anæsthesia and then falls at a rate determined by the combined fœtal and maternal metabolism, redistribution and excretion. It seems, therefore, that thiopentone may be used irrespective of the time delivery may take and that the longer the interval between the injection and delivery the lower the fœtal levels of thiopentone will be. Most workers, therefore, believe now that, as the fœtus cannot be extracted in under the maternal circulation time, the longer the time interval between the injection of the drug and the removal of the fœtus the greater will be the margin of safety. Thus, in the absence of fœtal distress undue speed is a disadvantage.[176-180] These results apply only to single injections of thiopentone for, with continuous or multiple injection techniques, the fœtal serum thiopentone levels will rise parallel to the maternal serum levels and the risk of respiratory depression in the baby will be increased.[174, 181] The consensus of opinion is, therefore, that the use of intravenous barbiturates for induction of anæsthesia should not impose a limit on the time taken for delivery and, because of the pleasant induction, relative freedom from vomiting and lack of neonatal depression when a single small dose of an intravenous barbiturate is used, that these drugs are valuable in obstetric anæsthesia.

Electroconvulsant Therapy. An intravenous anæsthetic along with a short-acting muscle relaxant drug is now generally employed for modified electroconvulsant therapy.[182, 183] A recent report[184] on the effect of thiopentone—between 100 mg and 500 mg—on blood pressure and heart rate showed that the rises following the shock were lessened by an increase in the dose of thiopentone. This was offset, however, by the disadvantages of prolonged duration of apnœa and unconsciousness following treatment. From a comparison of the use of relaxant-modified electroconvulsant therapy with and without thiopentone anæsthesia it was concluded that modification by means of suxamethonium chloride without anæsthesia is safer, less time consuming and less complex than modification by means of thiopentone and suxamethonium together.[185] Further, it was claimed that, although anxiety may occur in the patient during the injection of the suxamethonium, if the electrical stimulus is given early the duration of the anxiety is brief and there is no subsequent memory of the experience. In a similar series of cases reported by Little and Reid[186] it was found that the use of the relaxant significantly delayed the return of breathing, but that this was reduced by the addition of buthalitone and to a lesser extent by thiopentone. Further, while thiopentone delayed the recovery of consciousness following relaxant-modified electroconvulsant therapy, the period required for recovery from the effects of the relaxant was not significantly increased when buthalitone was employed. These authors concluded that, although the use of suxamethonium without an anæsthetic gives a satisfactory modification of the fit, better results were obtained when an intravenous anæsthetic was also given. They claim that buthalitone is superior to thiopentone for this purpose and this is supported by Frieze and Mather[187] who found that induction and recovery of anæsthesia was smoother and quicker with buthalitone than with any other intravenous agent used. It seems likely, however, that methohexitone will prove superior for this purpose.

Use of Intravenous Anæsthesia in Special Circumstances

Normal patients vary considerably in their sensitivity to the depressant effects of thiopentone and the skill and experience of the administrator is of more importance in determining the safety of an intravenous anæsthetic than the presence or absence of a pathological condition. Further, in some situations where an intravenous drug as the main anæsthetic agent would be unwarranted, it may be justified, when used carefully and in small dosage, for induction of anæsthesia only. In the presence of certain diseases, such as cardiac or renal failure, status asthmaticus, Addison's Disease or porphyria, or when the patient is receiving concurrent drug therapy, such as cortisone, the risks associated with an intravenous induction may be considerably increased. It is, therefore, important that the anæsthetist should be aware of the existence of any concurrent disease and of any drug treatment which the patient is receiving so that he can assess the risks involved and take appropriate steps to reduce these to a minimum.

Peripheral Circulatory Failure. Attention has again been drawn to the dangers associated with the use of thiopentone in patients suffering from traumatic shock.[188] Much smaller doses of all anæsthetics are needed in shocked patients and this is particularly true in the case of intravenous barbiturates used for the induction of anæsthesia when very small doses should be given until the patient just falls asleep to avoid circulatory collapse and to prevent over-dosage which may result in prolonged narcosis. Changes of posture, particularly sudden ones, are very liable to precipitate collapse in the shocked patient and the greatest care should be taken to move the patient very carefully and only when absolutely necessary. How-ever, provided these precautions are taken Wolfsen considered that thiopentone is an excellent drug for induction of anæsthesia in shocked patients.

Liver Disease. Although it is now established that the liver is the main site of breakdown of thiobarbiturates in the body, Zuck[189] concluded that thiopentone is relatively well-tolerated, if used with care, in jaundiced patients as its cerebral action is terminated by redistribution to non-nervous tissues and is not dependent on detoxication in the liver. With average doses, therefore, there is rarely prolongation of narcosis in the presence of liver disease unless the liver is very severely damaged, the administration prolonged, or very large doses of thiopentone have been administered.

Hæmophilia. Leatherdale[190] described a method of anæsthesia which he had found to be satisfactory in 60 operations for dental extraction in 28 hæmophilic patients. He pointed out that the use of local infiltration or nerve block analgesia is contra-indicated in hæmophilic subjects because of the bleeding which may result and that traumatic intubation could produce serious respiratory obstruc-tion due to hæmatoma formation. He recommended that an intra-venous drip should be set up an hour before operation and 1 litre of plasma given. All premedication, relaxant or intravenous anæsthetic drugs should be administered via the drip, the dosage of each being as small as possible to ensure that rapid recovery of reflexes and consciousness occur. He considered that the technique which he described might be applied equally well to any patient suffering from a disease characterized by a hæmorrhagic diathesis.

Dystrophia Myotonica. Several reports have recently appeared in the literature on the effect of thiopentone in patients suffering from dystrophia myotonica.[191-194] In all of these the patients showed extreme sensitivity to thiopentone manifested by profound depression of respiration amounting to apnœa. In one case[191] the apnœa following 500 mg of thiopentone lasted for 2 hours and spontaneous adequate respiration did not return until $3\frac{1}{2}$ hours after induction. This patient, a man aged 50, subsequently received a test injection of 50 mg of thiopentone which was followed by very marked depression of respiration without loss of consciousness. He had been admitted to hospital for the removal of a cataract and the presence of the myotonia was unsuspected before operation. The authors pointed out that, although dystrophia myotonica is rare, at least 50 per cent of these patients develop cataracts and it seems likely that anæsthetists may more often encounter patients with this disease if the present trend to general anæsthesia for ophthalmic surgery continues. Local analgesia was suggested as the method of choice for such cases, but if for any reason thiopentone is to be used it should be given in very dilute solutions, e.g. 1%, and the dose should be limited to not more than 100 mg. If a larger dose is given in error the patient may regain consciousness before respiration becomes adequate and artificial respiration must be maintained with nitrous oxide and oxygen and not with oxygen alone. It has also been pointed out that cardiac involvement is frequently present in these cases and that the damaged myocardium is very susceptible to single or repeated doses of thiopentone.[194] In a girl of 12, death occurred 45 minutes after an operation for correction of ptosis for which 200 mg of thiopentone had been administered for induction of anæsthesia. Although respiration appeared to be adequate during the operation, respiratory arrest occurred 30 minutes after her return to the ward and, despite inflation of the lungs and cardiac massage, she could not be revived. At autopsy the outstanding features were adipose and collagenous infiltration of the cardiac muscle and changes in the skeletal musculature typical of a muscular dystrophy.

Porphyria. The danger of precipitating an acute attack in porphyric patients by the use of intravenous barbiturates has again been stressed in recent reports.[195, 196] In known cases and where the condition is suspected in a patient with acute abdominal symptoms the use of these drugs is absolutely contra-indicated. In view of the rarity of the condition in Britain one must, however, agree with Dundee and Riding[197] that there seems little justification in withholding thiopentone from every patient having an emergency laparotomy, in whom the exact diagnosis has not been made, in the remote chance that the abdominal pain may be due to acute porphyria.

Induction of Anæsthesia in Young Children. Intravenous thiopentone has been advocated for the induction of anæsthesia in infants and small children. Payne[198] recommended the use of thiopentone in a dosage of 2·5 to 5 mg/lb as a 2·5% solution given slowly into an intravenous drip of $\frac{1}{5}$ normal saline for induction of anæsthesia in newborn infants for repair of œsophageal atresia and Booth, Nisbet and Wilson[199] consider that induction of anæsthesia by the intravenous route offers advantages for surgical emergencies in children. When the child was reasonably fit, anæsthesia was induced with a $2·5\%$ solution of thiopentone, the maximum dose being, in their hands, 20 mg/stone body weight. They found that in infants venepuncture was usually possible in one of the veins on the front of the wrist provided a sharp, new, No. 26 needle was used and a trained assistant held the wrist in the optimal position with the skin stretched and the veins congested. Hodges[200] studied the psychological effects of an intravenous induction of anæsthesia in 142 children, aged 3 to 12 years, who were undergoing removal of their tonsils and adenoids. Premedication consisted of 0·6 mg of atropine hypodermically or orally. During induction two observers classified the apprehensiveness of the patient into five grades. As a result of these observations, a postoperative follow-up study and replies to a questionnaire sent to parents after 2 to 3 months and again after $2\frac{1}{2}$ years it was found that three patients in the series showed psychic trauma attributable to the anæsthesia. He considered that the success of the method was attributable to the careful handling of the children and the intravenous method of inducing anæsthesia.

The value of intravenous thiopentone in dosage determined according to body weight for the induction of anæsthesia in children undergoing adeno-tonsillectomy has also received favourable comment from several other authors,[201, 202] although it was found that efficient venepuncture occasionally proved difficult in very small or in uncoöperative children.

Rectal Thiopentone. The rectal administration of thopentone in a 10% aqueous solution has been in use for some time, the accepted dosage being 1 G per 50 lb (22·7 kg) body weight. The method has achieved some popularity for inducing basal anæsthesia in young children who are thereby spared the anxiety of other forms of induction and has been used as the sole form of anæsthesia for various diagnostic and therapeutic procedures or, supplemented with local or inhalational anæsthesia, for surgical operations.[203] Satisfactory results have also been reported with rectal thiopentone solution followed by local infiltration with an analgesic drug in 83 children having dental treatment as outpatients.[204] Sixteen required supplementary anæsthesia with divinyl ether but all the children walked out of the dental surgery within an average of 34 minutes.

The difficulty of assessing accurately the amount of thiopentone retained when given in an enema has, however, led to the use of the drug in the form of rectal suppositories.[205-207] A high proportion of satisfactory results were achieved but the onset and recovery times were slower than with the suspension.

The use of rectal thiopentone in pædiatric anæsthesia is a satisfactory procedure but patients require careful watching and facilities must be readily available to deal with respiratory depression.

Intramuscular Thiopentone. Keown and Hitchcock [208] have described their experiences with intramuscular thiopentone in a series of more than 500 children to provide basal narcosis prior to regional block or inhalational anæsthesia or for diagnostic procedures, such as cardiac catheterization, angiocardiography and electroencephalography, with analgesia if required by infiltration of local anæsthetic solutions. An initial dose of 5 to 10 mg per lb body weight, depending on the general condition of the child and the dosage of other premedicant drugs given, was injected rapidly and deeply into the gluteal muscles through a wide bore needle. They considered that the use of a more dilute solution of thiopentone was less satisfactory as the bulk of solution was inconveniently large and the absorption rate slower. If the initial dose proved inadequate in 15 minutes, a second dose of 2 to 5 mg per lb was given into the opposite buttock. This technique was only used in children weighing less than 50 lb in whom intravenous administration is difficult as it is a less accurate method. Although the injection is quite painful, evidence of tissue irritation was only observed in one patient in whom a temporary neuropathy of the sciatic nerve followed a badly placed injection. A degree of respiratory or circulatory depression occurred in a small percentage of cases when the dose of intramuscular thiopentone was excessive or when the child was extremely ill or moribund. Dhruva[209] employing a similar dosage in 41 children did not observe any marked respiratory depression and considered that the danger of laryngeal spasm was much less with intramuscular than with intravenous thiopentone administration. This author injected 8 to 10 mg per lb of 5% thiopentone into the gluteal muscles on both sides and found that if this was mixed with hyaluronidase the child was asleep within 3 to 5 minutes but that the duration of anæsthesia was reduced.

A series of 1,018 children anæsthetized for cardiac catheterization has been reported[210] using the intravenous, rectal and intramuscular routes for administration of the anæsthetic. The authors considered that intramuscular thiopentone as a 5% solution was satisfactory for infants and children under 6 years. However, in young children who were quiet and had good veins a 1·25% solution was injected intravenously and when the cardiac catheter was still in position supplementary doses of this solution were injected through it, especially towards the end of a procedure begun with intramuscular thiobarbiturates. The anæsthetic was not injected when the tip of the catheter was in the ventricle or low in the atrium because of the danger of respiratory depression which was the major complication encountered in the series. Children aged 6 years or more were given a sleep dose of 2·5% thiopentone or thiamylal and no significant difference was observed between the two drugs.

Other investigators considered the injection of supplementary doses of thiopentone through an intravenous needle to be preferable to injection through the cardiac catheter as it avoided possible contamination, inadvertent injection of air and waste of time involved by the need to disconnect the catheter for injection of the drug.[211] After the child was asleep following the rectal administration of bromethol or thiopentone, venepuncture was carried out and a syringe containing 1·25% thiopentone sodium solution and one with isotonic saline were connected to the indwelling intravenous needle via a three-way stopcock or "Y" connection for use if additional thiopentone was required as the effect of the bromethol wore off. They noted a 4 to 5% fall in arterial oxygen saturation when supplementary injections of thiopentone were given. Adams and Parkhouse[212] found intravenous thiopentone in small doses satisfactory as an induction agent for children subjected to cardiac catheterization.

Intravenous Lignocaine

The use of intravenous lignocaine as a supplement to nitrous oxidethiopentone anæsthesia continues to receive favourable comment. The local analgesic may be given in dilute solution by continuous infusion or in 2% solution by intermittent injections. In one series of 400 surgical patients[213] an initial dose of 3 ml of 2% lignocaine was given, following induction with 300 to 500 mg of thiopentone, with 2 ml every 5 minutes for the first hour, 1 ml every 5 minutes for the second hour and 1 ml every 10 minutes for each succeeding hour in the average fit adult. The dosage was reduced to half in aged, toxic or juvenile subjects. Steinhaus and Howland[214] gave a dose of 2% lignocaine equivalent to the induction dose of $2\frac{1}{2}$% thiopentone and subsequently during maintenance intermittent injections of thiopentone and lignocaine in equal amounts were administered. These authors considered that one of the chief advantages of lignocaine as a supplement to thiobarbiturate and nitrous oxide anæsthesia was the suppression of pharyngeal and largyngeal reflexes without obvious respiratory depression and this has led other workers[215] to use intravenous lignocaine to reduce troublesome respiratory reflexes during ether anæsthesia. They found, however, that when 150 mg of 2% lignocaine was injected intravenously it produced a reduction of the alveolar ventilation which in some cases amounted to apnœa. In five patients from whom arterial blood samples were obtained before and after the administration of lignocaine three showed a significant rise in PCO_2 and a fall in pH. They concluded that the apparent improvement in respiratory pattern which had been observed after lignocaine was not due to increased ventilation but to quieter respiration from further respiratory depression. One limitation of the technique is the lack of muscular relaxation but this can be overcome by the addition of a specific muscle relaxant drug. All authors commented favourably on the rapid recovery, absence of nausea and vomiting and decreased demand for analgesics in the postoperative period following this type of anæsthesia but no doubt many of these effects were due to the light level of anæsthesia used.

The danger of toxic effects on the circulation or central nervous system which may occur with local analgesic drugs requires careful and constant supervision. In the dosage used the electrocardiogram revealed no marked alterations and in 11 patients in whom direct measurement of the arterial blood pressure was carried out no fall occurred and most showed a slight rise in pressure.[214] The well-known stimulant effects of local analgesics which result in convulsions were never observed when the doses of lignocaine and thiobarbiturates were balanced. However, signs of cortical irritation, manifested by visible muscle fasciculations or twitchings, were present in all 12 unanæsthetised volunteers who received 2 mg of lignocaine per minute for 25 minutes in a comparative study of intravenously given local analgesic agents.[216] Chloroprocaine was found to be least toxic and it is surprising that this agent has not achieved greater popularity as an intravenous supplement to thiopentone-nitrous oxide anæsthesia.

The effect of *prolonged storage* on thiopentone has been investigated by Nielsen and Spoerel.[217] A sample of thiopentone prepared in 1935 was compared, for anæsthetic potency and side-effects, with a fresh batch in animals and in patients undergoing minor operations. The results showed no signficant difference between the two samples in regard to depth and duration of anæsthesia and there were no undesirable effects. It appears therefore that thiopentone retains its potency and can be safely used after prolonged storage.

The *variations in concentration* at different levels in an ampoule of thiopentone which had been inadequately mixed during preparation have been studied by Rawstron and Margolin.[218] The results, though not unexpected, are interesting for it was found that even after keeping for 24 hours there was little diffusion between the bottom 5 ml and upper 15 ml in a 1 G ampoule. Thus, thiopentone solution from the top of the ampoule may well be insufficient to produce anæsthesia while that in the bottom 5 ml, which was found to contain 0·745 to 0·865 G of thiopentone, may easily produce serious overdosage if used under the impression that it was a 5% solution.

Intra-arterial Thiopentone

Although the danger of injecting thiopentone into an artery is well-known to all anæsthetists reports of this accident still appear in the literature from time to time. In several, despite obvious care, a small amount of thiopentone has been followed by ischæmic changes in the distal part of the limb necessitating amputation. A case reported by Forrester[219] emphasizes the increased risk of accidental intra-arterial injection in the presence of shock when arterial pulsation is reduced and the onset of pain following the injection of the first few mls of thiopentone may be delayed. The risk of entering an artery in the cubital fossa[220] and reports of anomalous and superficial arteries in the forearm[221] has led to the more general use of veins on the back of the hand for induction of anæsthesia with thiopentone and it is therefore disconcerting to read the report by Baillie[222] of two cases of accidental intra-arterial injection of thiopentone at this site. However, Stace[224] has drawn attention to the fact that when the drug is injected into contracted veins in the hand or foot the patient may complain of severe pain and blanching of the skin in a patchy distribution over an area both distal and proximal to the needle point may occur. The severity of the reaction is related to the pressure of injection and in severe cases may be followed by œdema of the skin or superficial necrosis. The writer suggested that in these cases the thiopentone had passed in a retrograde manner into the smaller veins and so into the capillaries and tissue spaces and that the concentration of thiopentone solution used did not alter the occurrence of the effect.

In the prevention of accidental intra-arterial injection of thiopentone emphasis continues to be laid on the avoidance of the cubital fossa as the site of injection and on the use of a 2·5% solution of thiopentone. Careful examination of the region for pulsations should be carried out before compression or a tourniquet is applied and a pause made after the injection of the first few mls and the patient asked if he feels any pain. Despite the above report the back of the hand is the safest place for the injection for, even if an inadvertent intra-arterial injection of thiopentone occurs in this area, because of the extensive collateral circulation it is less likely to have the disastrous consequence of such an injection higher in the limb.

The important investigation carried out by Kinmonth and Shepherd[224] in rabbits on the circulatory changes following intra-arterial thiopentone is of great practical interest to all anæsthetists. Injections of thiopentone (2·5%, 5% and 10%) were made, under a dissecting microscope, into the femoral artery of the rabbit and changes in diameter of the vessel measured. After the injection there was a rapid initial contraction of the whole length of the artery for about 30 seconds followed by a rapid return to normal and then slight dilatation which lasted for about one minute. No prolonged spasm was seen and the injection of a sodium bicarbonate buffer solution of the same pH as thiopentone caused no change in the diameter of the artery. The brief contraction and subsequent dilatation also occurred in animals in which the femoral nerve had been divided so that they were apparently due to a direct effect of the solution on the vessel and not mediated reflexly. Injections of vasodilator drugs such as procaine, tolazoline and papaverine, into the artery produced only a transient effect and, as the vasoconstriction due to thiopentone was in any case so short-lived, it appears unlikely from these investigations that it can play any significant part in the tissue necrosis which follows intra-arterial thiopentone. Studies on the effect of sympathetic denervation and high doses of heparin for several days on the extent of tissue loss in the rabbit ear which had been injected with intra-arterial thiopentone were also made by the same investigators. Both these measures produced a considerable reduction in the average area of tissue loss.

However, Burn[225] found that the addition of 25 to 50 mg of thiopentone to modified Ringer's solution perfusing the isolated ear of the rabbit caused constriction of the artery but that the same volume of perfusate adjusted to the same pH produced no change in the outflow. As pretreatment with reserpine or the injection of tolazoline abolished the constrictor action of thiopentone he concluded that the effect was due to the release of noradrenaline from the artery walls. In further experiments in which 0·04 ml of a 10% solution of thiopentone was injected subcutaneously into the tails of white mice it was found that the incidence of local ulceration and necrosis was significantly less frequent in reserpine-treated animals in comparison with the control animals and that the onset of gangrene of the tail was delayed, though the incidence was probably not reduced. Burn considered that the reduced tissue loss in the rabbit ear following sympathetic denervation, which was observed by Kinmonth and Shepherd, was due to the disappearance of noradrenaline, although the authors themselves suggested that it was the result of increasing the blood flow through the part which thereby discouraged clotting in damaged vessels.

It appears, therefore, that the release of noradrenaline from blood vessel walls following the injection of thiopentone may be responsible for local necrosis following extravenous injection and for the initial spasm following intra-arterial injection, but that the subsequent gangrene produced by the latter is due primarily to intimal damage and thrombosis. Thus, the injection of vasodilator drugs may be advantageous in reducing the initial spasm, but in every case where operation can be postponed intensive heparin therapy offers the best chance of avoiding tissue necrosis. When operation cannot be delayed, however, neurectomy of the sympathetic supply to the affected limb should be carried out surgically.

Analeptics

Many agents have been introduced which have been claimed to shorten the narcosis produced by barbiturates and which would, therefore, be of value in the treatment of barbiturate overdosage, or in reversing postoperatively the effects of therapeutic doses. Whatever the value of these agents in barbiturate poisoning their use in clinical anæsthesia would appear to be rather limited as barbiturates are now seldom employed as the principal anæsthetic agent for long operations, and, with the introduction of the shorter acting agents, the need for reversing the narcotic effect is very infrequent and probably limited to the occasional case of inadvertent overdosage.

Bemegride (Megimide) which is β-ethyl-β-methylglutarimide, was introduced as an antidote to barbiturate intoxication and has been the subject of several articles regarding its use to terminate thiopentone anæsthesia. Although it was observed that bemegride caused an alteration in the tissue distribution of pentothal-S 35 in the tissues of mice and suggested that the shortened sleeping time following the administration of bemegride might be due to its action in facilitating the excretion of sodium thiopentone in the urine,[226] it is now generally agreed that it probably exerts a non-specific analeptic action by stimulation of the reticular nuclei of the brain stem.[227-229]

Harrison and Bull[230] carried out a controlled trial in 160 patients undergoing minor gynæcological procedures under thiopentone anæsthesia. Bemegride was given intravenously, the initial dose being 50 mg and if no response resulted the same dose was repeated every minute to a total of 200 mg. The use of bemegride resulted in a mean shortening of the recovery time by 6 minutes compared to the control group, but there was a wide individual variation and overlapping with the control values. Two patients in the series developed convulsions following the administration of 200 mg of bemegride. These authors concluded that the drug appeared to be of no real value in shortening the recovery time after routine barbiturate anæsthesia, but that it may be of some use in cases of inadvertent overdosage with thiopentone. Wyke and Frayworth[229] from a study of 52 patients given repeated intravenous injections of 0·5% solution of bemegride, the initial dose averaging 50 mg, following thiopentone anæsthesia, found that it was an effective and safe antidote to barbiturate anæsthesia, increasing respiration and the return of reflexes, although there was little effect on full recovery of consciousness, while Waine and Dinmore[231] using doses of 2 mg of bemegride for each 5 mg of thiopentone injected, up to a maximum of 200 mg, observed that they could terminate anæsthesia rapidly in 88 per cent of patients. One patient in the latter series, who received a dose of 280 mg of bemegride, developed typical Jacksonian convulsion; amylobarbitone was given and there were no further sequelæ. O'Riordan and Breward[232] compared the efficacy of various analeptics in reversing thiopentone anæsthesia and concluded that the most effective were bemegride and a combination of bemegride with amiphenazole, which is only a weak antagonist of barbiturates when used alone. Mackett[233] compared the recovery time of 100 patients who received thiopentone (40 mg per stone body weight) with 100 cases receiving, in addition, 50 mg of bemegride at the termination of anæsthesia. He observed a significant shortening in the recovery time of 50 cases where the duration of anæsthesia did not exceed 4 minutes, but, where anæsthesia was more prolonged, there was less difference between the recovery times of the bemegride and control series. He does not recommend the routine use of bemegride to accelerate recovery from thiopentone anæsthesia. In contrast to these findings in two controlled clinical blind trials in which bemegride was used in a dosage of 50 mg following thiopentone anæsthesia, no significant difference in recovery time was detected between patients who received bemegride and those who received water or saline.[234, 235]

It has been claimed[236] that a thiopentone-bemegride mixture has several advantages over thiopentone alone, namely, reduced toxicity, less respiratory depression and shorter duration of action and that addition of bemegride up to a ratio of 1 : 3 does not affect the anæsthetic potency of thiopentone. The validity of these results has, however, been questioned on the grounds that the method was not sensitive enough to detect considerable decrease in the thiopentone potency.[237] In a further study, therefore, the electroencephalogram, a sensitive index of barbiturate narcosis, has been used to measure drug effect and as a servo-mechanism to control the intravenous administration of methohexitone which was used to maintain a constant electroencephalographic level in unpremedicated dogs. From the change in the methohexitone requirements following the administration of the thiopentone-bemegride mixture it was found that thiopentone was 1·51 times as potent as thiopentone plus bemegride.

Methyl Phenidate (Ritalin). This compound in methyl 1-phenyl-2-piperidylacetate. Gale[238] observed the effect of methyl phenidate on recovery from thiopentone-nitrous oxide anæsthesia in 262 patients and 108 controls following minor gynæcological operations. Methyl phenidate shortened recovery time to a statistically significant degree, the maximum effect being obtained with doses between 0·1 and 0·19 mg. per lb. body weight. He concluded that the drug was not a biological competitor of thiopentone, but a central nervous system stimulant. The value of this agent for hastening the recovery of ambulant dental patients and of patients undergoing minor surgery under barbiturate anæsthesia has been confirmed by other workers.[239, 240] They observed, however, a high incidence of euphoria, restlessness, mental agitation and headache following its administration in moderate doses and considered that these precluded its routine use following barbiturate anæsthesia. Recently, Roberts[241] has studied the value of the postoperative administration of methyl phenidate by a double blind method in 294 patients, 174 of whom received methyl phenidate and 120 normal saline. Analysis of the results indicated that there was no significant decrease in the awakening time of the methyl phenidate series, but the degree of respiratory stimulation due to the drug was statistically significant while blood pressure changes were minimal. Psychomotor stimulation occurred in both groups but was slightly more in the treated group than in the controls.

Gale[242] studied the comparative and additive effects of methyl phenidate and bemegride on recovery time in 696 patients who had undergone the uterine dilatation and curettage under thiopentone-nitrous oxide anæsthesia. Recovery times were significantly shorter after the combination of drugs than after either drug alone. O'Riordan and Marcus[243] noted that the arousal effects with bemegride, methyl phenidate and the combination of methyl phenidate and nikethamide were of comparable order. They commented that the arousal effect on the cerebral cortex occurred with all the drugs used but that the stimulant effect on respiration was most marked with the latter combination. While large doses of methyl phenidate may produce moderate and transient rises in blood pressure, in most reports clinical doses produced little change. However, the drug modifies the action of sympathomimetric agents, preventing the pressor effect of amphetamine and ephedrine but potentiating that of noradrenaline.[68, 244]

Ethamivan (Vandid) is N N-diethylvanillamide. In a preliminary communication Gardner[245] stated that ethamivan was more effective than nikethamide, bemegride or picrotoxin in bringing about a rapid return to full consciousness following thiopentone anæsthesia. In 6 out of the first 15 cases in which the drug was used, however, mild convulsions occurred. In the next 25 consecutive cases no untoward effects were observed and it was considered that the dosage was previously too large or that the drug had been given too quickly. Romagnoli and Diamond[246] also considered that side-effects, such as sneezing, coughing, itching and flushing, were the result of unduly rapid administration of concentrated solutions of ethamivan. They employed a 1% solution in normal saline given slowly over 3 minutes in a ratio of 1 ml of ethamivan : 1 ml of $2\frac{1}{2}$% sodium thiopentone. Of the 200 patients in their series no side-effects were noticed in 153. They found the drug to have useful arousal and respiratory stimulant activity in many types of central nervous depression including barbiturate, morphine, alcohol, ether and carbon dioxide narcosis. This non-specific respiratory and higher centre stimulant effect of ethamivan has been confirmed in 43 patients with barbiturate intoxication, chronic pulmonary emphysema and other clinical states associated with impaired ventilation.[247]

In view of the potent cortical stimulating effect of *lysergic acid diethylamide* (*L.S.D.*) investigations have been carried out to determine if this compound possessed an analeptic effect against thiopentone. Dobkin and Harland[248] carried out experiments in dogs and found that there was no statistically significant analeptic effect with L.S.D.-25 as determined by the time taken for dogs to raise their heads and rise on their paws following administration of thiopentone. In 55 female patients undergoing minor gynæcological procedures under thiopentone-nitrous oxide anæsthesia who were given 25 G of L.S.D.-25 immediately after the end of the anæsthesia no significant difference in the time required for awakening was noticed between this group and a similar group of fifty-five patients having the same anæsthetic, but receiving no analeptic.[249] In experiments on mice other investigators found that lysergic acid diethylamide prolonged pentobarbitone and hexobarbitone anæsthesia and demonstrated that pentobarbitone was a competitive inhibiter of L.S.D. metabolism in vitro.[250]

Phenyl-pyrrolidino-pentane, which is a synthetic derivative of papaverine, has been used as an analeptic agent following barbiturate anæsthesia and found to produce lightening of anæsthesia with marked respiratory stimulation increasing the depth of breathing and abolishing respiratory irregularity.[251]

Tacrine, which is 5-amino-1:2:3:4:-tetrahydroacridine (Tetra-hydroaminocrine, THA), has been used as a respiratory stimulant in anæsthesia and in barbiturate and morphine poisoning with beneficial effect[252, 253] but further work will be required to elucidate its true value.

A comparison of the analeptic activity against thiopentone of many new compounds including several recently introduced for the treatment of mental depression has been carried out by Dobkin.[254, 255] He considered that *Micoren* (a mixture of equal parts of N-crotomyl-α-ethyl aminobutyric acid diethylamide and N-crotonyl-α-propylaminobutyric acid dimethylamide) and *RP 8228* (1-phenyl-1-(2-piperidyl)-1-acetoxymethane) deserve extensive clinical trial to determine whether they have a higher therapeutic index in man than the combination of bemegride with amiphenazole or methyl phenidate. He also suggested that greater efficiency in the treatment of prolonged postanæsthetic unconsciousness might be derived from combining leptazole with micoren, RP 8228, beme-gride, pipradrol or ethamivan.

In conclusion, it seems that none of these analeptic agents is likely to find a place for routine use following barbiturate anæsthesia. However, in patients who have received inadvertent overdosage with thiopentone, the use of an analeptic drug which will augment respiratory exchange and bring reflex activity towards a normal level, may be indicated, although complete recovery of conscious-ness may not be achieved. If an attempt is made to bring these patients to a state of full wakefulness muscular twitching, exaggerated reflexes and mild convulsions may occur. The present trend in intravenous anæsthesia is towards the discovery of a short acting intravenous agent rather than to reverse the anæsthesia with an analeptic drug.

References

1. DUNDEE, J. W. (1955). *Anæsthesia*, **10**, 391.
2. SWERDLOW, M. (1958). *Brit. J. Anæsth.*, **30**, 2.
3. DUNDEE, J. W., and RIDING, J. E. (1955). *Brit. J. Anæsth.*, **27**, 381.
4. TOVELL, R. M., ANDERSON, C. C., SADOVE, M. S., ARTUSIO, J. F., PAPPER, E. M., COAKLEY, C. S., HUDON, F., SMITH, S. M., and THOMAS, G. J. (1955). *Anesthesiology*, **16**, 910.
5. DUNDEE, J. W., and RIDING, J. E. (1960). *Brit. J. Anæsth.*, **32**, 206.
6. DUNDEE, J. W., BARRON, D. W., and KING, R. (1960). *Brit. J. Anæsth.*, **32**, 566.
7. NOBES, P. (1955). *Lancet*, **2**, 1296.
8. RUDDELL, J. S. (1955). *Lancet*, **2**, 1138.
9. DAVIDSON, J., and LOVE, W. J., (1956). *Brit. J. Anæsth.*, **28**, 377.
10. DUFFIELD, J. R., and GINSBERG, H. (1957). *S. Afr. med. J.*, **31**, 128.
11. HENDERSON, A. G., and MACKETT, J. (1957). *Brit. med. J.*, **1**, 1095.
12. MURRAY, D. B. (1957). *Scot. med. J.*, **2**, 396.
13. YOUNG, D. S. (1956). *Proc. R. Soc. Med.*, **49**, 735.
14. DRUMMOND-JACKSON, S. L. (1956). *Brit. dent. J.*, **100**, 213.
15. MOSTERT, W. J., and DURHAM, F. J. (1957). *J. dent. Ass. S. Afr.*, **12**, 224.
16. LITTLE, A. F. M., and REID, A. A. (1957). *Lancet*, **1**, 1016.
17. ROSALES, K. J., DENNIS, R., and GILBERT, R. G. B. (1957). *Canad. Anæsth. Soc. J.*, **4**, 405.
18. SIMMONS, P. H. and BLANSHARD, M. S. (1957). *Brit. med. J.*, **2**, 1347.
19 WYANT, G. M., CHANG, C. A., and COCKINGS, E. C. (1959). *Canad. Anæsth. Soc. J.*, **6**, 108.
20. WYANT, G. M., DOBKIN, A. B., and AASHEIM (1957). *Brit. J. Anæsth.*, **29**, 194.
21. KANE, P. O., and STEPHENS, C. J. (1959). *Brit. J. Anæsth.*, **31**, 533.
22. SIMMONS, P. H., and CURWEN, M. P. (1960). *Brit. med. J.*, **1**, 32.
23. O'MULLANE, E. J. (1957). *Brit. J. Anæsth.*, **29**, 71.
24. KEÉRI-SZÁNTÓ, M., and LABARRE, J. (1957). *Canad. Anæsth. Soc. J.*, **4**, 338.
25. HENDERSON, A. G., and MACKETT, J. (1958). *Brit. J. Anæsth.*, **30**, 317.
26. ORKIN, L. R., MORALES, G. A., FUJITA, M., and GABUYA, R. L. (1958). *Anesthesiology*, **19**, 110.
27. IRWIN, S., STAFF, R. D., DUNBAR, E., and GOVIER, W. M. (1956). *J. Pharmacol.*, **116**, 317.
28. LINN, R. H., and TORMEY, W. C. (1958). *Oral Surg.*, **11**, 496.
29. FITZPATRICK, L. J., CLARIE, D. C., and MERSCH, M. M. (1956). *Anesthesiology*, **17**, 684.
30. BOONE, J. D., MUÑOZ, R., and DILLON, J. B. (1956). *Anesthesiology*, **17**, 284.
31. DUNDEE, J. W. (1956). *Thiopentone and other Thiobarbiturates*, p. 262. E. & S. Livingstone, Edinburgh.
32. O'HERLIHY, D. B., NISHIMURA, N., LITTLE, D. M., and TOVELL, R. M. (1956). *Canad. Anæsth. Soc. J.*, **3**, 326.
33. FLEMING, S. A., and ROBINSON, J. G. (1957). *Canad. Anæsth. Soc. J.*, **4**, 52.
34. GALE, A. S. (1957). *Anesthesiology*, **18**, 573.
35. REDISH, C. H., VORE, R. E., CHERNISH, S. M., and GRUBER, C. M. Jr. (1958). *Oral Surg.*, **11**, 603.
36. EGBERT, L. D., SECHZER, P. H., and ECKENHOFF, J. E. (1958). *Anesthesiology*, **19**, 656.

37. LITTLE, D. M. Jr., CRETEUR, C. A. J., and TOVELL, R. M. (1959). *Anesthesiology*, **20**, 177.
38. BLAKE, M. W., and PERLMAN, P. L. (1956). *J. Pharmacol.*, **117**, 287.
39. PAPPER, E. M., PETERSEN, R. C., BURNS, J. J., BERSTEIN, E., LIEF, P., and BRODIE, B. B. (1955). *Anesthesiology*, **16**, 544.
40. BARRON, D. W., and DUNDEE, J. W. (1961). *Brit. J. Anæsth.*, **33**, 81.
41. STOELTING, V. K., GRAF, J. P., and THEYE, R. A. (1960). *J. Ind. med. Ass.*, **43**, 477.
42. GIBSON, W. R., SWANSON, E. E., and DORAN, W. J. (1955). *Proc. Soc. exp. Biol.*, **89**, 292.
43. HEATON, C. E. (1956). *Curr. Res. Anesth.*, **35**, 522.
44. GRUBER, C. M. Jr., STOELTING, V. K., HICKS, M. L., and DOUGHTY, S. (1956). *Fed. Proc.*, **15**, 432.
45. GRUBER, C. M. Jr., STOELTING, V. K., FORNEY, R. B., WHITE, P. and DEMEYER, M. (1957). *Anesthesiology*, **18**, 50.
46. STOELTING, V. K. (1957). *Curr. Res. Anesth.*, **36**, 49.
47. WEYL, R., UNAL, B., and ALPER, Y. (1958). *Surg. Gynec. Obstet.*, **107**, 588.
48. WYANT, G. M., and CHANG, C. A. (1959). *Canad. Anæsth. Soc. J.*, **6**, 40.
49. GREEN, R. A., and JOLLY, C. (1960). *Brit. J. Anæsth.*, **32**, 593.
50. CHRISTENSON, G. R., HEBERT, C. L., and DRISCOLL, E. J. (1961). *Curr. Res. Anesth.*, **40**, 77.
51. EGBERT, L. D., and WOLFE, S. (1960). *Curr. Res. Anesth.*, **39**, 416.
52. WYANT, G. M., and BARR, J. S. (1960). *Canad. Anæsth. Soc. J.*, **7**, 127.
53. COLEMAN, J., and GREEN, R. A. (1960). *Anæsthesia*, **15**, 411.
54. TAYLOR, C., and STOELTING, V. K. (1960). *Anesthesiology*, **21**, 29.
55. DUNDEE, J. W., and MOORE, J. (1961a). *Anæsthesia*, **16**, 50.
56. MOORE, J., and DUNDEE, J. W. (1961a). *Brit. J. Anæsth.*, **33**, 3.
57. MOORE, J., and DUNDEE, J. W. (1961b). *Brit. J. Anæsth.*, **33**, 422.
58. DUNDEE, J. W., and MOORE, J. (1961c). *Anæsthesia*, **16**, 194.
59. MOORE, J., and DUNDEE, J. W. (1961c). *Anæsthesia*, **16**, 61.
60. DUNDEE, J. W., and MOORE, J. (1961b). *Brit. J. Anæsth.*, **33**, 382.
61. DUNDEE, J. W. (1961). *Practitioner*, **187**, 811.
62. LUNDY, J. S. (1955). *J. Amer. med. Ass.*, **157**, 1399.
63. LORHAN, P., HANSEN, J. M., and ARTHUR, W. J. (1957). *Anesthesiology*, **18**, 143.
64. TAIT, C. A., DAVIS, D. A., GROSSKREUTZ, D. C., and BONIFACE, K. J. (1956). *Anesthesiology*, **17**, 536.
65. COTTEN, M. DEV., and BAY, E. (1956). *Anesthesiology*, **17**, 103.
66. WYANT, G. M., KILDUFF, C. J., MERRYMAN, J. E., and DOBKIN, A. B. (1956). *Canad. Anæsth. Soc. J.*, **3**, 291.
67. ARTHUR, W. J., LOHRAN, P. H., and HANSEN, J. M. (1958). *Amer. Surg.*, **24**, 171.
68. PLUMMER, A. J., and YONKMAN, F. F. (1958). *Curr. Res. Anesth.*, **37**, 371.
69. GOLD, M. I. (1958). *Curr. Res. Anesth.*, **37**, 347.
70. FASTIER, F. N. (1958). *N.Z. med. J.*, **57**, 171.
71. SMITH, B., MCDERMOTT, T. F., and KOPPANYI, T. (1960). *Curr. Res. Anesth.*, **39**, 240.
72. STEPHEN, C. R., and DUVOISIN, P. M. (1960). *Anesthesiology*, **21**, 482.
73. GREIFENSTEIN, F. E., YOSHITAKE, J., DEVAULT, M., and GAJEWSKI, J. E. (1958). *Curr. Res. Anesth.*, **37**, 283.
74. JOHNSTONE, M., EVANS, V., and BAIGEL, S. (1959). *Brit. J. Anæsth.*, **31**, 433.
75. LEAR, E., SUNTAY, R., PALLIN, I. M., and CHIRON, A. E. (1959). *Anesthesiology*, **20**, 330.
76. COLLINS, V. J., GOROSBE, C. A., and ROVENSTINE, E. A. (1960). *Curr. Res. Anesth.*, **39**, 302.
77. MUIR, B. J., EVANS, V., and MULCAHY, J. J. (1961). *Brit. J. Anæsth.*, **33**, 51.
78. KURTZKE, J. F. (1961). *Neurology, Minneap.*, **11**, 390.

79. LABORIT, H., COIRAULT, R., DAMASIO, R., GAUJARD, R., LABORIT, G., FABRIZY, P., CHARONNAT, R., LECHAT, P., and CHARETON, J. (1957). *Presse Méd.*, **65**, 1051.
80. DELIGNÉ, P., DAVID, M., and TALAIRACH, J. (1959). *Anésth. Analg.*, **16**, 1012.
81. DUNDEE, J. W. (1958). *Brit. J. Anœsth.*, **30**, 409.
82. THUILLIER, M. J., and DOMENJOZ, R. (1957). *Anœsthesist*, **6**, 163.
83. THEOBALD, W., and DOMENJOZ, R. (1959). *Arzneimittel-Forsch.*, **9**, 285.
84. PULVER, R. (1957). *Anœsthesist*, **6**, 167.
85. PULVER, R., and LITVAN, F. (1960). *Arzneimittel-Forsch.*, **10**, 111.
86. SIMMER, H., and BECK, H. (1960). *Arzneimittel-Forsch.*, **10**, 660.
87. MERCIER, J., GAVEND, M., GAVEND, M. R., DESSAIGNE, S., and HUGUENARD, P. (1959). *Anésth. Analg.*, **16**, 979.
88. FREY, R., and HERRMANN, K. J. (1957). *Anœsthesist*, **6**, 170.
89. HENSCHEL, W. F., and JUST, O. (1957). *Anœsthesist*, **6**, 174.
90. FEURSTEIN, V. (1957). *Anœsthesist*, **6**, 177.
91. BOUREAU, J. (1959). *Anésth. Analg.*, **16**, 1061.
92. SWERDLOW, M. (1961). *Brit. J. Anœsth.*, **33**, 104.
93. DUNDEE, J. W., and HAMILTON, R. C. (1961). *Brit. J. Anœsth.*, **33**, 230.
94. P'AN, S. Y., GARDOCKI, J. F., HUTCHEON, D. E., RUDEL, H., KODET, M. J., and LAUBACH, G. D. (1955). *J .Pharmacol.*, **115**, 432.
95. LAUBACH, G. D., P'AN, S. Y., and RUDEL, H. W. (1955). *Science*, **122**, 78.
96. DAS, P. K., and ARORA, R. B. (1957). *J. Pharmacol.*, **121**, 149.
97. LERMAN, L. H., and PATON, W. D. M. (1960). *Brit. J. Pharmacol.*, **15**, 458.
98. LERMAN, L. H. (1956). *Brit. med. J.*, **2**, 129.
99. DENT, S. J., WILSON, W. P., and STEPHEN, C. R. (1956). *Anesthesiology*, **17**, 672.
100. HARBORD, R. P., and WILD, W. N. (1956). *Proc. R. Soc. Med.*, **49**, 487.
101. LOWLAND, W. S., BOYAN, C. P., and WANG, K-C. (1956). *Anesthesiology*, **17**, 1.
102. WEISS, K. S., and WALLACH, S. (1956). *Curr. Res. Anesth.*, **35**, 507.
103. GREISHEIMER, E. M., ELLIS, D. W., STEWART, G. H., MAKARENKO, L., and OPPENHEIMER, M. J. (1957). *Amer. J. Physiol.*, **190**, 137.
104. MURPHY, F. J., GUADAYNI, N. P., and DEBON, F. (1956). *J. Amer. med. Ass.*, **158**, 1412.
105. TAYLOR, N., and SHEARER, W. M. (1956). *Brit. J. Anœsth.*, **28**, 67.
106. BURSTEIN, C. L. (1956). *Curr. Res. Anesth.*, **35**, 476.
107. CLUTTON-BROCK, J. (1960). *Anœsthesia*, **15**, 71.
108. DUNDEE, J. W. (1960). *Brit. J. Anœsth.*, **32**, 450.
109. ANSBRO, F. P., BLUNDELL, A. E., SWEENEY, J. C. Jr., and PILLION, J. W. (1957). *J. Amer. med. Ass.*, **164**, 163.
110. BRYCE-SMITH, R. (1959). *Brit. J. Anœsth.*, **31**, 262.
111. HUNTER, A. R. (1957). *Anœsthesia*, **12**, 10.
112. GALLEY, A. H., and ROOMS, M. (1956). *Lancet*, **1**, 990.
113. WILSON, P. (1957). *Aust. N.Z. J. Surg.*, **27**, 135.
114. LANDAU, E. (1958). *Anœsthesia*, **13**, 147.
115. GALLEY, A. H., and LERMAN, L. H. (1959). *Brit. med. J.*, **1**, 332.
116. POTTS, M. W. (1959). *Anœsthesia*, **14**, 148.
117. PFLÜGER, H. (1957). *Med. Mitteil.* (Schering A. G., Berlin). No. 3.
118. TAYLOR, N. R. W., and WATSON, H. (1958). *Lancet.*, **2**, 300.
119. DOW, G. R. (1961). *Anœsthesia*, **16**, 207.
120. FELDMAN, S. A., ROBBIE, D. S., and MONRO, J. A. (1961). *Anœsthesia*, **16**, 217.
121. HARBORT, G. (1957). *Zbl. Gynäc.*, **79**.
122. KIVALO, I., and TAMMISTO, T. (1959). *Acta. anœsth. Scand. Suppl.*, **2**, 35.
123. STEDTFELD, G. (1957). *Anœsthesist*, **6**, 140.
124. OPDERBECKE, H. W. (1957). *Thoraxchirurgie*, **5**, 53.
125. GREWE, H. E., PIECHOWSKI, U., and ZUCKERT, D. (1958). *Chirurg.*, **29**, 121.

126. ROBERTSON, J. D., and WYNN WILLIAMS, A. (1961). Anæsthesia, 16, 389.
127. TAYLOR, W. (1959). Acta. endocr., Copenhagen, 32, 187.
128. MARK, L. C., BURNS, J. J., CAMPOMANES, C. I., NGAI, S. H., TROUSOF, N., PAPPER, E. M., and BRODIE, B. B. (1957). J. Pharmacol., 119, 35.
129. PRICE, H. L., DUNDEE, J. W., and CONNER, E. H. (1957). Anesthesiology, 18, 171.
130. PLOUGH, I. C., WALDSTEIN, S. S., BARILA, T. G., and GOLDBAUM, L. (1956). J. Pharmacol., 116, 486.
131. BRODIE, B. B., BERNSTEIN, E., and MARK, L. C. (1952). J. Pharmacol., 105, 421.
132. PRICE, H. L., and CONNER, E. H. (1959). Fed. Proc., 18, 1714
133. PRICE, H. L. (1960). Anesthesiology, 21, 40.
134. KEÉRI-SZANTO, M. (1960). Brit. J. Anæsth., 32, 415.
135. SOEHRING, K., FREY, H. H. and VÖLGER, P. (1955). Anæsthesist, 4, 162.
136. ANDERSON, E. G., and MAGEE, D. F. (1956). J. Pharmacol., 117, 281.
137. DUNDEE, J. W. (1955). Anæsthesia, 10, 391.
138. FREY, H. H. (1959). Arch. int. Pharmacodyn., 118, 12.
139. BRODIE, B. B. (1952). Fed. Proc. 11, 632.
140. DUNDEE, J. W., PRICE, H. L., and DRIPPS, R. D. (1956). Brit. J. Anæsth., 28, 344.
141. RICHARDS, R. K., and TAYLOR, J. D. (1956). Anesthesiology, 17, 414.
142. CLUTTON-BROCK, J. (1961). Anæsthesia, 16, 80.
143. DUNDEE, J. W. (1960). Brit. J. Anæsth., 32, 407.
144. ECKENHOFF, J. E., KNEALE, D. H., and DRIPPS, R. D. (1961). Anesthesiology, 22, 667.
145. BROWN, R. C., and LANDMESSER, C. M. (1961). Curr. Res. Anesth., 40, 275.
146. DOBKIN, A. B. (1960). Brit. J. Anæsth., 32, 424.
147. DOBKIN, A. B. (1960). Anesthesiology, 21, 292.
148. STARK, D. C. (1958). Anæsthesia, 13, 391.
149. STUART, P. (1958). Brit. J. Anæsth., 30, 524.
150. SCHOTZ, S., BLOOM, S. S., and HELMSWORTH, F. W. (1957). J. Amer. med. Ass., 163, 345.
151. BROWN, A. I. P., and SELLICK, B. A. (1955). Brit. med. Bull., 11, 174.
152. GRAY, T. C., and RIDING, J. E. (1957). Anæsthesia, 12, 129.
153. MOORE, A. (1956). Irish, J. med., 6th ser., 176.
154. DOBKIN, A. B., WEHLING, B., GROSS, G., and MENDELSOHN, H. (1955). Anæsthesia, 10, 328.
155. MACINTOSH, R. R. (1954). Anæsthesia, 9, 77.
156. KELSALL, P. D. (1954). Brit. J. Anæsth., 26, 182.
157. PINKERTON, H. H. (1957). Brit. J. Anæsth., 29, 421.
158. TOKER, P. (1955). S. Afr. med. J., 29, 40.
159. CHEATLE, C. A., and CHAMBERS, K. B. (1955). Anæsthesia, 10, 171.
160. LAMMERT, T. K. (1961). J. Amer. med. Ass., 175, 49.
161. REITMAN, J. S. (1957). J. Amer. med. Ass., 165, 943.
162. RIWCHUN, M. H. (1958). Curr. Res. Anesth., 37, 75.
163. BAUER, W. D. (1959). Curr. Res. Anesth., 38, 1.
164. EVANS, G. L. (1956). Brit. J. Anæsth., 28, 372.
165. CONDON, H. A. (1956). Brit. J. Anæsth., 28, 80.
166. HARPER, J. K. (1955). Proc. Wld. Congr. Anesth., Scheveningen, p. 253. Burgess, Minneapolis.
167. MOORE, J. G. (1958). Brit. J. Ophthal., 42, 723.
168. SANDIFORD, H. B. C. (1957). Brit. J. Anæsth., 29, 319.
169. GOLDSMITH, E. (1961). Anæsthesia, 16, 241.
170. HELLMAN, L. M., SHETTLES, L. B., MANAHAN, C. P., and EASTMAN, N. J. (1944). Amer. J. Obstet. Gynec., 48, 851.
171. COLLIER, H. (1956). Brit. J. Anæsth., 28, 130.
172. HAMER HODGES, R. J., BENNETT, J. R., TUNSTALL, M. E., and KNIGHT, R. F. (1959). Brit. J. Anæsth., 31, 152.

173. McKechnie, F. B., and Converse, J. G. (1955). *Amer. J. Obstet. Gynec.*, **70**, 639.
174. Crawford, J. S. (1956). *Brit. J. Anæsth.*, **28**, 146.
175. Marx, G. F. (1961). *Anesthesiology*, **22**, 294.
176. Steele, G. C. (1957). *Lancet*, **2**, 48.
177. Binham, W. (1957). *Anæsthesia*, **12**, 435.
178. Dundee, J. W. (1956). *Brit. J. Anæsth.*, **28**, 257.
179. Dance, C., and Ward, R. (1958). *Curr. Res. Anesth.*, **37**, 249.
180. Holmes, F. (1959). *Acta. anæsth. Scand., Suppl.*, **2**, 27.
181. Flowers, C. E. (1959). *Amer. J. Obstet. Gynec.*, **78**, 730.
182. Byrne, P. D. (1955). *Proc. Wld. Congr. Anesth., Scheveningen*, p. 207. Burgess, Minneapolis.
183. Steven, R. J. M., and Tovell, R. M. (1959). *Curr. Res. Anesth.*, **38**, 42.
184. Egbert, L. D., Dumas, P. A., Ginter, G. C., and Eckenhoff, J. E. (1959). *Anesthesiology*, **20**, 309.
185. Kelleher, J., and Whiteley, R. W. (1955). *Lancet*, **2**, 589.
186. Little, A. F. M., and Reid, A. A. (1957). *J. med. Sci.*, **103**, 270.
187. Frieze, M., and Mather, I. (1957). *Brit. med. J.*, **1**, 1305.
188. Wolfson, L. J. (1956). *Brit. J. clin. Pract.*, **10**, 783.
189. Zuck, D. (1957). *Brit. J. clin. Pract.*, **11**, 365.
190. Leatherdale, R. A. D. (1958). *Anæsthesia*, **13**, 27.
191. Bourke, T. D., and Zuck, D. (1957). *Brit. J. Anæsth.*, **29**, 35.
192. Hewer, C. L. (1957). *Brit. J. Anæsth.*, **29**, 180.
193. Lodge, A. B. (1958). *Brit. med. J.*, **1**, 1043.
194. Pachomov, N., and Caughey, J. E. (1958). *Aust. Ann. Med.*, **7**, 159.
195. Staples, W. G. (1959). *Med. Proc.*, **5**, 418.
196. Norris, W., and MacNab, G. W. (1960). *Brit. J. Anæsth.*, **32**, 505.
197. Dundee, J. W., and Riding, J. E. (1955). *Anæsthesia*, **10**, 55.
198. Payne, J. P. (1955). *Brit. J. Anæsth.*, **27**, 388.
199. Booth, A. J., Nisbet, H. I. A., and Wilson, F. (1960). *Anæsthesia*, **15**, 361.
200. Hodges, R. J. H. (1960). *Lancet*, **1**, 82.
201. Doughty, A. (1957). *Brit. J. Anæsth.*, **29**, 407.
202. McAlpine, D. F., and Bowering, M. W. (1958). *Canad. Anæsth. Soc. J.*, **5**, 61.
203. Benson, F., and Saarne, A. (1960). *Acta. Anæsth. Scand.*, **4**, 51.
204. Behrman, S. J., Mark, H. J., and Brown, A. A. (1955). *J. Oral Surg.*, **13**, 125.
205. Aladjemoff, L., Kaplan, I., and Gestash, T. (1958). *Anæsthesia*, **13**, 152.
206. Albert, S. N., Henley, E. E., Albert, C. A., and Eccleston, H. N. (1959). *Curr. Res. Anesth.*, **38**, 56.
207. Lowther, G. P. (1959). *Anæsthesia*, **14**, 100.
208. Keown, K. K., and Hitchcock, P. (1960). *Curr. Res. Anesth.*, **39**, 1.
209. Dhruva, A. J. (1960). *Curr. Res. Anesth.*, **39**, 236.
210. Keown, K. K., Fisher, S. M., Downing, D. F., and Hitchcock, P. (1957). *Anesthesiology*, **18**, 270.
211. Fieldman, E. J., Lundy, J. S., DuShane, J. W., and Wood, E. H. (1955). *Anesthesiology*, **16**, 868.
212. Adams, A. K., and Parkhouse, J. (1960). *Brit. J. Anæsth.*, **32**, 69.
213. DeClive-Lowe, S. G., Desmond, J., and North, J. (1958). *Anæsthesia*, **13**, 138.
214. Steinhaus, J. E., and Howland, D. E. (1958). *Curr. Res. Anesth.*, **37**, 40.
215. Siebecker, K. L., Kimmey, J. R., Bamforth, B. J., and Steinhaus, J. E. (1960). *Acta. Anæsth. Scand.*, **4**, 97.
216. Foldes, F. F., Molloy, R., McNall, P. G., and Koukal, L. R. (1960). *J. Amer. med. Ass.*, **172**, 1493.
217. Neilson, J. S., and Spoerel, W. E. (1959). *Curr. Res. Anesth.*, **38**, 29.
218. Rawstron, R. E., and Margolin, L. (1961). *N.Z. med. J.*, **60**, 209.
219. Forrester, A. C. (1959). *Anæsthesia*, **14**, 388.

220. STUART, P. (1955). *Brit. med. J.*, **2**, 1308.
221. RICHARDSON, W. W. (1956). *Brit. med. J.*, **2**, 754.
222. BAILLIE, T. W. (1958). *Brit. J. Anæsth.*, **30**, 373.
223. STACE, J. H. (1958). *Brit. J. Anæsth.*, **30**, 551.
224. KINMONTH, J. B., and SHEPHERD, R. C. (1959). *Brit. med. J.*, **2**, 914.
225. BURN, J. H. (1960). *Brit. med. J.*, **2**, 414.
226. ACHOR, L. B., GEILING, E. M. K., and DOMEK, N. S. (1956). *Curr. Res. Anesth.*, **35**, 534.
227. HAHN, F., and OBERDORF, A. (1957). *Arch. exp. Path. Pharmacol.*, **231**, 298.
228. ZAPATA-ORTIZ, V., DE LA MATA, R. C., and CAMPOS-ITURRIZAGA, A. (1959). *J. Pharmacol.*, **125**, 347
229. WYKE, B. D., and FRAYWORTH, E. (1957). *Lancet*, **2**, 1025.
230. HARRISON, G. G., and BULL, A. B. (1957). *S.Afr. med. J.*, **31**, 1225.
231. WAINE, T. E., and DINMORE, P. (1958). *Anæsthesia*, **13**, 324.
232. O'RIORDAN, E. F., and BREWARD, A. D. (1958). *Curr. Res. Anesth.*, **37**, 126.
233. MACKETT, J. (1959). *Anæsthesia*, **14**, 248.
234. THOMSON, T. J. (1958). *Brit. med. J.*, **1**, 976.
235. KAUFMAN, L. (1958). *Anæsthesia*, **13**, 43.
236. BENTLEY, G. A., and SAVIDGE, S. (1958). *Brit. J. Anæsth.*, **30**, 506.
237. BELLVILLE, J. W., MURPHY, T., and HOWLAND, W. S. (1960). *J. Pharmacol.*, **130**, 364.
238. GALE, A. S. (1958). *Anesthesiology*, **19**, 521.
239. CHRISTENSEN, R. O. (1958). *Oral Surg.*, **11**, 999.
240. PERCHESON, P. B., CARROLL, J. J., and SCREECH, G. (1959). *Canad. Anæsth. Soc. J.*, **6**, 277.
241. ROBERTS, H. (1961). *Canad. Anæsth. Soc. J.*, **8**, 257.
242. GALE, A. S. (1961). *Anesthesiology*, **22**, 210.
243. O'RIORDAN, E. F., and MARCUS, P. S. (1961). *Curr. Res. Anesth.*, **40**, 188.
244. GALE, A. S. (1959). *Curr. Res. Anæsth.*, **38**, 406.
245. GARDNER, E. K. (1958). *Brit. J. Anæsth.*, **30**, 155.
246. ROMAGNOLI, A., and DIAMOND, M. J. (1961). *Canad. Anæsth. Soc. J.*, **8**, 551.
247. SILIPO, S., HAGEDORN, C., ROSENSTEIN, I. N., and BAUM, G. L. (1961). *J. Amer. med. Ass.*, **177**, 378.
248. DOBKIN, A. B., and HARLAND, J. H. (1960). *Anæsthesia*, **15**, 48.
249. DOBKIN, A. B., PEARSON, J. L., and BARR, J. S. (1960). *Canad. Anæsth. Soc. J.*, **7**, 16.
250. BURTON, R. M., SODD, M. A., and GOLDIN, A. (1957). *Arch. int. Pharmacodyn.*, **13**, 83.
251. SNIPER, W. (1961). *Brit. J. Anæsth.*, **33**, 414.
252. SHAW, F. H., and BENTLEY, (1952). *Nature, Lond.*, **169**, 712.
253. SHAW, F. H. (1960). *Brit. J. clin. Pract.*, **14**, 23.
254. DOBKIN, A. B. (1960). *Anæsthesia*, **15**, 146.
255. DOBKIN, A. B. (1960). *Anæsthesia*, **15**, 273.

CHAPTER 3

MUSCLE RELAXANTS

H. C. CHURCHILL-DAVIDSON

*Radio-active Muscle Relaxants—Types of Neuromuscular Block—
Neuromuscular Block — Measurement — Variations — Present
Position of d-Tubocurarine—Present Position of Suxamethonium
(Succinylcholine) New Muscle Relaxants—Abnormal Responses
to Muscle Relaxants*

THE neuromuscular junction might well be described as one of the
cross-roads of medicine, because it is here that anatomist, biochemist,
physiologist and clinician all meet in a common interest. Until
recently, a knowledge of function has steadily outdistanced the
revelation of anatomical structure, but current studies with the
electron microscope have made considerable headway in reducing
this gap. New techniques involving the use of micro-electrodes that
are so small that they can be placed within the lumen of a single cell
are also contributing to our knowledge of this structure. To the
anæsthetist, however, the most significant advances probably lie in
the use of muscle relaxant drugs that can be labelled with radio-
active atoms and so traced throughout the body to their ultimate
destination.

Radio-active Muscle Relaxants

Radio-active d-tubocurarine would be an ideal agent, but unfortunately it has not been possible to produce this compound
because its corresponding tertiary alkaloid d-tubocurarine (which is
necessary for the process) has not yet been discovered. A potent non-
depolarizing ^{14}C-Toxiferin has however been prepared and extensive
studies carried out both in the cat and the mouse.[1] Fig. 3 shows the
effect of this compound when injected into the mouse and depicts its
uptake by the diaphragmatic muscle. Immediately after apnœa has
occurred the animal is killed, the diaphragm is removed and then
placed in direct contact with an X-ray film. Two to six months later
the contact film is developed and the end-plates can be clearly seen
arranged as a circular band or halo around the central tendon of the
diaphragm.[2] Using this technique it is possible to distinguish individual end-plates and also to assess how many molecules of curarine

are bound to a single end-plate. These results suggest that only a few highly differentiated receptors—widely distributed in the muscle—are actually occupied by the muscle relaxant.

To study the localization of depolarizing drugs decamethonium with six radio-active methyl groups was synthesized.[2] Using the same technique the autoradiographs again demonstrated the direct action of these drugs on the end-plate. But there were some important differences. The density of the end-plate regions after decamethonium was so much greater than after curarine that it appeared that 50

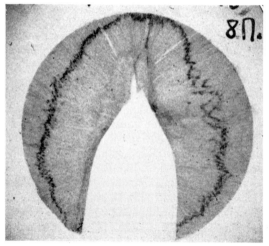

FIG. 3. Effect of C^{14}-Toxiferin on mouse diaphragm (Waser[2])

times as many molecules had been taken up by the receptors. Furthermore, the clear-cut picture of the halo of end-plates as seen with curarine was not apparent (Fig. 4). There was always a blurred appearance in this region, suggesting that the decamethonium was diffusing into the muscle cell. This evidence is in agreement with that of Taylor[3] who used another labelled depolarizing drug closely related to decamethonium—I-131 iodocholinium dichloride. The significance of these findings will be discussed in greater detail later (see dual block).

On the basis of these observations Waser[2] suggests that the receptor site is a pore in the synaptic membrane. It could be visualized as a folding of the protein substance so that there is a pore at the entrance and within there is an anionic wall to which the quaternary

N-groups become attached and nearby an esteratic site which holds the acetylcholine esterase.

It must be remembered that all non-depolarizing drugs (like d-tubocurarine) are large bulky molecules, whereas the depolarizing agents (like succinylcholine) are slim molecules. If it is assumed that the receptor site is in fact a pore on the synaptic membrane guarding the entrance to a fold of receptor protein then it is easy to understand how the large molecules of d-tubocurarine merely cover the pores of the end-plate and prevent acetylcholine entering. On the other hand,

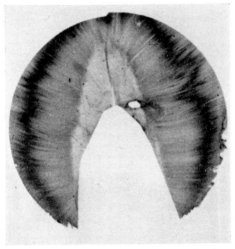

FIG. 4. Effect of C^{14} decamethonium on mouse diaphragm (Waser[2])

the slim depolarizing molecule can readily pass through the pore to obtain a bonding with its receptor site. Later these depolarizing drugs may penetrate deeper and come to lie within the muscle cell.

The Receptor Substance. Chagas, Bovet and Sollero[4] used a labelled gallamine triethiodide in the electric eel in an attempt to isolate the receptor substance. They then extracted the tissue that was bound with the radio-active material and concluded that this was the receptor material. They believe it to be a complex amino polysaccharide containing acetylglucosamines resembling some of the hyaluronic acids. Other workers[5, 6] have isolated a protein from the end organ of the electric eel, and they find that it shows many of the characteristics of the receptor substance *in vivo*.

Types of Neuromuscular Block

Nomenclature. There has been considerable confusion in the literature over the use of terms to denote the various types of relaxant drug and neuromuscular block. This has arisen because there has never been any general agreement amongst authors upon precise terminology. Bovet and his colleagues[7] first suggested the division of relaxant drugs into two simple groups—the pachy and leptocurare. This gained little favour and likewise the use of the term "competitive inhibitor" was never popular when describing the mode of action of d-tubocurarine because many were quick to point out that even the depolarizing drugs probably competed with acetylcholine for the same receptors.

There is now fairly general agreement in the use of the term "depolarizing drugs" to denote those acting like acetylcholine, whereas those acting like d-tubocurarine are usually referred to as "non-depolarizers" or as "anti-depolarizers". A further complication arose from the finding that a depolarization block, if continued, nearly always resulted in a change-over to a non-depolarizing block. The end-product of this block is termed a "dual" or "bi-phasic" block, the use of the term "mixed block" having been virtually abandoned except to describe the chaos resulting from mixing drugs with different actions!

Recently Linssen[8] made an extensive study of the various muscle relaxant drugs. For this work he used isolated strips of the frog's rectus abdominis muscle and the nerve-muscle preparation of the cat and chicken. The results suggest that it is no longer possible to divide the muscle relaxant drugs into two simple groups—those that depolarize and those that act by non-depolarization.

One relaxant drug of particular interest is dioxahexodecane (Prestonal). First introduced into clinical anæsthesia by Frey,[9] it enjoyed only a short spate of popularity owing to its vagal blocking and histamine releasing activity. Considerable speculation took place about its precise mode of action and as to whether or not the neuro-muscular block could be reversed by anticholinesterase drugs.

Linssen[8] found that dioxahexodecane not only enhances the neuromuscular blocking properties of d-tubocurarine but also those of succinylcholine. Normally a depolarizing type of drug antagonizes the block of a non-depolarizer and vice versa. Dioxahexodecane produces neuromuscular block in its own right, yet it enhances both types of block. It produces a flaccid paralysis in the chick, just like d-tubocurarine, yet the neuromuscular block in the cat is not reversible by anticholinesterase drugs (e.g. neostigmine). On the basis of this evidence Linssen suggests that this drug acts differently from both succinylcholine and d-tubocurarine.

In attempting to describe this new type of neuromuscular block it is necessary to view the action of drugs at the motor end-plate as a whole. Drugs having an affinity for specific receptors and at the same time producing an intrinsic activity are able to generate a stimulus which leads to an effect. The stimulus is by definition directly proportional to receptor occupation. The relation between the stimulus and

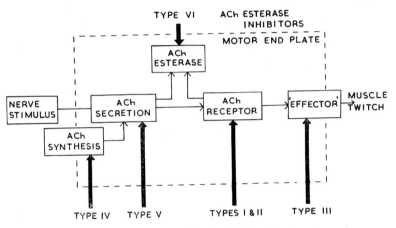

FIG. 5 (after Linssen, 1961). Diagram of mode of action of various types of neuromuscular blocking drugs (↑) on the motor end-plate (⸇⸇⸇⸇)

Thus:

Type I   The depolarizing drugs such as succinylcholine and decamethonium.

Type II   The non-depolarizing drugs such as d-tubocurarine and gallamine triethiodide.

Type III The "non-competitors" which have an affinity to other receptors than those of acetylcholine and which are "non-competitive" antagonists of acetylcholine. The only example to date of this group is dioxahexadecanium (Prestonal).

Type IV   Drugs which block the *synthesis* of acetylcholine in the myoneural junction, such as hemicholinium.

Type V   Drugs which block the *release* of acetylcholine in the myoneural junction, such as magnesium ions and botulinus toxin.

Type VI   Drugs which inhibit acetylcholine esterase. Thus neostigmine, if given in sufficient dosage, can produce a depolarization block due to the accumulation of acetylcholine.

the effect may be complex and often not known in detail. In the case of the motor end-plate this relationship (termed "effector") includes all the stages from the occupation of the receptor by acetylcholine right up to the ultimate effect, i.e. the muscle twitch. Part of the effector, therefore, is located within the end-plate and the remainder in the muscle fibre and muscle membrane.[8]

Thus, drugs may develop their actions at the end-plate in a number of ways. First, by an interaction with specific receptors and by mimicking the action of an endogenous substance, e.g. decamethonium and suxamethonium. Secondly, by an interaction with specific receptors but without having the ability to mimic the action of an endogenous substance, e.g. d-tubocurarine chloride and gallamine triethiodide. In the third instance it is necessary to postulate that drugs may interact with some other receptors different from the specific ones yet still be capable of influencing the final effect. Such receptors may be termed "non-competitive" in that they are not specific for acetylcholine but their occupation is still capable of producing neuromuscular block. Dioxahexadecanium is believed to act by having an affinity for these "non-competitive" receptors.[8]

Furthermore, as a result of this work it has also been possible to postulate that there are two different ways of interfering with the release of acetylcholine. First, magnesium ions and botulinus toxin block the release of acetylcholine at the presynaptic membrane in the myoneural junction. Secondly, hemicholinium blocks the synthesis of acetylcholine in the myoneural junction probably by interfering with the transport mechanism of choline. Linssen[8] has detailed six basic types of "curariform" drug that are capable of producing neuromuscular block by a separate mechanism (Fig. 5).

Benzoquinonium hydrochloride ("Mytolon"), synthesized by Cavallito and his colleagues[10] is another drug which enjoyed a short period of clinical popularity only to wane rapidly as the marked vagal stimulant properties became apparent. Furthermore, its mode of action was incompletely understood.[11] From his experiments in animals Linssen[8] concluded that this drug had two actions. First, it produced a non-depolarizing type of block, and secondly, it was a potent inhibitor of acetylcholine esterase. Here, therefore, is a drug which possesses two actions at the neuromuscular junction, and each of these is antagonistic to the other. It seems hardly surprising that it has not become more popular.

Although all these new facts have not yet been confirmed in man, it would now seem possible to define six types of neuromuscular block, as outlined in the following table:

Mechanism	Example
1. Depolarization	Succinylcholine
	Decamethonium
2. Non-depolarization	d-tubocurarine
	Gallamine triethiodide
3. Non-acetylcholine	
(a) Release	Mg or botulinus toxin
(b) Synthesis	Hemicholinium
4. Dual (biphasic)	Repeated doses of a depolarizing drug
5. Non-competitive	Dioxahexadecanium (Prestonal)
6. Anti-cholinesterase	Neostigmine
	Edrophonium

Neuromuscular Block

Since the introduction of the muscle relaxants into clinical anæsthesia the great bulk of the investigation of these drugs has been carried out in animals. Unfortunately, there is no single species that responds to these relaxant drugs in exactly the same manner as man. This has led to considerable confusion in the literature, because some authors have erroneously assumed that such direct comparison is possible. During recent years, however, many attempts have been made to obtain data on the activity of these drugs from direct observations on conscious volunteers and patients. Some of these investigations are outlined below.

Measurement of Neuromuscular Block. Any investigation of comparative muscle-strength before and after the administration of a relaxant drug could be crudely described as a method of measuring the effectiveness of the drug in the dosage given. Nevertheless, if the subject retains his volitional powers during the experiment he can at will either rise to Olympian heights of strength or merely slacken off because he is bored. For this reason, all measurements made on conscious subjects with their volitional powers intact are open to a wide margin of error.

A study is often made of the tidal volume of respiration. This method is commonly chosen because the anæsthetist is primarily concerned with ventilation, but it is sometimes erroneously assumed that if the tidal volume in an anæsthetised patient is depressed the relaxant drug must be responsible. The danger of this hypothesis cannot be emphasised too strongly. Respiratory activity not only depends on the state of conductivity at the neuromuscular junction of the particular muscles of respiration, but also upon the sensitivity of the respiratory centre. If one is not very careful such drugs as morphine and thiopentone, which are powerful respiratory depressants, must of necessity become classified as relaxant drugs.

The only certain method of accurately studying neuromuscular transmission is to stimulate the main nerve fibre and record the resultant contraction of the muscle either electrically or mechanically. The principal methods of measuring neuromuscular transmission are outlined below.

(a) *Volitional Measurements*. The relative value of such measurements has already been discussed above, but in combination with other more specific measures they may be found useful. The instrument most commonly used is the ergograph (Fig. 6). The time taken to produce "fatigue" of muscle power is measured when a rhythmical

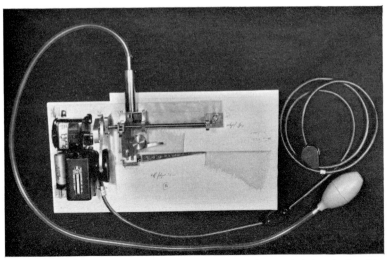

Fig. 6. The Recording Ergograph. The grip-strength is recorded electrically with the aid of a direct-writer. (Greene *et al.*[12])

maximal effort of grip-strength is made. The effect of a particular dose of relaxant drug or known pathological state can be assessed.

(b) *Involuntary Measurements*. Such techniques ensure that the patient, whether conscious or unconscious, cannot influence the power of the muscle contraction. This can only be achieved by applying a suitable electrical stimulus to a main nerve trunk and so compelling every muscle fibre supplied by that nerve to contract. The resultant muscle contraction can then be measured either mechanically or electrically.

MECHANICALLY. The leg muscles are most commonly used in this technique, but it is equally applicable to the muscles of the upper limb if required. Cutaneous electrodes are placed either over the medial popliteal nerve or the motor point of the tibialis muscle. A supramaximal stimulus is then delivered to ensure that every motor nerve fibre carries the stimulus, and the depression of the forefoot with each mechanical contraction is recorded with the aid of a strain-gauge and a pen recorder (Fig. 7).[13]

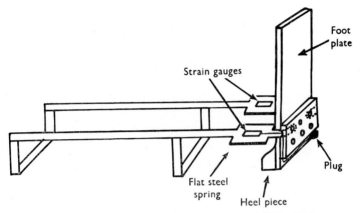

FIG. 7. Diagram of the caliper. The leg is placed in the caliper and the degree of depression of the foot plate following motor nerve stimulation is measured.
(Cannard and Zaimis, 1959)

ISOLATED MUSCLE PREPARATIONS. A similar principle for recording the mechanical contraction of isolated pieces of muscle has also been developed by Dillon and his colleagues.[14, 15] Using this technique, small pieces of muscle—such as the intercostals—are taken and placed in saline which is slightly modified by Krebs solution. The muscle is attached at both ends to a recording device so that any change in tension can be noted. Since it is impossible to remove the motor nerve intact with the muscle-specimen, this method relies upon using a specially designed stimulator which emits stimuli of such short duration that they do not excite the muscle fibre directly but are picked up by the nerve fibrils and thus a muscle contraction is brought about through the medium of the neuromuscular junction. Using two different durations of stimulus it is possible to excite the muscle fibres alternately through the neuromuscular junction and by a direct action on the fibre.

With this technique it is possible to study the effects of various drugs not only on neuromuscular transmission but also directly on the muscle fibre itself. Furthermore, the effects of these drugs in both normal and pathological states can be compared. The principal disadvantage of such a method applies to all isolated-specimen techniques in that the tissue is not being perfused at the time of study and therefore is without a satisfactory blood supply.

ELECTRICALLY. This technique comprises stimulating a motor nerve and recording the electrical discharge from the affected muscle —i.e. electromyography. It is particularly suitable for studying neuromuscular transmission in both conscious and anæsthetised subjects.[16]

It is essential that all nerve fibres supplying a particular muscle group convey a stimulus, and this is achieved by applying a current greater than that required to excite every nerve fibre (supramaximal

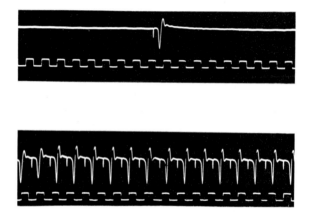

FIG. 8. Normal action potential

stimulus). Since the neuromuscular junction obeys the "all or none" law, every muscle fibre supplied by that nerve must undergo a contraction. This mechanical shortening gives rise to an electrical discharge similar to that seen on the electrocardiogram when the heart muscle contracts. A group of 150–300 muscle fibres all contracting synchronously gives rise to an electrical discharge which is called an "action potential". When displayed on the electromyograph it is possible to see the point at which the stimulus arrives at the nerve-ending followed by a pause during the passage of the stimulus from nerve to muscle, and then the explosion of electrical activity as all the affected muscle fibres contract.

The height of—or, more correctly, the surface area included by—the action potential is directly related to the number of muscle fibres that are functioning. Thus, as a muscle relaxant is administered, so the height or area of the action potential is diminished, until finally, when complete paralysis develops, only a straight line remains.

The technique of electromyography is particularly sensitive to even minute changes in neuromuscular transmission and is therefore very useful for studying the changes produced by the different relaxant drugs.

The Pattern of Neuromuscular Block. (*a*) *Depolarization Block.* This is the type of neuromuscular block that follows the administration of acetylcholine or of such an agent as suxamethonium; and four principal electromyographic characteristics can be demonstrated in man.[17] First, successive stimuli lead to a response of the muscle which is well sustained whether the rate of stimulation be fast (tetanic) or slow (twitch). Secondly, after a period of tetanic stimulation there

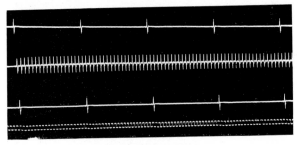

Fig. 9. Depolarization block
(Churchill-Davidson *et al*.[17])

is no obvious improvement in the conduction of a single stimulus (i.e. no post-tetanic facilitation) (Fig. 9). Thirdly, the drug produces isolated discharges of a whole group of fibres which can occasionally be seen as fasciculations. This third type of response is particularly well demonstrated after an intravenous dose of suxamethonium, but it can also be recorded in a more modified form after other depolarizing agents such as decamethonium and hexamethylene biscarbaminoylcholine.[16]

Finally, if an anti-cholinesterase drug (neostigmine 2·5 mg) is given after a small dose of a depolarizing drug, a potentiation of the block with an increase in muscle weakness is found.

CLINICAL SIGNIFICANCE. These changes, as observed electromyographically, are characteristic of a depolarization type of neuromuscular block and most of them can be observed clinically without the aid of any complex apparatus. A peripheral nerve-stimulator is, however, essential. The most convenient muscles for the anæsthetist to study are those in the hand, as the upper limb is usually readily accessible during any operation, particularly when an intravenous infusion is being used.

The ulnar nerve—either in the bicipital groove at the elbow or where it lies superficially at the wrist—is a particularly suitable nerve to stimulate because of the characteristic "*main en griffe*" position taken by the fingers. Stimulation of the ulnar nerve trunk reproduces this position whereby the main flexion appears in the fourth and fifth digits. Two features of a depolarization block can be particularly well demonstrated provided the paralysis is not complete.

1. Well-sustained successive stimuli, whether the rate of stimulation be fast or slow (Fig. 10).

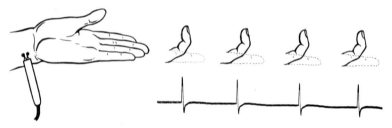

FIG. 10. Mechanical movement of fingers in a depolarization block (Churchill-Davidson, H. C., and Wise, R. P., (1960). *Brit. J. Anæsth*, **32**, 384.)

2. Absence of post-tetanic facilitation.

Furthermore, the administration of a short-acting anti-cholinesterase drug (edrophonium 10 mg) will produce a momentary increase in the depth of paralysis. Such therapy, however, is quite unnecessary (and may even be harmful) if the other characteristic responses of depolarization have already been observed.

(*b*) *Non-depolarization Block*. This type of block is seen after the administration of d-tubocurarine chloride and gallamine triethiodide. The main characteristics, as seen electromyographically, are in direct contrast to those observed for a depolarization block. First, both twitch and tetanic rates of nerve stimulation lead to a successive failure or "fade" in the response of the muscle fibres (Fig. 11). Secondly, after a burst of tetanic stimulation there is a brief period lasting about 2–3 minutes wherein neuromuscular transmission is dramatically improved, i.e. post tetanic facilitation.

A possible theoretical explanation of this phenomenon is that

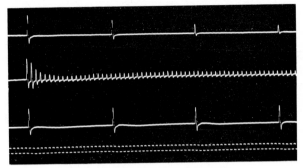

FIG. 11. Non-depolarization block
(Churchill-Davidson *et al.*[17])

during the period of rapid stimulation there is an increased production and liberation of acetylcholine molecules which persists for
a short period after the tetanus has ceased. This type of response is
not seen in a case of pure depolarization block because even though
a severe paresis may be present and the height of the action greatly
dimished, there is no "fade" on tetanic stimulation and therefore no
improvement (post-tetanic facilitation) on resumption of a slow rate
of stimulation.

Thirdly, there is no recordable contraction of muscle fibres or
fasciculations before the onset of paralysis. And finally, this type of
block is partially or completely counteracted by an anti-cholinesterase
drug.

Using an isolated human nerve-muscle preparation (Dillon,[18]) it
has been possible to demonstrate a failure of neuromuscular transmission (indirect stimulation) after d-tubocurarine while the direct
stimulation of the muscle fibre remains unaffected (Fig. 12). This is a

HUMAN INTERCOSTAL MUSCLE

COMPETITIVE NEUROMUSCULAR BLOCK BY d - TUBOCURARINE

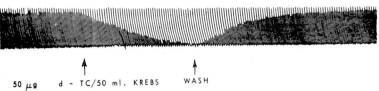

50 μg   d - TC/50 ml. KREBS   WASH

FIG. 12. (Dillon, J. B. Personal communication)

modern version in man of the classical experiments of Claude Bernard over a hundred years ago with the sciatic-gastrocnemius preparation of the frog.

CLINICAL SIGNIFICANCE. Again these changes can be recognized as mechanical contractions of the affected muscles and are particularly well seen in the response of the fingers upon stimulation of the ulnar nerve. Two features are particularly easy to recognize. First, the characteristic "fade" after both slow and fast rates of stimulation (Fig. 13) and secondly, the brief but dramatic period of improvement in neuromuscular transmission after a burst of tetanic stimulation (post-tetanic facilitation).

With these various techniques it is now possible to differentiate between a depolarization and a non-depolarization type of neuro-

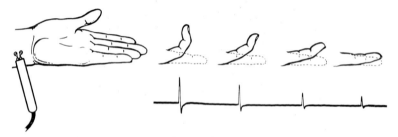

FIG. 13. Mechanical movement of fingers in a non-depolarization block.

muscular block that is present at any time even when the type of the relaxant drug is not known. Most of the relaxant drugs in clinical use can now be classified into two types—by their acting either as "depolarizers" or as "non-depolarizers". This simple classification should prevent the confusion over their mode of action that was showing signs of arising when some authors described drugs as acting in a "mixed" manner. It is essential for an anæsthetist using relaxant drugs to know the precise type of block that is present, for the administration of an anticholinesterase would be of great benefit in one case and extremely harmful in the other.

Recently a further study of these types of neuromuscular block has revealed that under specific conditions certain alterations in the degree or type of block can be produced.

Variations in Neuromuscular Block

Dual Block. The fact that a depolarization block in man can graduually undergo a change from one of pure depolarization to that

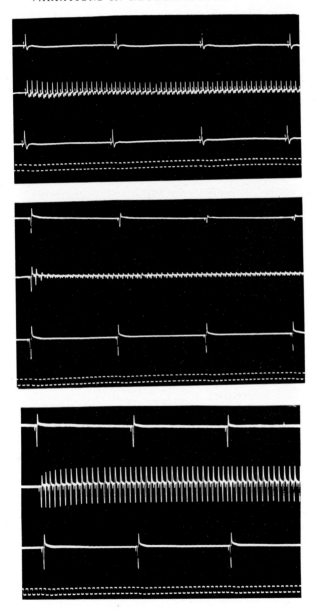

FIG. 14. a. b. c. (Churchill-Davidson *et al.*[17])

resembling non-depolarization is now established.[17] Electromyo-graphically the changes in this process can be described as first a neuromuscular block with the signs of depolarization (Fig. 14 (a)), followed by a period of tachyphylaxis, i.e. a gradually diminishing response to the same dose of relaxant drug. Then comes a period in which there is an increasing inability to sustain the fast rates of stimulation. At first this affects only the very fastest rates, but gradu-ally this "fade" appears at slower rates until finally it is well-estab-lished at even slow rates of stimulation (Fig. 14 (b)).

Once a dual block has become fully established it can readily be reversed by an injection of neostigmine (2·5 mg) (Fig. 14 (c)).

Clinically, a dual neuromuscular block is difficult to recognize without the aid of a peripheral nerve-stimulator. Nevertheless, its presence should be suspected in any patient who has received a large

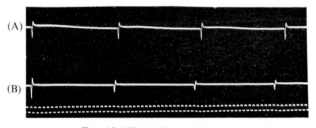

Fig. 15. (Churchill-Davidson et al.[17])

infusion of a depolarizing drug. Fig 15 is an example of the response to slow (twitch) stimulation in a patient receiving a continuous in-fusion of succinylcholine. Note how successive potentials are well maintained after the initial dose of 50 mg (A) but how after 1·5G (B) there is a marked fade which denotes the presence of a non-depolarizing type of block.

A dual block is particularly likely to occur in any patient who has received an infusion of suxamethonium exceeding 1G. It is not often seen in patients receiving less than 0·5G except in two specific instances. First, patients who have a low blood volume, dehydration and electrolyte imbalance are liable to show this change much earlier than normal patients. Secondly, those patients with an atypical form of plasma cholinesterase usually remain paralysed for a very long time after a single dose of succinylcholine, and on recovery the signs of a dual block are often observed. This response is attributed to the almost complete absence of enzymatic destruction of the drug causing these patients to behave in a similar manner to their more normal brethren who have received a very large dose of the drug.

It is true to say that a depolarization block in man will always eventually turn into a non-depolarization type of block. A dual block is rarely seen after a single dose of a depolarizing drug but electro-myographically minor degrees of this change can often be recognized. Clinically it should always be suspected if the patient does not show a steadily increasing improvement in muscle strength. For example, after an injection of suxamethonium, respiratory activity usually begins in a limited form within two to four minutes; once the first signs of movement are visible, a full tidal volume is established within a further two minutes. If a dual block is present one of the characteristic signs is a very slow improvement in respiratory activity, and a persistent "tracheal tug" is commonly observed. With the longer-acting depolarizing drugs such as decamethonium a much longer recovery period is to be anticipated. Unfortunately a slow recovery phase from a depolarizing drug is not diagnostic of a dual block because a persistent "tracheal tug" may signify the presence of a mechanical obstruction in the bronchial tree. However, if a dual block is suspected the application of a peripheral nerve-stimulator will immediately reveal the presence or absence of this state. A well-sustained muscle response with no post-tetanic facilitation denotes a depolarization block whereas a successive "fade" in the response with marked post-tetanic facilitation reveals the presence of a non-depolarization block. If there are signs of the latter, then an injection of an anti-cholinesterase drug should be given with confident assurance that neuromuscular transmission will be improved. Alter-natively, if there is a vigorous response of the hand muscles on electrical stimulation then the possibility that the muscle relaxant is not the cause of the inadequate ventilation must be considered.

Mechanism of Dual Block. This type of neuromuscular block was first observed in animals. [19, 20] A similar type of block has also been demonstrated in man following large and repeated doses of a de-polarizing drug. [17] A block with many of these characteristics following only a single dose of a depolarizing drug has also been observed in patients with myasthenia gravis[21] and in apparently normal neonates during the first few weeks of life. [22]

The exact mechanism of this type of block is still unknown but much progress has been made by the studies of Taylor and his colleagues[23] using radio-active iodocholinium in the rabbit lumbrical preparation. The block produced by decamethonium always occurs in two phases with an intervening period during which there is recovery of neuromuscular transmission. The first phase of the block is characteristic of depolarization and is of rapid onset and of short duration. If curare is given prior to the decamethonium it will inhibit the uptake of the decamethonium molecules and so prevent the block taking place. The second phase of the block does not show the signs of depolarization but resembles that produced by curare itself in that it is antagonised by anti-cholinesterases, potassium ions and a fall in temperature, but it differs from a curare-block only in that it takes 5–10 times as long to develop.

This delay in development of the second phase appears to be related to the penetration of the muscle fibre by the labelled depolarizing drug.[3] Curare does not appear to have any action in preventing the molecules from leaving the fibre once access has been attained, suggesting that the entrance and exit of the depolarizing drug are by different means.

In these experiments the muscle fibre was able to take up large quantities of the labelled depolarizing drug and this uptake was closely associated with the development of a non-depolarizing type of block. Furthermore, an anti-cholinesterase drug given once a large quantity of depolarizer had been stored led to an immediate improvement in neuromuscular transmission despite the fact that the muscle was unable to rid itself of the drug. This suggests that neuromuscular transmission depends upon the state of affairs prevailing at the end-plate irrespective of the condition of the interior of the fibre, though the actual performance of the muscle fibre may be altered.

Muscle Temperature. A lowering of the muscle temperature, such as occurs during hypothermia, leads to an increase in the duration and intensity of a depolarization block whereas it diminishes the effect of a non-depolarization block. A reduction of body temperature of 5° C led to a fourfold prolongation of the period of the paralysis. Conversely, rewarming reduces the intensity and duration of a depolarization block but increases only the degree of block due to the non-depolarizing drugs, without affecting the duration.[24]

Clinically these findings probably are rarely of great consequence in causing a marked prolongation of paralysis. This is because large doses of relaxant drugs are seldom required in the patient undergoing deep hypothermia, for once the first few degrees of body temperature have fallen the amount of anæsthetic and relaxant drugs required becomes correspondingly less. Such drugs are often required at the start of anæsthesia when the body temperature is around normal, but though cold may potentiate or oppose the action of these drugs, on rewarming the degree of neuromuscular block should be returned to normal. Nevertheless, this evidence emphasises the need for special caution in the administration of relaxant drugs in the presence of alterations in body temperature. In clinical practice no marked alteration in response has been reported, but it is known that the neuromuscular block produced by d-tubocurarine is readily reversible at a body temperature of 30–31° C.

Carbon Dioxide. Little is known of the effect of variations of the carbon dioxide tension of the blood (Pco_2) in man on neuromuscular transmission. Nevertheless, in the cat a rise in Pco_2 opposes the activity of suxamethonium, decamethonium and gallamine but enhances the action of d-tubocurarine.[25] The precise reason for this phenomenon is unknown.

Present Position of d-Tubocurarine

Despite the fact that d-tubocurarine is used extensively throughout the world, there is a surprising lack of clinical investigation of this drug. However, whatever is lacking in fundamental investigation is more than compensated for by the wealth of hypotheses and theories that surround this drug.

There are four principal points of interest concerning its use in man. First, does it liberate histamine in significant quantities? Second, does its ganglion-blocking activity ever lead to serious hypotension? Third, does it have a central depressant action? And finally, are there occasions when the block produced by d-tubocurarine is not reversible by neostigmine—i.e."neostigmine-resistant curarization"?

Unfortunately, owing to the dearth of data on this subject, none of these questions can be answered with certainty. Nevertheless, Gray and Wilson[26] in a questionnaire sent to one-third of the anæsthetists in the United Kingdom, found that 96 per cent preferred the use of a non-depolarizing relaxant for prolonged muscular relaxation. About half of those questioned admitted they had observed hypotension after d-tubocurarine, but interestingly enough an even greater number claimed to have seen it after gallamine triethiodide and succinylcholine.

Histamine release or ganglion-blockade following d-tubocurarine would have one most important effect in the anæsthetized patient—namely hypotension. The fact that since the introduction of d-tubocurarine over 17 years ago there is not one single substantiated case of acute hypotension due to d-tubocurarine causing sudden death suggests that the hypotension, when it occurs, is seldom serious enough to be fatal. From a clinical viewpoint, however, there can be few anæsthetists who have not observed a fall in systemic pressure following a dose of d-tubocurarine. It is particularly liable to occur in cases of essential hypertension with severe arteriosclerosis, but if the d-tubocurarine is administered slowly (over a five-minute period) the fall in pressure is seldom more than mild. Furthermore, if hypotension does occur following d-tubocurarine it is not long-lasting, the systolic pressure tending to start to rise again after a few minutes.

The case of the central action of d-tubocurarine is even more obscure.

Hersey and his colleagues,[27] using a crossed-circulation technique to the brain, found that most of the commonly used relaxants caused depression of the central nervous system. They state that "the dosage required to produce central respiratory arrest or depression was found to approximate closely to that required to produce a peripheral myoneural block in the donor body". In direct contrast to this finding is the evidence of Smith et al.[28] who received $2\frac{1}{2}$ times the paralysing dose of d-tubocurarine without any demonstrable central action, and also more recently, the findings of Davidson and Eyal[29] that 200 mg of succinylcholine given intramuscularly in man produced apnœa for nearly ten minutes yet the subject was "acutely aware of his surroundings!"

Nevertheless, though the evidence in man does suggest a lack of depression of levels of consciousness with the relaxant drugs, it does not exclude a specific depressant action on the respiratory centre. Paton and Zaimis (1952),[30] working with animals, however, found no change in the phrenic nerve action potentials following either d-tubocurarine or decamethonium until asphyxia had supervened.

Much of the evidence for a passage of d-tubocurarine across the blood-brain barrier has been reviewed by Paton.[31] He reached the conclusion that "it seems somewhat improbable that d-tubocurarine is ever likely to have a significant central action in practice".

Neostigmine-resistant curarization still remains a mystery, for to date there is no authenticated case in the literature demonstrating, first, that neuromuscular block was present and, secondly, that neostigmine had failed to improve neuromuscular transmission. The matter must await further investigation.

Present Position of Suxamethonium (Succinylcholine)

In direct contrast to the paucity of clinical investigation of d-tubocurarine, in recent years a whole wealth of information on the action of succinylcholine has become available. This can best be considered under separate headings:

Muscle Pains. The incidence of pain or stiffness in skeletal muscle of adults developing on the day following the injection of intravenous succinylcholine is now well established. In ambulant patients about 60–70 per cent are afflicted, whereas if the patient is confined to bed after the injection the incidence drops to about 10 per cent.[32-35] Despite suggestions to the contrary, the work of Burtles[36] and Parbrook and Pierce[37] has shown that there is no significant diminution in the incidence of these pains if suxethonium as opposed to suxamethonium is used. Bush and Roth[38] have pointed out that in children of 5–14 years of age the overall incidence was only 10 per cent even when the patients were ambulant. In the group of 5–9 years old it was only 3 per cent.

Most authors are now in agreement that a small dose of a non-depolarizing drug (3 mg d-tubocurarine, or 20 mg gallamine triethiodide) given at least 4 minutes before the succinylcholine, will prevent or seriously modify these muscle pains. However, such a practice may occasionally give rise to a prolonged reaction and therefore cannot be recommended for general clinical use.

Dual Block. The mechanism and incidence of this condition have already been discussed. It now seems quite certain that if the depolarizing drugs are used in large doses in man the characteristics of the neuromuscular block always eventually undergo a change so that finally a non-depolarization type of block ensues. The total dose required and the duration of paralysis are obviously interrelated but there is a fairly wide variation amongst patients. Nevertheless, the larger the dose of the depolarizing drug used, the more likely is the development of dual block.

In clinical practice the principal disadvantage of a dual block is that unless special facilities are available it is often difficult to diagnose with certainty, yet it may be the principal reason for a prolongation of the muscle paresis. Until it is fully established the use of anti-cholinesterase drugs may only make matters even worse.

For this reason the clinical use of the long-acting depolarizing drugs has largely been abandoned in favour of the greater consistency of action of the non-depolarizing group of drugs, which are also readily reversible. Suxamethonium, a short-acting depolarizing drug, is still widely used for producing profound muscular relaxation of limited duration but the continuous intravenous infusion almost invariably leads to a dual block if the operation lasts long enough. The popularity of this drug even for short periods of paralysis is likely to be short-lived if a non-depolarizing drug of equivalent duration is ever discovered.

In order to overcome the objection to using large doses of succinyl-choline and thereby avoiding much of the risk of the onset of dual block, Foldes and his colleagues[39] in the United States have championed the combination of succinylcholine and a specific anti-cholinesterase, hexafluorenium bromide (Mylaxen). This latter drug inhibits the enzymatic breakdown of suxamethonium but, unlike neostigmine, the muscarinic side-effects such as salivation and bradycardia are minimal. The initial recommended dose of hexa-fluorenium is 0·5 mg/kg followed by an initial dose of 0·2 mg/kg of suxamethonium. Hexafluorenium delayed the onset but markedly prolonged the duration of neuromuscular effects of suxamethonium so that only one-seventh to one-fifth of the normal dosage was required.

Despite the possible advantages of this technique, most anæs-thetists in the United Kingdom have favoured the use of a non-depolarizing drug for prolonged muscular relaxation since this type of block can always be readily reversed by an anti-cholinesterase if and when required.

Action on the Eye

Dillon and his colleagues[15] have reported that the administration of succinylcholine to a patient undergoing intra-ocular surgery may produce a serious complication in that it increases the intra-ocular tension and thus in cases of glaucoma might precipitate damage to the optic nerve fibres, with the possibility of permanent damage and blindness. From their investigations in both man and the cat they concluded that this rise of intra-ocular pressure was due to a "con-tracture", (as opposed to contraction) of the extra-ocular muscles.

The rise in ocular tension occurs in both adults and children with an average increase in pressure of about 7·5 mm Hg.[40]

Björk, Halldin and Wåhlin[41] have demonstrated that succinyl-choline causes a retraction of the eyeball (enophthalmos) despite the fact that the extraocular muscles appear by electromyography to be paralysed. Furthermore, whilst succinylcholine produces enophthal-mos in the rat, noradrenaline leads to exophthalmos, and the two drugs are antagonists. These results suggest that succinylcholine is acting on the smooth muscle.[41, 42] In man the smooth musculature in the orbit is normally considered to be of only rudimentary importance, but when the skeletal muscles are paralysed it is quite possible that this smooth muscle contracts and brings about enophthalmos and a rise in intra-ocular tension. In clinical practice a slight rise in intra-ocular tension is rarely of great significance, but this evidence suggests the use of succinylcholine in cases of severe glaucoma to be contra-indicated.

Cardiac Effects. The fact that succinylcholine produced a brady-cardia in children[43] received little attention until it was demonstrated that this slowing of the heart rate could actually lead to a temporary "cardiac arrest".[44, 45, 46] The arrhythmias following the injection of succinylcholine appear to be related to the size of the dose used and are not often seen after the inital injection but are commonly observed if large subsequent doses are given.[46] These cardiac irregularities can be prevented by the prior administration of atropine sulphate (1 mg).

Placental Transmission. A method for detecting small concentrations of suxamethonium in serum[47] has been used to study the possible passage of this drug across the placental barrier. It was found that when doses less than 300–500 mg of suxamethonium were used there was no detectable placental transmission, but when higher doses were used "small but definitely detectable quantities were found."[48] None of the infants, however, appeared to be affected by the presence of this drug in the cord blood.

Relation to Plasma Cholinesterase. The enzymatic breakdown of suxamethonium by plasma cholinesterase to succinylmonocholine and then to succinic acid and choline is now well-known. Occasionally however, a patient is encountered who is unable to destroy suxamethonium in this manner, and a long period of apnœa ensues. The incidence of a prolonged response to suxamethonium in clinical practice is about 1 : 2,400 cases.[49] Originally it was assumed that even in those patients without any cholinesterase activity at all, the suxamethonium would nevertheless be destroyed by alkaline hydrolysis in about three times the time normally taken by plasma cholinesterase.[50] Kalow,[51] however, estimates that less than 5 per cent of the suxamethonium in the body at any given time will be destroyed by alkaline hydrolysis per hour. Great interest, therefore, has centred upon those patients who do not destroy suxamethonium quickly. It has now been shown that there are two types of serum cholinesterase in man which behave differently towards suxamethonium.[52] Both types are inherited and must be regarded as normal variants, although they do not occur with equal frequency.[53] The rare form has been called atypical esterase, and in a survey of the Canadian population about 1 in every 2,800 patients was found to possess only this atypical type of esterase.[51] The principal difference between the normal and the atypical esterase is that whereas both esterases are capable of destroying suxamethonium, only the normal esterase is capable of doing this when the concentration of suxamethonium in the blood is low. Hence, if a patient with atypical esterase receives a dose of suxamethonium, the dilution caused by the blood volume rapidly causes a drop in its concentration below the effective level of the atypical esterase. Since it can now no longer destroy the suxamethonium this drug continues to circulate and the patient remains paralysed. In short, the essential difference between these two enzymes is merely one of degree, namely the normal esterase can function at concentrations which are impossible for the atypical esterase.

Plasma cholinesterase levels are normally determined by the Warburg apparatus and the estimation is both difficult and tedious; but the introduction of a test paper incorporating a similar principle has been found both simple and accurate enough for clinical purposes.[54] Using this method it is possible to decide quickly whether the patient has a low plasma cholinesterase or not. Like all the other esterase estimations, however, it will not differentiate those patients who have a low esterase value because they possess only the atypical esterase from those who have a low value due to inadequate liver function.

This differentiation requires a special test of its own. Kalow and Genest[55] have shown that these two conditions—an atypical esterase or a low normal esterase—behave differently in the presence of a local analgesic agent—dibucaine (cinchocaine: "Nupercaine"). Thus dibucaine inhibits almost completely the normal enzyme, irrespective of whether its activity value is high or low. In direct contrast the atypical esterase is hardly inhibited at all by dibucaine. These facts are sometimes expressed as a dibucaine number (DN), so that a person with a normal type of esterase would be described as having a DN of 70–80 per cent, whereas a patient with nothing but atypical esterase has a DN of 16–25 per cent. or less.

Lehmann and Silk[56] have demonstrated convincingly how the family history of a patient with atypical esterase can be traced. The transfer of the "defective gene" from parent to child can best be shown in a study of pseudo-cholinesterase levels in a whole family.[57] Normal pseudo-cholinesterase level is 60–120 units.

Those persons with a high value of pseudo-cholinesterase (i.e. 90 or more) are presumed to have inherited two normal genes (i.e. are normal homozygotes). Those with values on the low side of normal 40–90 units, however, are believed to have inherited dissimilar genes (heterozygote), one gene from one parent being normal and the other gene from the other parent being atypical. In the event of two

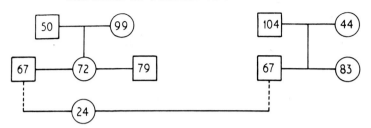

heterozygotes marrying, one of their offspring may inherit two atypical genes (abnormal homozygote).

However, it must not be assumed that all patients having a low pseudo-cholinesterase (Ps.Ch.) level have necessarily inherited an atypical gene, because this does not take into account those patients who have a low enzyme activity due to malnutrition or liver damage. The only satisfactory method of differentiating between an inherited and an acquired low pseudo-cholinesterase is with the aid of the dibucaine test. Thus, only those patients with two atypical genes will show a really low dibucaine number. This situation is best exemplified in the Table below, where the values expressed for both Ps.Ch. and dibucaine are merely given as approximates.

	Ps.Ch. esterase units	Dibucaine number % inhibition
Normal homozygote (two normal genes)	60–120	70–85
Normal homozygote (liver damage)	8–59	70–85
Heterozygote (one normal and one abnormal gene)	26–90	50–65
Heterozygote (liver damage) ..	8–40	50–65
Abnormal homozygote (two abnormal genes)	8–35	16–25

Lehmann (1962).[58]

It will be seen from the above table that in the case of the abnormal homozygote who has inherited two atypical genes, the value for pseudo-cholinesterase is always found to be low. It is, in fact, just this type of patient that produces the really low values for pseudo-cholinesterase level and gives the dramatically long periods of apnœa following succinylcholine.

New Muscle Relaxants

During the past few years there have been only two new relaxant drugs of merit—namely c-Toxiferine I and hexamethylene biscarbaminoylcholine bromide (Imbretil). Both these drugs have a long action, and the fact that they have not received world-wide acclaim is probably due to their possessing only a marginal improvement value (if any) over the other more tested compounds in general clinical use, e.g. d-tubocurarine and suxamethonium.

C-Toxiferine I is one of the many alkaloids isolated from calabash curare that have neuromuscular-blocking properties. The pharmacological actions of this drug were first investigated by Waser[59] and it was subsequently used in man.[60-62]

Toxiferine is a bis-quaternary ammonium compound that is unstable in solution and therefore must be mixed with saline immediately before use. It is the most potent neuromuscular blocking agent yet known, since 2–3 mg will produce a non-depolarization block in the average adult which will last two to three times as long as d-tubocurarine. Because of its high potency it is relatively free from side-effects, and causes neither hypotension nor histamine-release. The neuromuscular block is reversed by anti-cholinesterase drugs.

Despite these obvious advantages, however, the extremely long action makes its use in clinical practice difficult, for it is seldom possible to predict at the outset of an operation that full muscular relaxation will certainly be required for at least $1-1\frac{1}{2}$ hours. More information on the reversibility of this relaxant drug by neostigmine is required, because in clinical practice it does not appear that the neuromuscular block is readily reversible when the concentration of toxiferine at the end-plates is high. Hence the insistence on allowing a long time-interval to elapse between the last dose of toxiferine and the attempt to reverse its action. Similarly, subsequent doses extend the period of apnœa or muscle paresis and therefore should not be given within one hour of the close of the operation. These time limits make its clinical use awkward in the normal course of surgery, but if there is certain knowledge of the precise duration of a long operation, then its relative lack of side-effects may be found useful.

The main value of this drug would appear to lie in the treatment of such diseases as tetanus or poliomyelitis, where prolonged muscular relaxation with the absence of circulatory effects is so important.

Hexamethylene 1-6 biscarbaminoylcholine bromide (Imbretil) was synthesised by Klupp et al.[63] and was subsequently used extensively in Europe. At first it was believed to have some properties of depolarization and some of non-depolarization, but subsequent studies have shown that it is a true depolarizing agent like decamethonium and large doses will lead to a dual block which is then readily revers-

ible with neostigmine.[64] The drug is longer-acting than d-tubocurarine but shorter-acting than toxiferine. Dripps and his colleagues,[65]
in a clinical investigation of this drug, commented on the "relatively
high incidence of respiratory inadequacy seen at the conclusion of
the operation and persisting into the immediate post-operative
period".

Hexamethylene would not appear to have any great advantage over
the more familiar long-acting depolarizing drug decamethonium.

The clinical need for a new non-depolarizing drug of short action
is great[66] but though many attempts have been made to isolate such
a compound, up to the present no suitable drug has become available
for use in man.[49, 67, 68]

Abnormal Responses to Muscle Relaxants

Occasionally a particular muscle relaxant fails to work in the
predicted manner, and the possible reasons for this "prolonged
effect" continue to interest anæsthetists. Fortunately the occasions
when a "prolonged apnœa" develops are extremely rare and the
incidence diminishes steadily as fresh information upon the action of
the relaxant drugs becomes known.[69-72]

Two important advances have been made in recent years. First, it
has been possible to single out and identify people with a "myasthenic syndrome", which is a separate clinical entity from myasthenia
gravis. Secondly, with the use of a peripheral nerve stimulator it is
now possible to diagnose the precise degree and type of neuromuscular block that is present in a particular patient, and thus to
determine whether anti-cholinesterase therapy will be of benefit or
not.

1. "Myasthenic Syndrome". This is sometimes loosely referred to
as "carcinomatous neuropathy". Originally it was thought that there
was a close relationship between cases of bronchial carcinoma and
myasthenia gravis (Anderson *et al.*).[73] This view is now known to be
wrong. Although at a quick glance there are some similarities between myasthenic syndrome and myasthenia gravis, a closer look
reveals a wide discrepancy. Lambert[74] was the first to describe
myasthenic syndrome and Wise[75] has studied the action of the
various relaxant drugs in this condition.

Myasthenic syndrome is essentially a condition of peripheral
muscle weakness developing in a patient with a bronchial carcinoma.
The finding of this type of peripheral weakness in the absence of
obvious evidence of neoplasm is sufficient to stimulate an intensive
search for its presence. The characteristic of the peripheral muscle

weakness is that the muscle power improves on effort, so that a patient may actually comment that for a brief period he feels stronger the more he tries to perform a particular task. Nevertheless, the essential clinical feature of this condition is muscle weakness. Whatever the ætiology of this condition, these patients are extremely sensitive to both types of muscle relaxant (depolarizer and non-depolarizer) and the inadvertent administration of one of long-acting drugs may results in many hours of "prolonged apnœa".

Electromyography is needed to differentiate this condition from myasthenia gravis. There are, however, two characteristic signs which are necessary for the diagnosis of myasthenic syndrome. First, on slow (twitch) stimulation (supramaximal) of a motor nerve the resultant action potential of the corresponding muscle fibres is found to be of a low voltage variety (i.e. very small). Often it is only one-fifth of the normal size. Secondly, rapid (tetanic) stimulation of the motor nerve leads to a gradual "growth" of succeeding action potentials until these are many times the size of the original. This response is diagnostic of myasthenic syndrome and is in direct contrast with the "fade" in successive responses seen in myasthenia gravis.

In a clinical assessment of the effect of relaxant drugs in cases of myasthenic syndrome Wise[75] has clearly demonstrated the sensitivity of these cases to both the depolarizing and the non-depolarizing drugs.

Clinically, if this condition is suspected and diagnosed by electromyography, a thorough search for the presence of a bronchial carcinoma must be made. Often only a small chest shadow may be

Myasthenic syndrome	*Myasthenia gravis*
1. Peripheral muscle weakness.	Peripheral and bulbar muscle weakness.
2. Always associated with bronchial carcinoma	Rarely associated with bronchial carcinoma.
3. Very sensitive to depolarizing drugs	Resistant to depolarizing drugs.
Very sensitive to non-depolarizing drugs.	Very sensitive to non-depolarizing drugs.
4. Muscle power *improves* temporarily with exercise.	Muscle power *fatigues* steadily with exercise.
5. Electromyography:	
A characteristic "growth" of the action potential	A characteristic "fade" of the action potential.
Small voltage single potential.	Large voltage single potential.
Muscle biopsy.	
Non-specific degeneration of motor end-plates.	Specific pattern of disintegration at motor end-plates.

V. MacDermot (1961).[76]

found on X-ray. Nevertheless, extreme caution must be used in anæsthetizing such patients, particularly for such a simple procedure as bronchoscopy, and the use of muscle relaxants should always be avoided.

The principal differences between myasthenic syndrome and myasthenia gravis are detailed on p. 106.

2. Diagnosis and Treatment of Prolonged Apnœa. This matter has already been discussed in detail elsewhere[71]. There are, however, certain points which require re-emphasis. When faced with the situation of a patient who will not breathe spontaneously at the end of an operation, the first point that must be settled is whether, in fact, there is *central* depression of the respiratory centre or whether the failure to breathe is due to paralysis of the *peripheral* musculature. This can only be achieved with the aid of a peripheral nerve stimulator. Thus, if the corresponding muscles contract vigorously it can be assumed that the muscle relaxant is not the principal cause of the apnœa or inadequate respiration, and a search must be made elsewhere. Alternatively, if there is no response at all, an excessive degree of muscular paralysis is present.

Once it has been established whether the muscle relaxant is at fault or not, it is then possible to diagnose the precise type of block that is present. This is done by observing the pattern of movement of the fingers with particular emphasis on whether there is a "fade" of successive responses and the presence or absence of post-tetanic facilitation (see p. 89). If the response shows the characteristics of a non-depolarization block with both "fade" and post-tetanic facilitation then a dose of anti-cholinesterase (neostigmine) and atropine is indicated. Provided there is satisfactory improvement it can be repeated, but the total dose of neostigmine should not exceed 5 mg.

In the event of a depolarization block being present the signs will be those of a "sustained" response without either fade or facilitation. In this case no anti-cholinesterase drug should be given but, armed with infinite patience, the anæsthetist must continue to ventilate the patient adequately until neuromuscular transmission recovers. There is no evidence to support the contention that any muscle relaxant *per se* is capable of producing a fatal outcome.

References

1. WASER, P., SCHMID, H., and SCHMID, K. (1954). Resorption, Verteilung und Ausscheidung von Radio-calebassen-curarin bei Katzen. *Arch. int. Pharmacodyn.*, **96**, 386.
2. WASER, P. G. (1960). The cholinergic receptor. *J. Pharm. Pharmacol.*, **12**, 577.

3. TAYLOR, D. B. (1961). Personal communication.
4. CHAGAS, C., BOVET, D., and SOLLERO, L. (1953). Curarisation musculaire et curarisation electrique chez le poisson Electrophorous electricus. *C. R. Acad. Sci.* (*Paris*), **236**, 1997.
5. EHRENPREIS, S. (1961). The isolation and identification of the acetylcholine receptor protein from electric tissue of Electrophorous electricus. *Proc. of the Symposium on Comparative Biolectrogenesis*, p. 379. Amsterdam, Eisevier Publishing Co.
6. NACHMANSOHN, D. (1959). Drug action at the myoneural junction. *Anesthesiology*, **20**, 421.
7. BOVET, D., BOVET-NITTI, F., GUARINO, S., LONGO, V. G., and FUSCO, R. (1951). Recherches su les poisons curarisants de synthese. *Arch. int. Pharmacodyn.*, **88**, 1.
8. LINSSEN, G. H. (1961). *Curariform Drugs*. Gedrukt door drukkerij Thoben, Nijmegen.
9. FREY, R. (1956). A Short-acting muscle relaxant: Prestonal (G 25178). Preliminary report. (*Proc. World Congr. Anesthesiologists*, Scheveningen, September 1955). Minneapolis: Burgess Publishing Co.
10. CAVALLITO, C. J., SORIA, A. E., and HOPPE, J. O. (1950). Amino and ammonium alkylaminobenzoquinones as curarimimetic agents. *J. Amer. chem. Soc.*, **72**, 2661.
11. WYLIE, W. D., and CHURCHILL-DAVIDSON, H. C. (1960). *A Practice of Anæsthesia*. Lloyd-Luke (Medical Books) Ltd., London.
12. GREENE, R., RIDEOUT, D. F., and SHAW, M. L. (1961). Ergometry in the diagnosis of myasthenia gravis. *Lancet*, **2**, 281.
13. CANNARD, T. H., and ZAIMIS, E. J. (1959). The effect of lowered muscle temperature on the action of neuromuscular blocking drugs in man. *J. Physiol.*, **149**, 112.
14. DILLON, J. B., FIELDS, J., GUMAS, T., JENDEN, D. J., and TAYLOR, D. B. (1955). An isolated human voluntary muscle preparation. *Proc. Soc. exp. Biol.* (*N. Y.*), **90**, 409.
15. DILLON, J. B., SABAWALA, P., TAYLOR, D. B., and GUNTER, R. (1957). Action of succinylcholine on extra-ocular muscles and intra-ocular pressure. *Anesthesiology*, **18**, 44.
16. CHURCHILL-DAVIDSON, H. C., and CHRISTIE, T. H. (1959). The diagnosis of neuromuscular block in man. *Brit. J. Anæsth.*, **31**, 290.
17. CHURCHILL-DAVIDSON, H. C., CHRISTIE, T. H., and WISE, R. P. (1960). Dual neuromuscular block in man. *Anesthesiology*, **21**, 144.
18. DILLON, J. B. (1961). Personal communication.
19. JENDEN, D. J., KAMIJO, K., and TAYLOR, D. B. (1951). The action of decamethonium (C.10) on the isolated rabbit lumbrical muscle. *J. Pharmacol. exp. Ther.*, **103**, 348.
20. ZAIMIS, E. J. (1953). Motor end-plate differences as a determining factor in the mode of action of neuromuscular blocking substances. *J. Physiol.*, **122**, 238.
21. CHURCHILL-DAVIDSON, H. C., and RICHARDSON, A. T. (1953). Neuromuscular transmission in myasthenia gravis. *J. Physiol.* (1953) **122**, 252.
22. CHURCHILL-DAVIDSON, H. C., and WISE, R. P. (1961). Unpublished work.
23. TAYLOR, D. B. (1959). The mechanism of action of muscle relaxants and their antagonists. *Anesthesiology*, **20**, 439.
24. ZAIMIS, E. J., CANNARD, T. H., and PRICE, H. L. (1958). Effects of lowered muscle temperature on neuromuscular blockade in man. *Science*, **128**, 34.
25. PAYNE, J. P. (1958). Influence of carbon dioxide on neuromuscular blocking activity of relaxant drugs in the cat. *Brit. J. Anæsth.*, **30**, 206.
26. GRAY, T. C., and WILSON, F. (1959). The development and use of muscle relaxants in the United Kingdom. *Anesthesiology*, **20**, 519.
27. HERSEY, L. W., GOWDEY, C. W., and SPOEREL, W. (1961). Central effects of five muscle relaxants. *Canad. Anæsth. Soc. J.*, **8**, 335.

28. SMITH, S. M., BROWN, H. O., TOMAN, J. E. P., and GOODMAN, L. (1947). Lack of cerebral effects of d-tubocurarine chloride. *Anesthesiology*, **8**, 1.
29. DAVIDSON, J. T., and EYAL, Z. (1961). Intramuscular suxamethonium. *Anæsthesia*, **16**, 227
30. PATON, W. D. M., and ZAIMIS, E. J. (1952). Methonium compounds. *Pharmacol. Rev.*, **4**, 219.
31. PATON, W. D. M. (1959). The effects of muscle relaxants other than muscular relaxation. *Anesthesiology*, **20**, 453.
32. CHURCHILL-DAVIDSON, H. C. (1954). Suxamethonium (succinylcholine) chloride and muscle pains. *Brit. med. J.*, **1**, 74.
33. MORRIS, D. D. B., and DUNN, C. H. (1957). Suxamethonium chloride administration and post-operative muscle pain. *Brit. med. J.*, **1**, 383.
34. FOSTER, C. A. (1960). Muscle pains that follow administration of suxamethonium. *Brit. med. J.*, **2**, 24.
35. LAMOUREAUX, L. R., and URBACH, K. F. (1960). Incidence and prevention of muscle pain following the administration of succinylcholine. *Anesthesiology*, **21**, 394.
36. BURTLES, R. (1961). Muscle pains after suxamethonium and suxethonium. *Brit. J. Anæsth.*, **33**, 147.
37. PARBROOK, G. D., and PIERCE, G. F. M. (1960). Comparison of postoperative pain and stiffness between suxamethonium and suxethonium. *Brit. med. J.*, **2**, 579.
38. BUSH, G. H., and ROTH, F. (1961). Muscle pains after suxamethonium chloride in children. *Brit. J. Anæsth.*, **33**, 151.
39. FOLDES, F. F., HILLMER, N. R., MOLLOY, R. E., and MONTE, A. P. (1960). Potentiation of the neuromuscular effect of succinylcholine by hexafluorenium. *Anesthesiology*, **21**, 50.
40. CRAYTHORNE, N. W. B., ROTTENSTEIN, H. S., and DRIPPS, R. D. (1960). The effect of succinylcholine on intraocular pressure in adults, infants and children during general anesthesia. *Anesthesiology*, **21**, 59.
41. BJÖRK, A., HALLDIN, M., and WÅHLIN, Å. (1957). Enophthalmos elicited by succinylcholine. *Acta anæsth. Scandinav.*, **1**, 41.
42. WÅHLIN, Å. (1960). Clinical and experimental studies on effects of succinylcholine. *Acta anæsth. Scandinav.*, Suppl. V, p. 9.
43. LEIGH, M. D., McCOY, D. D., BELTON, M. K., and LEWIS, G. B. (1957). Bradycardia following intravenous administration of succinylcholine chloride to infants and children. *Anesthesiology*, **18**, 698.
44. MARTIN, K. H. (1958). *Simposio Internazionale su curare curarosimili e curarizzante. Venice*, 1958. *XI Congress*. Atti Societa Italiana di Anestesiologia.
45. BULLOUGH, J. (1959). Intermittent suxamethonium injections. *Brit. med J.*, **1**, 786.
46. LUPPRIAN, K. G., and CHURCHILL-DAVIDSON, H. C. (1960). Effect of suxamethonium on cardiac rhythm. *Brit. med. J.*, **2**, 1774.
47. KVISSELGAARD, N., and MOYA, F. (1961a). Estimation of succinylcholine blood levels. *Acta anæsth. Scandinav.*, **5**, 1.
48. KVISSELGAARD, N., and MOYA, F. (1961b). Investigation of placental thresholds to succinylcholine. *Anesthesiology*, **22**, 7.
49. CHURCHILL-DAVIDSON, H. C. (1961). The changing pattern of neuromuscular block. *Canad. Anæsth. Soc. J.*, **8**, 91.
50. FOLDES, F. (1957). *Muscle Relaxants in Anesthesiology*. Charles C. Thomas, Springfield, Illinois.
51. KALOW, W. (1959). The distribution, destruction and elimination of muscle relaxants. *Anesthesiology*, **20**, 505.
52. KALOW, W. and DAVIES, R. O. (1958). The activity of various esterase inhibitors towards atypical human serum cholinesterase. *Biochem. Pharmacol.*, **1**, 183.

53. LEHMANN, H., SILK, E., and LIDDELL, J. (1961). Pseudocholinesterase. *Brit. med. Bull.*, **17**, 230.
54. CHURCHILL-DAVIDSON, H. C., and GRIFFITHS, W. J. (1961). Simple test-paper method for the clinical determination of plasma pseudocholinesterase. *Brit. med. J.*, **2**, 994.
55. KALOW, W., and GENEST, K. (1957). A method for the detection of atypical forms of human serum cholinesterase; determination of dibucaine numbers. *Canad. J. Biochem. Physiol.*, **35**, 339.
56. LEHMANN, H., and SILK, E. (1961). Familial pseudocholinesterase deficiency. *Brit. med. J.*, **1**, 128.
57. KAUFMAN, L., LEHMANN, H., and SILK, E. (1960). Suxamethonium apnœa in an infant. *Brit. med. J.*, **1**, 166.
58. LEHMANN, H. (1962). Personal communication.
59. WASER, P. G. (1950). Pharmakologie einiger Reinalkaloide aus Calebassencurare. *Helv. physiol. pharmacol. Acta.*, **8**, 342.
60. WASER, P. G., and HARBECK, P. (1959). Erste Klinische Anwendung der Calebassenalkaloide Toxiferin I und Curarin I. *Der Anæsthesist*, **8**, 193.
61. FREY, R., and SEEGER, R. (1961). Experimental and clinical experience with toxiferine. *Canad. Anæsth. Soc. J.*, **8**, 99.
62. FOLDES, F. F., WOLFSON, B., and SOKOLL, M. (1961). The use of toxiferine for the production of surgical relaxation. *Anesthesiology*, **22**, 93.
63. KLUPP, H., KRAUPP, O., STORMANN, H., and STUMPF, C. (1953). Uber die pharmakologischen Eigenschaften einiger Polymethylen-Dicarbaminsaure-Bischolinester. *Arch. int. Pharmacodyn.*, **96**, 161.
64. CHRISTIE, T. H., WISE, R. P., and CHURCHILL-DAVIDSON, H. C. (1959). Hexamethylene 1:6 biscarbaminoylcholine bromide. A new synthetic muscle relaxant. *Lancet*, **2**, 648.
65. DRIPPS, R. D., HANKS, E. C., NGAI, S. H., OECH, S. R., PAPPER, E. M., and SECHZER, P. H. (1959). A clinical study of the muscle relaxant, Imbretil. *Anesthesiology*, **20**, 646.
66. CHURCHILL-DAVIDSON, H. C. (1958). *Simposio Internazionale su curare curarosimilie e curarizzante. Venice, 1958. XI Congress.* Atti Societa Italiana di Anestesiologia.
67. HAINING, C. G., JOHNSTON, R. G., and SMITH, J. M. (1959). Neuromuscular blocking agents of short duration. *Nature*, **183**, 542.
68. COLLIER, H. O. J., GLADYCH, J. M. Z., MACAULEY, B., and TAYLOR, E. P. (1958). Some new neuromuscular blocking agents. *Nature*, **182**, 1424.
69. PATON, J. W. (1958). Possible causes of prolonged apnœa. *Anæsthesia*, **13**, 253.
70. CHURCHILL-DAVIDSON, H. C. (1956). Neuromuscular block in man. *Anesthesiology*, **17**, 88.
71. CHURCHILL-DAVIDSON, H. C. (1959). Causes and treatment of prolonged apnœa. *Anesthesiology*, **20**, 535.
72. FOLDES, F. F., RENDELL-BAKER, L., and BIRCH, J. H. (1956). Causes and prevention of prolonged apnœa with succinylcholine. *Curr. Res. Anesth.*, **35**, 609.
73. ANDERSON, H. J., CHURCHILL-DAVIDSON, H. C., and RICHARDSON, A. T. (1953). A case of bronchial neoplasm with myasthenia. *Lancet*, **2**, 1291.
74. LAMBERT, E. H., ROOKE, E. D., EATON, L. M., and HODGSON, C. H. (1959). Myasthenic syndrome occasionally associated with bronchial neoplasm. *Myasthenia gravis*, p. 362. Charles C. Thomas, Springfield, Illinois.
75. WISE, R. P. (1962). Personal communication.
76. MACDERMOT, V. (1961). Personal communication.

CHAPTER 4

HYPOTHERMIA*

B. A. SELLICK

History—Purpose and Uses of Hypothermia—Temperature Control and Measurement—Principal Physiological Changes— Changes in the Cardio-vascular System—Methods of Inducing Hypothermia—Rewarming—Anæsthesia for Hypothermia—Surface Induced Hypothermia—Postoperative Considerations.

HYPOTHERMIA may occur spontaneously in neonates whose heat regulating mechanism is not fully established, in hypothyroidism; on exposure to excessive cold when the compensating mechanisms of decreased heat loss and increased heat production are exhausted, or under the influence of anæsthetic and other drugs which disturb the heat regulating mechanism and in shock.

INDUCED HYPOTHERMIA

Induced generalized hypothermia, about which this chapter is mainly concerned, can be defined as the deliberate lowering of body temperature by physical means.

It should not be confused with "hibernation" which is a condition foreign to the human species, nor with "hibernation anæsthesia" which is a term applied to the decreased metabolism and slight lowering of body temperature following the use of mixtures of opiates and phenothiazine derivatives—the "lytic" cocktail.[1]

History. The local numbing effect of cold has always been known. Its first recorded use in surgery was by Baron Larrey, Napoleon's surgeon, who amputated frozen limbs in the battle of Eylau in Poland in 1807. Deliberate refrigeration for the amputation of limbs was not undertaken until 1942 by Allen.

In 1798 James Currie, a Liverpool surgeon, investigated total body hypothermia in man in relation to survival after shipwreck in cold seas.

Deliberate total body cooling was first attempted by Smith and Fay in 1938 in an attempt to slow the growth of inoperable carcinoma. To Bigelow of Toronto must go the credit of investigating the clinical possibilities of hypothermia and his classic paper in 1950 on the relationship of oxygen consumption to body temperature in

* Further detailed reference to this subject will be found in other chapters.

the anæsthetized dog was the starting point for the use of hypothermia in surgery.

For further details of the history of hypothermia the reader is referred to: Allen, F. M. *et al.* (1942), *J. Internat. Coll. Surg.* March/April, 125; Fay, T. *et al.* (1939), *J.A.M.A.* **113,** 653; Currie, J. (1797), "Medical Reports on the effects of Water Cold and Warm as a Remedy in Fever and Febrile Diseases, whether applied to the Surface of the Body or used as a Drink."

The Purpose and Uses of Hypothermia. The purpose of inducing hypothermia is to reduce metabolism of the vital tissues of the body to enable them to withstand reduced or absent circulation for greater periods than can be tolerated at normal temperatures (see Table 1).

At 37° C the cells of the cerebellum and the cerebral cortex which are the most susceptible tissues of the body to oxygen lack can withstand no more than 3 minutes anoxia without irreversible damage. At 15° C this period is prolonged to 50 minutes. At 30° C at which temperature for many reasons (see below) the majority of hypothermia cases are conducted, the brain can safely withstand a period of 10 minutes' circulatory arrest.

TABLE I

° C	Depth of Hypothermia	Period of safe circulatory arrest
37° C	Normothermia . . .	3 minutes
37°–32° C	Mild hypothermia . .	3–8 minutes
32°–28° C	Conventional hypothermia .	8–15 minutes
28°–18° C	Deep hypothermia . .	15–45 minutes
18°– 0° C	Profound hypothermia . .	45– ? minutes
Below 0° C	Super cooling . . .	? minutes

TABLE II

USES OF HYPOTHERMIA

1. Peripheral Vascular Surgery

    1. Resection of aneurysm.
    2. Arterial grafting.
    3. Endarterectomy.
    4. Organ transplant.

2. Neuro-Surgery

    1. Resection of berry aneurysm.

    2. Cerebral tumours.

    3. Protection of brain from effects of induced hypotension.

3. Cardiac Surgery

    1. Repair of cardiac lesions under direct vision.

    2. Reduction of cardiac rate and irritability.

    3. Combined with extracorporeal circulation to facilitate prolonged exclusion of heart from circulation.

4. Miscellaneous Therapeutic Uses

    1. Treatment of cerebral œdema or ischæmia following head injury, cerebral infarct, anoxic episode.

    2. Treatment of chronic anoxia in association with respiratory poliomyelitis or irreversible shock.

    3. Treatment of malignant disease.

The uses of hypothermia are summarized in Table II. The uses in neurology and neuro-surgery are covered in the chapter on neuro-surgical anæsthesia and this chapter will deal primarily with its use in cardiac and cardio-vascular surgery.

Temperature Control and Measurement

To facilitate discussion it is usual to divide the body into a superficial layer or "shell" consisting of skin, subcutaneous tissue, fat, muscle and bone and a deep "core" of vital tissues comprising structures contained within the skull, thorax and abdomen.

The core structures are those most susceptible to anoxia and it is the primary purpose of induced hypothermia to reduce their temperature. Core temperature is normally maintained within narrow limits by the activity of the heat regulating centre of the hypothalamus, whereas the shell has a more labile temperature particularly towards the surface. The shell insulates the core if heat conservation is required or transmits heat if it is to be dissipated through the skin. These functions are dependent upon the degree of dilatation of the superficial vessels which determine the amount of heat which is carried to the skin from the body core.

Even at normal temperature there is a temperature gradient between the core and the skin; it is useless to assess core temperature from thermometers placed superficially.

The most useful temperatures to record are those of mid-œsophagus and the naso-pharynx. Oral and rectal thermometers are difficult to maintain in position and frequently give misleading readings. The proximity of the œsophagus to the heart and great vessels result in its temperature closely following that of blood, which during either surface or blood stream cooling will at first be colder than the rest of the core structures.

The naso-pharyngeal temperature reflects cooling of tissues distal to the heart and is a convenient guide to the temperature of the brain. During cooling and rewarming the œsophageal temperature precedes the naso-pharyngeal and only during periods of temperature equilibrium are the two identical.

The "After-drop". The temperature gradient built up during the application of cold to the surface of the body results in a continued loss of heat from the core to the shell after the patient has been removed from the cold environment or even if surface rewarming has begun. This "after-drop" may be 2°–6° C and its control is one of the essential features of any method of surface cooling.

Rate of Cooling. Cardiac arrhythmias during hypothermia (q.v.) are an expression of the reduced temperature of the myocardium. In blood stream cooling the return of cold blood into the great veins or right atrium can rapidly cool the myocardium to a dangerous level and impair circulation long before the rest of the vital tissues of the body are cooled.

As all cold venous blood returning from the skin in surface cooling passes first through the right side of the heart a similar condition can occur if an excessive rate of cooling is permitted. The rapid transfusion of cold blood during surgery may cause a sudden drop in an already cold myocardium and initiate ventricular arrhythmias. To apply cold too rapidly to the surface of a warm vaso-dilated patient immediately after induction of anæsthesia may produce a sudden drop in myocardial temperature, particularly in small patients. A gradual introduction to the cold environment is safer.

Blood stream cooling must also be induced slowly to prevent disturbances of cardiac rhythm impairing circulation. When extra-corporeal circulation is used as a means of inducing profound hypothermia the effect of cooling on the myocardium is of less importance as the circulation is being maintained artificially.

Clinical experience shows that a rate of cooling of 1° C in 5 minutes is well tolerated by the heart.

Thermometers. Four types of thermometers are used in current clinical practice.

Mercury in glass. The standard clinical thermometer is useless because of its limited range and the necessity for repeated shaking. Lotion thermometers (National Physical Laboratory tested) of the range 0°–50 °C are valuable for measurement of temperatures of the cooling or re-warming media and for calibrating electrical thermometers. Glass thermometers are unsuitable for insertion into the œsophagus but in emergency (i.e. failure of electrical apparatus) can be used for measuring naso-pharyngeal temperatures if great care is exercised in inserting the thermometers via the nose.

Vapour Pressure Thermometers. The vapour pressure exerted by a volume of volatile liquid contained within a bulb is carried by a length of capillary tubing to a distant pressure gauge. The standard car radiator thermometer is of this type and it provides a convenient method of measuring temperature at a distance from the site of the bulb. The size of bulb precludes its use in the naso-pharynx or in a child's œsophagus. Vapour pressure does not bear a direct relationship with temperature and this makes calibration and reading more difficult.

Thermo-couple Thermometers. The E.M.F. generated by a bi-metal junction such as constantan and platinum is related to temperature and can be measured on a sensitive galvanometer. The thermocouple itself can be made very small and the sensitive end easily inserted into the naso-pharynx or œsophagus or after sterilization into the tissues of the body. Frequent calibrations are needed if accuracy in the clinical range is to be maintained.

Thermistor Thermometers. A small bead of resistance material is welded between two platinum wires. The resistance of this bead is related to the temperature and can be measured by means of a Wheatstone bridge circuit giving a direct linear reading on the scale over the usual clinical range of 10°–40° C. These thermometers are more stable than the thermo-couples and have proved more reliable.

For further details of thermometers see "The Measurement of Temperature" by P. Cliffe. *Anæsthesia*, 1962. Vol. 17, No. 2, p. 215.

PRINCIPAL PHYSIOLOGICAL CHANGES

Oxygen Consumption. Exposure to cold in the intact animal causes a great increase in heat production and oxygen consumption, due mainly to violent shivering. When the heat regulating mechanism is depressed by disease, drugs or anæsthesia and particularly if muscular activity is abolished by curare, exposure to cold causes a decrease in oxygen consumption parallel to the fall in body temperature.

Bigelow[2] showed that this relationship was linear, and in dogs at 30° C oxygen consumption was approximately 75 per cent normal, at 25° C, 50 per cent, and at 20° C only 25 per cent.

Actual measurements of human cerebral oxygen consumption have been made by Stone.[3] He found that the effect of hypothermia on cerebral metabolism is more marked, for example, at 30° C oxygen consumption is 39% and at 28° C is 35% normal. He also found that shivering greatly increases cerebral oxygen consumption and suggested that cerebral ischæmia in the presence of shivering is particularly dangerous.

The carriage of oxygen by blood in the hypothermic state is not significantly altered although cold blood carries more oxygen in solution. The shift of the oxygen dissociation curve to the left due to cold is counteracted by the high carbon dioxide level due to its increased solubility.

Tissue utilization of oxygen is not depressed below the metabolic requirements as was proved by Bigelow[2] who showed that no oxygen deficit occurred during cooling. This should not be confused with the effect of a period of prolonged circulatory occlusion under hypothermia when some oxygen deficit will occur.

Carbon Dioxide. The increased solubility of carbon dioxide in cold blood leads to a fall in pH. Elimination via the lungs keeps pace with carbon dioxide production and there is no CO_2 retention as a result of hypothermia itself, but, during periods of circulatory arrest, of course, tissue CO_2 accumulates. Rapidly changing pH has been blamed for cardiac irregularities during hypothermia particularly when these have coincided with manipulation of the heart. There is some evidence that a constant slightly raised P_{CO_2} or a slightly reduced P_{CO_2} maintained by the degree of ventilation reduces the incidence of arrhythmia.

Central Nervous System. Hypothermia in the unanæsthetized subject leads to loss of consciousness at a body temperature between 28°–30° C. In the anæsthetized the potentiation and delayed elimination of drugs maintains unconsciousness at 30° C for long periods after inhalational anæsthesia has been withdrawn and consciousness returns only on rewarming.

Cerebral blood flow is reduced because of the increased viscosity of blood, increased resistance of cerebral vessels due to cold induced vaso-constriction and the lowered cardiac output. This is a possible explanation of the reduction in brain volume that occurs during hypothermia for neuro-surgery.

The respiratory centre is depressed by hypothermia and respiration becomes progressively slower but not markedly shallower until respiratory arrest occurs at a temperature of 18°–20° C.

Liver Function. Many activities of the liver are depressed. The detoxification of drugs and their elimination are seriously impaired. The conjugation of morphine is particularly affected and accounts for the increased sensitivity to opiates of cases undergoing hypothermia. Metabolism of acids is impaired. Prothrombin formation is reduced and there is a decreased coagulability of blood.

These effects are largely reversible on rewarming but as shown by Brewin and Neil[4] if circulatory occlusion causes a high venous pressure, damage may result from hepatic congestion and delayed recovery of liver function follows. In particular this may lead to persistant acid/base disturbances.

Renal Function. Renal blood flow and glomular filtration are both diminished. At temperatures below 30° C there is a secretion of dilute urine. This water diuresis lasts only as long as the period of hypothermia and there is a return to the usual post-operative oliguria. Following profound hypothermia, below 20° C, the diuresis may persist into the post-operative period. Decreased renal activity reduces the ability of the body to maintain acid/base equilibrium.

Acid/Base Equilibrium. Hypothermia is responsible for disturbances in acid/base equilibrium. Cold reduces ionization and this in turn reduces the buffering capacity of hæmoglobin and the plasma proteins. The relatively less efficient bicarbonate/carbonic acid buffer system cannot deal with imbalance and as a result small changes in acid/base balance lead to a relatively large change in pH.

Acidosis which tends to be a feature of hypothermia is caused in at least four ways. Carbon dioxide is more soluble in cold blood and any respiratory insufficiency will increase still further the P_{CO_2}. There is an increase in the formation of fixed acids, particularly lactic acid as a result of shivering, anoxia, surgical trauma and anæsthesia and there is a decreased break down of them due to impaired liver function. Depression of renal activity prevents elimination of acid.

The persistence of acidosis after operation is an important cause of continuing circulatory difficulties.[5] Alkali reserve may be well below normal after operation and infusions of bicarbonate or sodium lactate may be needed to restore acid/base equilibrium.

Electrolyte Changes. The most important change occurring in hypothermia is a rise in serum potassium. This rise in potassium is increased by anoxia but even more so by the transfusion of stored blood in which anærobic metabolism leads to a high potassium and low pH.

During heart surgery the period immediately following resumption of circulation is one of particular danger in this respect. Anoxic tissue metabolism leads to marked acidæmia chiefly due to lactic acid and retained carbon dioxide and whilst this is beginning to circulate it is frequently necessary to restore blood volume by transfusion. A high potassium level when associated with a low pH is particularly dangerous and marked depression of cardiac activity may result. There are few other changes in electrolytes except in the serum sodium which may fall (see below).

Blood Sugar. Carbohydrate metabolism is deranged partly by the effect of liver metabolism and by decreased insulin formation, and a rise in blood sugar occurs. It has been stated[5] that the infusion of glucose solutions during hypothermia is dangerous. The accumulation of glucose in the extra cellular fluid as a result of slow metabolism draws water from the cells by osmosis. Dilution of extra cellular fluid dilutes the serum sodium level which falls rapidly and may lead to further cardio-vascular disturbances.

Effects on the Cardio-Vascular System

Peripheral Vessels. Surface cold causes arteriolar constriction and veno-spasm. The skin capillaries exposed to extremes of cold are paralysed and filled with oxy-hæmoglobin giving a characteristic cherry-red colour.

Spasm of peripheral blood vessels during surface or blood stream cooling makes the measurement of blood pressure by the auscultatory method extremely difficult and an oscillometric method is preferable. Blood pressure rises in the early stages of cooling because of increased peripheral resistance, but later falls when cold depresses cardiac activity.

The Heart. The most significant physiological disturbances of hypothermia are on the heart. It is the factor limiting the depth to which hypothermia can be safely induced when circulation is not maintained artificially. There is an increasing bradycardia as temperature falls. This bradycardia can be overcome by the administration of atropine down to 30° C but atropine is less effective below 30° C. Initially the cardiac output remains high. Diastole is prolonged in the slow heart and there is increased filling and a larger stroke volume. At temperatures approaching 30° C atrial fibrillation commonly occurs. This arrhythmia is usually of little significance, reverting in most cases to sinus rhythm on rewarming.

Below 30° C there is an increasing risk of ventricular fibrillation particularly if the heart is being stimulated by surgery. The mechanism of the onset of ventricular fibrillation is not certain but many factors have been blamed. The work of Malmajac[6] suggests that it is primarily a cardiac ischæmia due to fall in blood pressure and he has found that if blood pressure is maintained by a continuous infusion of adrenaline the onset of ventricular fibrillation is delayed until much lower temperatures are reached.

The electrocardiographic changes of impending ventricular fibrillation are a widening of the QRS complex and ST depression suggestive of coronary ischæmia. In practice the injection of adrenaline into the heart to increase its tone during ventricular fibrillation is a valuable preliminary to electrical defibrillation. A continuous infusion of adrenaline following defibrillation is a valuable method of maintaining adequate function. Other causes of cardiac arrhythmia are hyperkalæmia, sudden pH changes, sudden Pco_2 changes and citrate intoxication (see below). To these may be added the increased viscosity of cold blood particularly in the polycythæmic patient.

In surface and veno-venous cooling conventional hypothermia (28°–30° C) is a compromise. The risk of ventricular fibrillation at this temperature is small and a period of 10 minutes' circulatory occlusion can be safely tolerated.

If circulation is maintained artificially by cardiac or cardiopulmonary by-pass then the heart may be cooled to much lower levels before fibrillation starts. If circulation to the rest of the body is maintained the heart itself may be cooled to complete arrest either by direct perfusion of the coronary vessels or by the application of crushed ice. The perfusion of the heart subsequently by warmed blood enables it to be restarted. These techniques allow prolonged exclusion of the heart from the circulation for the purposes of intracardiac surgery, particularly repair of aortic valves.

Blood Volume. Hypothermia causes hæmo-concentration by the shift of water from the plasma to the interstitial compartment. During shivering there is also a passage of water into the muscle cells. These blood volume changes are seldom clinically evident during hypothermia to conventional levels.

Loss of circulating blood volume is far more frequently due to hæmorrhage. Cold blood if transfused rapidly may cause undue local cooling of the heart with dangerous results, and should be rewarmed first. Stored blood not only has a high potassium and low pH but in most cases has been collected in citrate solution. The hypothermic patient is unable to metabolize citrate and together with the low level of ionised calcium there is an ever present risk of citrate intoxication. The typical electrocardiographic change—prolongation of the Q.T. interval—is an indication for the administration of ionisable calcium in the form of calcium gluconate or chloride.

In some centres other anti-coagulants such as heparin or egludate are preferred to citrate to avoid this complication.

METHODS OF INDUCING HYPOTHERMIA

Surface Cooling. The application of cold to the surface of the body is the simplest method and refrigerated blankets, immersion in cold water, application of ice bags, wind tunnel and electric fans are all well tried methods.

Surface cooling is suitable for induction of conventional hypothermia ($28°–30°$ C) and is valuable for intracardiac procedures of limited duration. It is the method of choice for the closure of uncomplicated secundum type atrial septal defects and for the relief of simple valvular pulmonary stenosis. The limit of 10 minutes' circulatory arrest excludes this method for more prolonged intracardiac procedures. It is also indicated for peripheral vascular surgery where periods of inadequate circulation or circulatory arrest can be expected such as resection of aneurysm and arterial grafting. (See p. 163 for detailed technique.)

Internal Cooling. The intra-gastric balloon of Khalil[7] perfused by ice cold water has been used as a means of inducing hypothermia. It has found some favour in controlling hyper-pyrexia in children but it is not a practical method in adults.

Pleuro-pericardial application of cold saline has been used to reduce temperature, particularly the local temperature of the heart. Ice arrest of the heart can be achieved by packing the pericardium with sludged ice.[8] For induction of whole body hypothermia this method is inadequate.

Blood Stream Cooling. (*a*) *With Spontaneous Circulation*. The arterio-venous cooling coil[9] provides a neat method of cooling, particularly in experimental animals. Cannulation of the femoral artery and vein and the spontaneous flow of blood from one to the other via a cooling coil provides a method of blood stream cooling which does not require a thoracotomy.

Veno-venous cooling[10] can only be employed during thoracotomy. It is a rapid and controllable method of inducing hypothermia for heart surgery. Venous blood is withdrawn from a cannula in the superior vena cava and pumped through a cooling coil and returned to the inferior vena cava. Disadvantages of veno-venous cooling are its complexity which precludes its use for non-thoracic surgery, and rapid cooling of the myocardium increases the risk of cardiac arrhythmia.[11]

(*b*) *Assisted Circulation*. Cardio-pulmonary bypass using a pump oxygenator permits profound hypothermia to be induced without impairment of circulation. Profound hypothermia can also be induced by cardiac bypass as described by Drew.[12] In this method blood is withdrawn from the left atrium, cooled and pumped into the femoral artery. A second cannula withdraws blood from the right atrium and this is pumped into the pulmonary artery which is also cannulated. When the body temperature reaches 15° C both circuits are discontinued and up to 50 minutes' surgery is performed within the heart during total circulatory arrest. The cannulation is then restored to enable rewarming.

METHODS OF REWARMING

Spontaneous re-warming at room temperature takes many hours because of the slow return to normal metabolism. This slow return to normal temperature is of value after cerebral surgery or after an anoxic episode and helps to prevent the development of cerebral œdema. The risk of continued hypothermia in a patient with an abnormal heart precludes slow spontaneous re-warming.

Radio-frequency Re-warming. This method[13] by placing the patient in a diathermy field, e.g. by use of a diathermy coil or pads around the patient's pelvis, is slow but warms the deep tissues of the body. Owing to a risk of deep burns it is not entirely satisfactory.

Surface Re-warming. This is a simple and satisfactory method of re-warming from conventional levels of hypothermia. Immersion in a bath of warm water gives the maximum surface area for heat exchange. Re-warming by water blankets during cardiac surgery as described below reduces the duration of hypothermia without affecting its depth. This enables the lag in re-warming to be overcome by the time surgery is completed.

Internal Re-warming. The intragastric balloon may be perfused with warm water but the surface area offered for heat exchange is very small.

Flooding the pericardium with warm saline during thoracic surgery rewarms the heart itself which may have become unduly chilled or have developed dangerous arrhythmias. It is used as a means of rapid re-warming of the heart to enable defibrillation to be attempted electrically. As a means of re-warming the whole body it is ineffective.

Blood Stream Re-warming. The methods described for blood stream cooling can also be used for re-warming and are essential when profound hypothermia has been induced by means of extra-corporeal techniques.

ANÆSTHESIA FOR HYPOTHERMIA

The basic principle of anæsthesia during hypothermia is that adequate depth must be maintained to prevent reaction to cold. Shivering must be prevented and vaso-constriction reduced to a minimum. In view of the potentiation of anæsthetics at low temperatures and the slow elimination of intravenous or intramuscularly administered drugs, the main anæsthetic should be inhalational to facilitate its elimination once hypothermia has been established. In this way minimum drugs are present in the blood stream during circulatory interruption and this is of particular importance during cardiac surgery to avoid unnecessary myocardial depression.

Efficient ventilation must be maintained throughout. During thoracotomy, respiration is controlled and it is an advantage to maintain slight over-ventilation. If patients are breathing spontaneously respiratory acidosis is inevitable.

Light anæsthesia only is required for rewarming and nitrous oxide/oxygen alone will prevent shivering.[14]

A METHOD OF SURFACE INDUCED HYPOTHERMIA

A method of hypothermia for cardiac and peripheral vascular surgery of which the author has had experience approaching 500 cases is described below:

Premedication. Promethazine 25 mg, pethidine 100 mg and Scopolamine 0·4 mg is the standard dose for a 10-stone adult. These doses are varied according to the size and fitness of the patient. In small children below 50 lb body weight thiopentone suppositories or a solution of 5 % thiopentone in a dose of 20 mg per lb body weight has proved a very satisfactory method of basal narcosis.

The reduction of shivering by chlorpromazine makes it a valuable drug for inducing hypothermia in the conscious patient but it is an unsatisfactory drug for cardiac surgery because of its adrenolytic action and the unpleasant tachycardia that sometimes occurs.

Induction of Anæsthesia. In poor risk cases pre-oxygenation is indicated and in the seriously incapacitated, such as patients with the tetralogy of Fallot and other cyanotic heart disease, it is essential to place the patient in an oxygen tent for at least 12 hours before operation.

Thiopentone in small doses, given slowly up to a total of 5 mg per kilo body weight, is used for induction in adults. In conscious children who are "needle shy" an inhalational induction of nitrous oxide, halothane or cyclopropane with a high oxygen content may enable venipuncture to be performed later without distress.

The patient is then curarized and intubated. Thermistor thermometers are placed in the œsophagus to the level of the nipple line and in the naso-pharynx. Electrocardiograph leads are attached to all four limbs and an oscillometric blood pressure cuff applied to one arm. An intravenous cannula is inserted.

Maintenance of Anæsthesia. When induction is complete, and full controlled respiration is established, ether is added to secure adequate depth and to maintain vaso-dilatation. Halothane may be used in small concentration for this purpose and has the advantage of being non-explosive. It is, however, a hypotensive drug and can cause excessive bradycardia.

Induction of Hypothermia. Preliminary records are made of the patient's temperature, blood pressure, pulse and E.C.G. These are repeated at 5 minute intervals. The patient is then immersed in a bath of water at 20° C. The head and hands are kept out of the water by means of slings. Once the patient is in the water and no untoward effects have occurred from the immediate effects of cold, ice is added to bring the temperature of the bath down to, and maintain it at 10° C in adults and 15° C in children. This temperature differential produces an adequate rate of cooling. Use of colder water has disadvantages; it causes intense superficial vaso-constriction which actually slows heat exchange and the shell of the body is excessively cooled so that on removal from the bath an unpredictable and dangerous "after-drop" may occur. It is possible at very low temperatures for circulatory disturbances of the digits to occur.

The patient is frequently massaged and kneaded during the period of cooling to prevent stagnation of blood in dependant parts. Frequent stirring of the water assists heat exchange. The buoyancy of water reduces the pressure on the posterior surfaces of the body and exposes these areas for heat exchange.

Additional curare is added to eliminate any evidence of shivering and further ether given if superficial vaso-constriction or excessive "goose-pimples" are seen. After 5–15 minutes depending on the size of the patient, the body temperature begins to fall; the œsophageal temperature drop preceding the nasopharyngeal. After a further period of 5–10 minutes the rate of cooling increases and then becomes constant. Any flattening of the cooling curve at this stage indicates some reaction to cold and appropriate drugs are given.

When the œsophageal temperature reaches 32° C the patient is removed from the bath, dried and placed on the operating table between water blankets (q.v.). At this point both ether and nitrous oxide are discontinued and ventilation with 100% oxygen only is carried out until re-warming has begun.

Using this technique and placing the patient from the cold bath between water blankets kept at a temperature of 35°–40° C a predictable "after-drop" of 2° C takes place. Temperature equilibrium is reached within 10 minutes in a child and perhaps 20–25 minutes in an adult. After that time the temperature remains constant at approximately 30° C plus or minus ½° for a period varying between 10 minutes and 1 hour, again depending on the size of the patient. It then begins to climb slowly. During the period of temperature equilibrium the heart is exposed and the intracardiac procedure performed whilst circulation is occluded.

If a longer period is required at 30° C as for example in a difficult anastomosis for vascular surgery, then the water blankets are maintained at 30° C when hypothermia will be prolonged indefinitely.

Following completion of the intracardiac or vascular surgery rewarming can be speeded by raising the temperature of the water in the blankets. This can safely be raised to 42° C. In practice by the time surgery is completed body temperature has usually returned to 32° C.

On completion of surgery a dressing is applied to the wound and the patient is returned to a warm bath at 42° C. At the same time 50% nitrous oxide is added to ventilate the patient during the period of re-warming.

Re-curarization. At low temperatures curare is less effective and there may be generalized muscular stiffness and attempts to breathe. On re-warming to 32° or 33° full curarization reappears.

When the patient has been re-warmed to 35° C he is taken from the bath, dried and returned to bed. Residual curare is then reversed with atropine and neostigmine.

Post Operative Considerations

The particular points in the post operative period following hypothermia are:

Temperature. There is frequently an overshoot of temperature following hypothermia. Once metabolism is re-established it tends to be over active and pyrexia may follow within 12 hours. Excessive rise in temperature is treated by tepid sponging.

Shivering. Patients who have not fully re-warmed by the time consciousness is regained may complain of feeling cold and shivering may be a feature. Unless the patient is seriously ill no steps need to be taken to control this other than by application of warmth.

Circulatory Effects. Following hypothermia there is circulatory instability and the patient should be nursed flat for at least 8 hours post-operatively. Postural changes for the purposes of physiotherapy, etc., should be made slowly to prevent postural hypotension and sitting these patients up must be done gradually to avoid falls in blood pressure.

Acid/Base Imbalance. The acid/base imbalance may persist post operatively. If circulatory difficulties are experienced from this cause as confirmed by estimations of alkali reserve, etc., infusions of sodium bicarbonate or sodium lactate may prove necessary to restore balance, although in the vast majority the return of normal liver and kidney function restores equilibrium.

Post Operative Analgesia. The post hypothermic patient is unduly sensitive to the opiate drugs and these must be given in small doses to prevent risk of circulatory depression and dangerous levels of hypotension. For example, in an adult a dose of intramuscular pethidine of 100 mg might well drop the blood pressure to unrecordable levels for 4 hours. It is, therefore, preferable to give all analgesic drugs in very small doses intravenously and repeat only when circulatory effects have returned to normal.

In small children aspirin suppositories gr 2–5 have proved a useful analgesic.

References

1. LABORIT, H., et al. (1952). Presse Med., **60**, 206.
2. BIGELOW, W. G., et al. (1950). Amer. J. Physiol., **160**, 125.
3. STONE, H. H., et al. (1956). Surg. Gyn. and Obst., **103**, 313.
4. BREWIN, E. G., and NEIL, E., et al. (1955). Guy's Hosp. Rep., **104**, 177.
5. WYNN, V. (1954). Lancet, **2**, 575.
6. MALMAJAC, C. (1961). J. de Physiol. (Par), **53**, 415.
7. KHALIL, H. H. (1958). Lancet, **1**, 1092.
8. ROSS, D. (1961). Lancet, **2**, 293.
9. DELORME, E. J. (1952). Lancet, **2**, 914.
10. ROSS, D. (1954). Lancet, **1**, 1108.
11. GRAHAM, G. R. (1955). Brit. Heart J., **17**, 577.

12. DREW, C. E., *et al.* (1959). *Lancet*, **1,** 745.
13. BIGELOW, W. G. (1952). *Canad. J. Med. Sci.*, **30,** 185.
14. CLUTTON BROCK, (1959). *Brit. J. Anæsth.*, **31,** 210.

See also:

COOPER and ROSS (1960). *Hypothermia in Surgical Practice*. Cassell.
British Medical Bulletin (1961). Hypothermia and the effects of cold. Vol. 17 No. 1.

Chapter 5

ANÆSTHESIA FOR NEUROSURGERY

Robert I. W. Ballantine

*General Anæsthesia (Spontaneous and Controlled Respiration)—
Methods of lowering Intracranial Pressure—Head Injuries—
Radiological Investigations—Anæsthesia and Analgesia with
Patient-Coöperation.*

Many problems still exist for the neurosurgical anæsthetist, but in recent years an increased awareness of these problems and greater interest in this speciality has led to many advances. In the past the neurosurgical case was often left to a junior who was only expected to intubate the patient and maintain anæsthesia. With improved training in anæsthetic and research methods and a changed attitude of mind, the anæsthetist has increased his responsibility and the scope of his work, so that with new drugs and the application of modern anæsthetic techniques he is not only helping his patients but also extending the frontiers of surgery and facilitating the work of his surgical colleagues.

This is particularly true in neurosurgery, for it is here that the surgeon has two great problems, raised intracranial pressure, and the risk of severe hæmorrhage. It is from an effort to reduce these that the main advances have occurred in the last five or six years, with the use in neurosurgical anæsthesia of vascular hypotension, hypothermia, controlled respiration and improved dehydration therapy. At the same time the anæsthetist has realized the importance of attention to the small details and safety of the basic techniques, without which the refinements are not only useless but hazardous.

Finally, and as a result of his interest and application, the anæsthetist has become an indispensable member of the team, in whom the surgeon has confidence. This is of fundamental importance during neurosurgical operations. The respiratory and cardiovascular patterns may be changing from moment to moment as the vital centres are affected by surgery and pressure changes, and the anæsthetist by his knowledge of the effects of the anæsthetic drugs and his careful monitoring of the patient may be able to help in the assessment of the situation.

Before discussing these advances and the present position of neurosurgical anæsthesia in detail it may not be thought superfluous to emphasize that good anæsthesia requires that the following must be avoided:[1]

1. Respiratory obstruction.
2. Reflex respiratory effects such as coughing, straining and breath holding.
3. Inadequate respiratory activity from depressing and paralysing drugs.
4. Anoxia and carbon dioxide accumulation.
5. Incorrect posture.
6. Increased respiratory resistance from anæsthetic apparatus.
7. The use of toxic explosive drugs, or those that raise intracranial pressure.
8. Delay in replacing blood loss.
9. Deep anæsthesia with delayed recovery of consciousness post-operatively.

GENERAL ANÆSTHESIA

Until recently the importance of maintaining spontaneous respiration during neurosurgical operations has been stressed[1], as it provides an indication of the integrity of the patient's vital functions.[2] In some units it is now the practice to use complete curarization and controlled respiration in an effort to reduce the bulk of the brain.[3-6] These techniques will be considered separately.

Spontaneous Respiration

Premedication. The basic principles of premedication in these cases have not changed and heavy sedation is avoided in the following:[1]

(a) All patients with a raised intracranial pressure.
(b) Head injuries.
(c) Patients to be operated upon in the prone, sitting or steep reverse Trendelenburg position.

These patients are given atropine or scopolamine (hyoscine) alone. Other cases receive either papaveretum or pethidine and scopolamine.

The phenothiazine derivatives are used if hypothermia is to be induced, but for routine use tachycardia, postural hypotension and prolonged post-operative drowsiness have proved a disadvantage. Hunter[7] in a preliminary trial has found the combination of pecazine (Pacatal) with phenobarbitone encouraging. When pre-operative sedation is not contraindicated in young children, then trime-prazine tartrate[8, 9] (Vallergan) may be used in the form of the syrup (Vallergan Forte) 2 hours before operation in a dosage of 1·5 mg per lb.[10] This drug has anti-emetic and anti-histamine properties but children are easily awakened post operatively after its use.

Patients undergoing hypophysectomy[11] require special preparation as follows: 200 mg cortisone acetate is given daily by intramuscular injection for 2 days before operation and continued for 5 days after. On the 6th and 7th days the dose is reduced to 150 mg intramuscularly once a day, or 50 mg by mouth 8-hourly. On the 8th and 9th days 100 mg is given intramuscularly each day, or 50 mg by mouth 12-hourly. Subsequent maintenance is then reduced to 25 mg by mouth daily. If bilateral adrenalectomy has already been performed then in addition an intravenous drip of dextrose saline with 100 mg hydrocortisone hemisuccinate is required during the operation and possibly afterwards.

Occasionally if the intracranial pressure is very high pre-operatively, a ventricular drain may be inserted before the patient reaches the anæsthetic room, or dehydration therapy with 50% sucrose or 30% urea started intravenously before induction of anæsthesia.

Induction. If the intracranial pressure is known to be high the head end of the trolley is raised before induction. The minimum dose of $2\frac{1}{2}\%$ thiopentone is used for induction unless the patient is already unconscious, when either no anæsthetic is required, or nitrous-oxide and oxygen may be used from the start followed by trichlorethylene or halothane, and suxamethonium for intubation. In the case of head injuries the danger of aspiration of blood and C.S.F. from the mouth and pharynx, or of regurgitated stomach contents, must be remembered and the necessary precautions taken.

Normally, following thiopentone, 25–40 mg of suxamethonium is injected and the lungs inflated with oxygen prior to spraying the trachea with 5 ml of 4% lignocaine hydrochloride (Xylocaine). Some[2] prefer to use 75–100 mg of suxamethonium to allow a longer period of reflex suppression so that the topical analgesia will be more effective and the presence of the tube less likely to cause straining and a consequent rise in cerebral venous pressure. For the same reason, others[12] use d-tubocurarine chloride or gallamine triethiodide (Flaxedil) for intubation, so that when the respiration becomes adequate anæsthesia is already stabilized.

The advantage of suxamethonium is that it gives such complete relaxation that the trachea can be thoroughly sprayed with analgesic solution and the largest endotracheal tube passed without trauma. The disadvantages are:

(i)   The period of apnœa and possible rise in arterial and venous pressure.

  (ii) The possibility of prolonged apnœa.

  (iii) The muscle fasiculations and possible rise in intracranial pressure acompanying these.

  (iv) Post operative muscle pains.[13, 14]

  (v) The possibility of straining when the drug wears off.

Intubation. The introduction of flexometallic oral endotracheal tubes is a great advance, particularly in neurosurgical anæsthesia. In

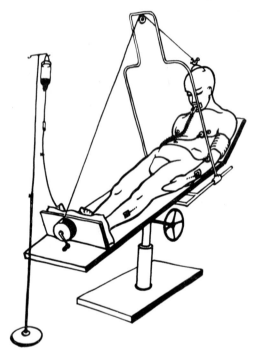

Fig. 16. Posterior fossa exploration.

many cases the head has to be flexed (Fig. 16) and may be rotated as well. The airway is of fundamental importance in this branch of anæsthesia and is almost inaccessible once the operation is in progress. In the past, using rubber or portex tubes, the maintenance of a perfect airway was a nightmare for the neurosurgical anæsthetist.[15] The largest size tube that can be passed easily should be used, and it has been found that the tubes with the wire spirals are superior to the nylon reinforced variety. The tubes are lubricated with lignocaine ointment and are examined carefully to see that the spirals have not become bent, the layers of latex separated or bubbles formed.[16] It is an advantage to use tubes with the bevels removed[1] (Fig. 17) and with a modified suction union so that the catheter mount and cork will fit either limb. When the head is fully flexed (Fig 16.) the anæsthetic tubing can then be attached to lie conveniently on the chest. Rendell-Baker[17] uses a straight endotracheal connector for use in cerebral angiography and posterior fossa operations.

Cuffed flexometallic tubes and pharyngeal packs are used when

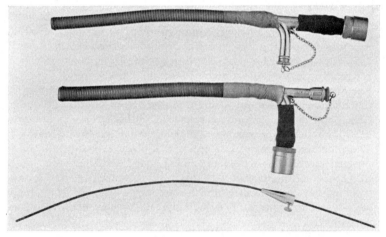

Fig. 17. Flexometallic endotracheal tubes with bevels removed. Short catheter mounts attached to different limbs of modified suction unions. (Medical and Industrial Equipment Ltd.). Talley copper wire introducer (Talley Anæsthetic Equipment Ltd.).

there is the possibility of regurgitation of stomach contents as in head injuries or the prone position, and when the air sinuses may be opened or controlled respiration used.

Maintenance. Once spontaneous respiration has returned anæsthesia is maintained with nitrous oxide 6 litres per minute and oxygen 2 litres per minute and minimal trichlorethylene or halothane using a semi-closed circuit and Magill re-breathing attachment with the valve fully open.

Since its introduction trichlorethylene has been used during neurosurgical anæsthesia in concentrations of 0.5% or less, with success. The great advantage of this drug is that it will provide hours of quiet, light, non-explosive anæsthesia without respiratory depression, or hypotension. If it is turned off before the end of the operation the patient will recover consciousness quickly and quietly with little laryngeal spasm or coughing. Its disadvantages are well known. It tends to cause ventricular ectopic beats[1] and tachypnœa, particularly in children, and may not settle the difficult, plethoric type of patient. There is still a place for trichlorethylene in neurosurgery, although halothane is now an alternative inhalation agent.

Halothane was studied pharmacologically by Raventós[18] and has been used clinically since 1956,[19-26] and its use in neurosurgical anæsthesia has been described.[27-31] It is advisable to use halothane with the Fluotec (Cyprane) vaporizer in a semi-closed circuit in the same way as trichlorethylene. Although this is an expensive method, it is safer than using this powerful drug in a closed circuit, particularly as little muscular relaxation is required during neurosurgery. It is equally safe but less expensive to use the Fluotec with a total flow rate of 4 litres per minute with either a circle or to-and-fro absorber in the semi-closed circuit. Atropine is used before halothane for it has been pointed out that in conventional dosage hyoscine has little blocking action on the cardiac vagus and is not a suitable alternative.[32] The potential hazard of combining halothane with subcutaneously injected adrenaline has been mentioned,[27] and while there is no doubt that E.C.G. changes occur with this drug[1] it seems likely that it is the combination of adrenaline and factors which increase sympathetic activity, such as respiratory depression with hypercarbia, which must be avoided.[33]

Initially, 1·5% halothane by volume may be required to stabilize anæsthesia, but thereafter 0·5% to 1·0% is sufficient to maintain smooth anæsthesia. After opiate premedication, shallow respiration with the danger of hypercarbia may develop, but after the light premedication customary in neurosurgical patients, this is unusual. Tachypnœa does occur but is less common than with trichlorethylene and is equally well controlled with doses of 10–20 mg of pethidine.

Hypotension is the main danger with halothane, and appears to be due mainly to the peripheral dilatation of blood vessels.[34] Provided the blood pressure is recorded continuously and not allowed to fall below 80 mm of mercury this danger may be turned to advantage in neurosurgical work where some degree of hypotension is desirable. If the blood pressure does not fall then oozing may be increased by the peripheral vasodilatation. When severe hæmorrhage is expected then halothane is combined with ganglion blocking agents to achieve controlled hypotension.[1, 34] If the operation necessitates a steep reverse Trendelenburg position (Fig. 16) it is safer to use trichlorethylene and avoid postural hypotension.

At the conclusion of light halothane anæsthesia patients wake up quickly but during the recovery of consciousness may exhibit muscle tremors, laryngeal spasm and coughing which spoil an otherwise smooth anæsthetic.

It is in anæsthesia for infants and children that halothane is seen at its best and represents a real advance. Nitrous oxide, oxygen and

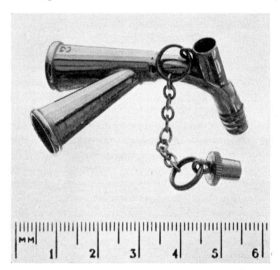

Fig. 18. Pædiatric suction union for use with T-piece.
(Ballantine, R. I. W. (1961). *Anæsthesia*, **16**, 502.)

halothane may be used for induction, with relaxation of the masseters and good intubating conditions following quite quickly. Halothane is then continued for the maintenance of anæsthesia with a semi-closed circuit or Ayre's T-piece,[35] depending on the size of the child. Alternatively induction may be with ethylchloride and open ether, or nitrous oxide, oxygen and ether. In older children, halothane may be used as in adults, following intubation with thiopentone and suxamethonium.

When using the T-piece circuit the suction union[36] illustrated (Fig. 18) will be found useful as the inspiratory and expiratory tubing lie in the horizontal plane and do not interfere with the drapes.

It is important to have an under-water or similar safety valve on the inflow side of the T-piece circuit so that any obstruction to the expiratory side developing under the drapes will become obvious at once,[1] and also to have some means of inflating the lungs should this become necessary.

Trichlorethylene or halothane used as described will provide satisfactory anæsthesia for almost every neurosurgical operation or investigation, but there are anæsthetists who, while favouring spontaneous respiration, prefer to avoid the use of these halogenated drugs. This is probably because of their well known vasodilator properties and cardiovascular effects. The maintenance of anæsthesia will then depend on the use of intravenous narcotic or analgesic drugs to supplement nitrous-oxide anæsthesia. Pethidine has proved useful in this respect,[2, 37] in spite of its respiratory depressant properties, having an analgesic and anti-cholinergic effect and providing some sedation in the post-operative period. It has been suggested that a total dose of 125 mg in the unsedated patient should not be exceeded in a major craniotomy, 50–70% of this dose being given during the first part of the operation which involves raising the bone flap.

The main advantage of spontaneous respiration is that its changing pattern can be related to altered physiological and surgical effects within the brain and give warning of potential danger that may be avoided. In addition it should be possible with the simple methods described, to ensure that the patient ventilates himself satisfactorily without undue resistance from apparatus and thus maintains a fully active thoracic pump action. The disadvantage of general anæsthesia with spontaneous respiration is that it does not lower intracranial pressure or reduce brain bulk, by itself.

Controlled Respiration

Method. The use of pethidine 50-100 mg for premedication combined with atropine or scopolamine (hyoscine) is permissible if the respiration is to be controlled, provided that neither the patient's level of consciousness nor respiration is depressed before operation. Induction is with $2\frac{1}{2}\%$ thiopentone followed in the adult by 20–30 mg of d-tubocurarine chloride. The lungs are inflated, the trachea sprayed with 4% lignocaine hydrochloride and a cuffed oral flexometallic tube passed. Maintenance of anæsthesia is with nitrous-oxide and 30% oxygen, with small doses of pethidine or pethilorfan as required. Full curarization is continued and positive-negative phase ventilation is carried out with a pulmo-flator which will provide a negative pressure of 5 cm of water. The use of a pharyngeal pack to provide an air tight fit is preferred to a cuffed tube by some anæsthetists[6] as being less traumatic in long operations, others taking the precaution of using both. It is important to ensure that spontaneous respiration does not suddenly return and give rise to bucking and straining. To avoid this it may be necessary to give d-tubocurarine at the rate of approximately 10 mg per half-hour. Alternatively the respiration may be taken over by hand from time to time to assess the degree of curarization.

The advantages of controlled respiration are that[1]:

  (i) Intracranial tension is low.
 (ii) Recovery from anæsthesia is immediate.
(iii) Post-operative brain swelling is reduced.
 (iv) Volatile anæsthetic agents are avoided.
  (v) Blood loss is reduced, although the blood pressure may not be low.
 (vi) Adequate oxygenation and carbon dioxide elimination are maintained even in the presence of central respiratory depression.
(vii) The effects of the face down position are minimized.
(viii) Post-operative vomiting is less.
 (ix) The possibility of straining during anæsthesia is reduced, provided curarization is maintained.

The reasons given for the lowered intracranial pressure and reduced brain bulk vary. There are those who use positive pressure alone, and believe that hyperventilation and consequent lowering of CO_2 tension, with increase in cerebral arteriolar tone and resistance reduce tissue fluid formation. They consider that the vasoconstriction resulting from hypocapnia more than counterbalances the possible obstacle to the venous flow.[38] Against this it has been shown that positive atmospheric pressure inflation will produce a rise in pressure in the fourth ventricle.[39] The intrathoracic pressure in paralysed patients receiving intermittent positive pressure respiration from respiratory pumps has been shown to be raised.[40-42] and the return of blood from the peripheral veins into the chest thus obstructed.

Hunter[43] believes that the lowered intracranial pressure during controlled respiration is related primarily to the administration of the relaxant and thus to the abolition of straining which might raise the intracranial venous pressure.

If a negative pressure of 5–10 cm of H_2O is applied to the trachea between inspirations the mean intrathoracic pressure can be reduced almost to that in the normal subject breathing spontaneously.[41] Most anæsthetists are agreed that if controlled respiration is to be used in neurosurgery then better conditions are obtained by the use of a negative phase and that this is due to:[44]

(i) The greater tidal volume and more efficient over-ventilation achieved.

(ii) The reduction in venous pressure which can sometimes be produced.

Marshall[44] warns that in the patient with chronic bronchitis and emphysema the high and prolonged pressure needed to inflate the lungs may raise the venous pressure and cause intracranial engorgement. In patients with large tumours and very high intracranial pressure also, vigorous overventilation may produce little effect.

The majority of anæsthetists who favour controlled respiration do not use the method for posterior fossa operations. In the sitting position (Fig. 16) operation conditions are usually good and it is in these cases particularly that respiratory changes may give information of value to the surgeon working close to the vital centres.

While the use of controlled respiration in neurosurgery remains a controversial subject and while most anæsthetists would agree that it should not be used indiscriminately there is no doubt that it can be of great help, particularly when used in combination with other methods. It has been suggested that it is primarily indicated in patients showing even slight respiratory depression and those in whom the vascular component of encephalic tension predominates.[38]

Whatever technique is used the recording of blood pressure, pulse rate and when possible the E.C.G. should be a routine. Aids to the monitoring of the patient's vital functions are available in the form of pulsometers, respirometers and spirometers.

On occasion electroencephalography is of value for determining the depth of anæsthesia; as an aid in the assessment of the condition of a limited area of cortex during the surgery of aneurysms, and in the tracing of epileptic foci.[1]

An intravenous drip is set up in every major case using a disposable plastic giving set, and the value of accurate estimation and replacement of blood loss in the neurosurgical case has become recognised in recent years.

METHODS OF LOWERING INTRACRANIAL PRESSURE

In addition to the use of controlled respiration there are other methods available for lowering the intracranial pressure:

(i) Ventricular drainage.

(ii) Spinal drainage.

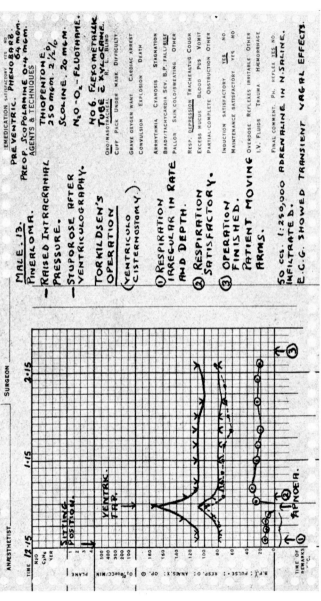

Fig. 19. Anæsthetic chart showing the respiratory and cardiovascular effects of a rising intracranial pressure and the immediate value of ventricular tap.

(iii) Dehydration therapy.
(iv) Hypothermia.
(v) Controlled hypotension.
(vi) Posture.

Ventricular Drainage

This is the most direct and effective method but can only be done rapidly if burr holes are present or a bone flap raised. In most cases requiring craniotomy ventriculography burr holes have already been made. The ventricles can be tapped rapidly if, for example, a rising pulse rate or respiratory failure should follow induction of anæsthesia (Fig. 19).

Spinal Drainage

This has been used during hypophysectomy[45] and in other types of intracranial surgery when it seemed appropriate, but is now rarely employed.

Dehydration Therapy

For many years hypertonic infusions have been used in the treatment of cerebral œdema and raised intracranial pressure. These solutions act by raising the crystalloid osmotic pressure of the plasma and thus removing water from the interstitial fluid and tissues.

Sucrose. Until recently 100 ml of 50% sucrose injected intravenously has been the solution of choice.

Urea. In 1958 Javid[46] recommended the use of urea, and this has become regarded as more effective than any other solution in the reduction of intracranial pressure.[47]

A 30% solution of urea made up in invert sugar solution or 5–10% dextrose is given by intravenous injection in a dosage of 1·0–1·5 G urea per kg of body weight. The infusion is begun either before or immediately after induction of anæsthesia and run at a rate of about 60 drops per minute, or more quickly if a greater effect is required for a shorter time. The maximum effect is said to occur within 1 to 2 hours and to persist for from 3 to 10 hours.

Urea reduces brain bulk quite dramatically and therefore makes the surgical approach much easier and less traumatic. The dura may be quite slack even in cases of expanding lesions within the brain,[47] and the post-operative condition of the patients noticeably improved. The solution may also be useful outside the operating theatre in lightening coma due to cerebral œdema both pre- and post-operatively. The use of urea in the management of head injuries has also

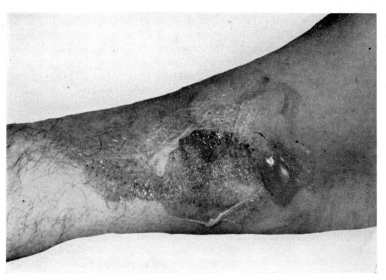

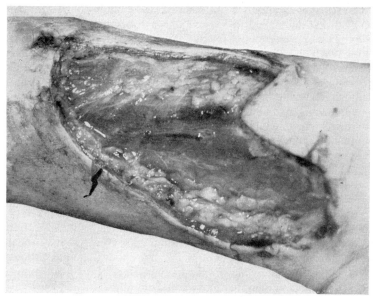

Fɪɢ. 20. Tissue necrosis following extravenous leakage of urea.
(Small, J. M. (1960). *Lancet*, **1,** 1252.)

Above: One day after operation. Commencing necrosis.
Below: One month after operation. Resulting ulcer.

been described.[48] In these cases it may be of value as an aid to decompressive procedures and where generalized cerebral œdema exists. It is definitely contraindicated in head injuries when there is intracranial bleeding or the suspicion of an intracranial clot, as it may mask the true picture by improving the patient's condition and giving a false sense of security. In these circumstances it has been stressed[48] that the preliminary exploration for bleeding should be made before using urea.

When used during craniotomy bleeding may be increased during the early stages. This is partly venous as the dura falls away from the skull when this is opened, and partly a generalized arterial ooze probably resulting from an increased blood volume and raised blood pressure.

Very great care is required with the practical details of urea administration. A few ml of the solution injected into the tissues will produce superficial blister formation, and a larger amount of solution leaking extravenously has resulted in serious tissue necrosis[48, 49] (Fig. 20). The irritant nature of the solution is such that thrombosis may occur. It has been suggested[48] that if a cut-down is necessary then a polythene catheter should be passed well up the vein, so that there is not too high a concentration of solution at one point. This applies also in patients with a poor peripheral circulation. Normally it is best to use a simple intravenous needle and cannula, to make absolutely certain it is in the vein, and then to raise the limb slightly on a pillow. It is quite common for the vein to become swollen and hard beyond the needle point, but this resolves without complications.

If urea is required in the post-operative period and gastric feeding has been established then it can be given and is effective by mouth in a dose of 12 G in 100 ml of water with orange or milk added, three times a day.

A urethral catheter should be passed at the start of the urea infusion and released regularly to avoid bladder distension. The blood urea should be estimated, and intravenous urea withheld if there is impaired renal function. It is possible that the increased circulating fluid volume resulting from urea infusion might overload the patient with a diminished cardiac reserve.[48] Urea increases the urinary excretion of sodium and chlorides, and to a lesser extent potassium. These findings are relevant to neurosurgical operations and particularly hypophysectomy.[50]

It has been suggested that a barrier to the entry of urea into the brain exists, that urea therefore passes into the brain more slowly than into other tissue and thus a concentration difference between plasma and brain urea is maintained and water withdrawn from the brain tissue.[47, 48] Others[44] believe that if the blood is made hypertonic then the blood supply to the brain is such that an apparently selective action on brain tissue would be expected without any blood-brain barrier being necessary.

There is no doubt that the use of urea in appropriate conditions and combined with controlled respiration or other methods of lowering intracranial pressure represents an advance in neurosurgical practice.

Plasma. Hypertonic plasma was introduced in 1938[51] to produce a sustained fall of intracranial pressure. More recently triple plasma has been recommended[52] in severe head injuries:

(*a*) To prevent cerebral œdema.
(*b*) To treat surgical shock.
(*c*) To reverse coning.

The solution is made up by mixing the dried plasma of 3 pints of blood with 400 ml of sterile water. The use of sucrose, urea, 10% dextran and plasma has been described to combat the cerebral œdema that follows acute hypoxia.[53, 54]

Magnesium Sulphate. The rectal use of 50% magnesium sulphate is still of value for gradual and prolonged decompression. The procedure may be repeated twice daily and the maximum effect is evident after three or four days.[1] In patients with signs of cerebral irritation a solution with a sedative action, such as magnesium sulphate has been suggested as the natural choice.[44]

Fluid Intake. In addition to the active dehydration methods mentioned the fluid intake is restricted before and after operation in cases of raised intracranial pressure.

Hypothermia

In 1950 McQuiston[55] introduced the idea of lowering the body temperature during anæsthesia for cardiac surgery, and in 1953[56] this was applied to neurosurgical cases as well. Since then there have been many reports of the value of hypothermia in neurosurgery.

Hypothermia lowers the metabolism of the brain so that its oxygen requirements are temporarily diminished and it is better able to tolerate a reduced circulation. Rosomoff and Gilbert[57] observed a reduced brain volume when experimenting with hypothermia in dogs and gave the following figures:[58]

(*a*) Cerebral blood flow decreased at a rate of 6·7% per degree centigrade.

(b) At 25° C metabolism and blood flow were one-third of the pre-cooling level.

(c) Reduction in the brain volume of 4·1 % at 25° C which in man would amount to a change of 55 ml.

(d) The C.S.F. pressure decreased at a rate of 5·5 % per degree centigrade.

There is no doubt that there is some reduction of brain bulk during hypothermia which will be of help in a certain proportion of neurosurgical procedures, but hypothermia is used primarily when it is known that the blood supply to part of the brain is to be temporarily cut off or reduced. The length of time and degree of protection afforded at 30° C (86° F) by temporary occlusion of, say, the middle cerebral artery are indefinite. Clamps have been applied for up to 15 minutes without ill effects.[59, 60] Rarely, the same artery has been permanently occluded at normal temperatures without damage. In practice the circulation to the brain is reduced as little as possible and for as short a time as possible.[39] Hypothermia will give some protection from the effects of vascular spasm that accompany rupture of an aneurysm or surgical approach to it, although not reducing the degree of spasm.

Hypothermia affords a greater margin of safety when hypotensive drugs are used, and some believe that hypothermia should always accompany the use of controlled hypotension.[60, 61]

In addition to its effects on metabolism, brain bulk and C.S.F. pressure, hypothermia will reduce cerebral œdema, and is therefore of value when this complicates the neurosurgical case. Following brain injury in hypothermic animals it has been found that there is a reduction in the extent of the inflammatory reaction, and a more rapid repairative response.[62] Hypothermia has been used in head injuries[52, 63, 64] and as a therapeutic measure in massive cerebral hæmorrhage[1, 29, 65] in an effort to protect the brain from the ischæmic pressure effects of cerebral œdema and to reduce cerebral volume.

Indications. The extent to which hypothermia is employed varies considerably in individual units. It would seem to have two definite indications during operation:[1]

(a) Aneurysms. Middle cerebral artery: anterior communicating artery.

(b) Large angiomata and meningiomata. (When severe hæmorrhage is expected).

There are other more controversial, but possible indications—

(c) Cases in which such great difficulty is expected that every possible aid must be used.[44]

(d) When hypotension is to be induced.

(e) Operations in the region of the mid-brain or hypothalamus.[66]

(f) Pyrexias of brain stem origin, when the temperature may either be lowered to normal or below.

(g) Massive cerebral hæmorrhage.

(h) Head injuries.

(i) Following acute hypoxia.

Technique. Many methods have been described and no doubt have their particular advantages. The following technique is similar to that introduced by the Liverpool neurosurgical team[60] and has proved simple and effective.[1]

Premedication is with chlorpromazine, promethazine and pethidine, up to 50 mg of each by deep intramuscular injection 2 hours before anæsthesia. The dosage is regulated by the size and general condition of the patient. Atropine is added when halothane is to be used.

Anæsthesia is induced with thiopentone suxamethonium and halothane in the usual way and once the patient is cooled maintenance is with nitrous oxide and oxygen alone. Oesophageal, nasopharyngeal and rectal thermometers are inserted, and E.C.G. and sphygmomanometer leads applied. An intravenous drip is set up.

The patient is lifted on to a second trolley and placed on ice bags already in position. The rest of the body is covered with ice bags and a fan turned on. Every few minutes the position of the bags is changed and the underlying tissues kneaded and massaged. Any evidence of shivering is an indication for chlorpromazine 10 mg intravenously. The E.C.G. is watched continuously and someone is always ready to perform cardiac massage if ventricular fibrillation should develop.

When the temperature has fallen to 33° C (91·4° F) the patient is removed from the ice, dried and placed on a special blanket on the operating table through which warm or cold water can be circulated Sorbo pads are placed under the scapulæ, buttocks and heels. The average time taken to reach 33° C (91·4 F) using this method has been 45 minutes.

The optimum temperature for neurosurgical work is 30° C (86° F) and the after drop usually brings the temperature to this level during the first part of the operation. Some degree of temperature control is afforded by circulating cold or warm water at not more than 42° C (107·6° F) through the blanket (Fig. 21.)

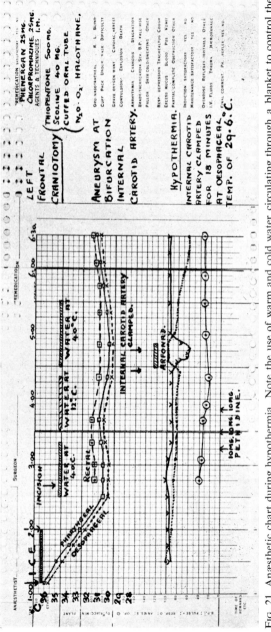

Fig. 21. Anæsthetic chart during hypothermia. Note the use of warm and cold water circulating through a blanket to control the final temperature.

At 30° C (86° F) the pulse rate is usually slow and the blood pressure variable. It is suggested that attempts should not be made to increase the pulse rate.[62] During hypothermia the ejection and relaxation phases of the ventricle are prolonged, and provided the pulse remains slow ventricular filling and coronary flow are satisfactory. If they are shortened by increasing the pulse rate ventricular failure and fibrillation may follow.

If hypotension is required for a short period to facilitate the surgery, then trimetaphan (Arfonad) is used (Fig. 21).

Care is taken to replace blood as it is lost as patients compensate poorly during hypothermia.[59] At the same time it must be remembered that the transfusion of stored bank blood is not without danger

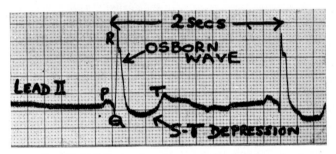

Fig. 22. E.C.G. showing changes during hypothermia.

because of its acidotic properties and potassium content. The slow transfusion of freshly collected blood, and the avoidance of large deficits requiring rapid replacement, is the ideal.[62] Similarly if ventricular fibrillation should occur during hypothermia the high potassium content and effect on pH of old-bank blood may be disastrous. It is doubtful whether calcium ion, which is normally recommended in rapid transfusion of the normothermic patient, should be used during hypothermia, as it may precipitate ventricular fibrillation. Bleeding, from prolongation of the clotting time, has not been a problem in these patients.

The E.C.G. changes associated with hypothermia are shown in Fig. 22.

After operation the patients are returned to bed and covered with blankets in the usual way, a rectal thermometer being left in position. No active measures are taken to rewarm the patient. Sometimes if cerebral œdema is anticipated in the post-operative period or there is pyrexia from disturbance of the heat-regulating centre then hypothermia is continued.

Ventricular fibrillation. While this is unlikely to occur at temperatures above 28° C (82·4° F) in patients with normal hearts, it is the most serious complication of hypothermia, and the E.C.G. must be watched constantly. The use of hyperventilation to reduce the tendency to ventricular fibrillation has been advocated.[67, 68] Others[1, 69] have had no case of ventricular fibrillation in several hundreds of neurosurgical cases using hypothermia and spontaneous respiration, and it seems likely as Gray suspects[69] that it is the avoidance of sudden changes in pH that is important.

Boba[62] goes further and argues that if carbon dioxide is removed by mechanical ventilation then compensation is brought about by the production and retention of fixed acids, or the dumping of fixed bases and a reduction in the size of the available buffer base. This is a dangerous state of affairs as the metabolic acidosis of hypothermia and particularly of shivering and rewarming is poorly tolerated. He believes that the blood pH and CO_2 combining power should be estimated regularly, and that the problem of acid-base balance in hypothermia is essentially one of detecting and preventing acidosis, and conserving an adequate buffer reserve.

Nevertheless as the advantages of controlled respiration in neurosurgery become more widely recognized, there is little doubt that this will be used during the induction and maintenance of hypothermia as in thoracic surgery.

Differential Brain Cooling. Experimental attempts have been made to cool the brain without cooling the rest of the body.[59, 70, 71] Kristiansen[72] has used selective brain cooling in man with promising results. Blood from the common carotid artery is diverted along a cannula by means of a roller pump through a cooling coil, a filter and a bubble trap and thence to the internal carotid artery via a second cannula. The apparatus is primed with 300 ml of heparinized blood and shortly before starting the extracorporeal circulation, heparin and trimetaphan (Arfonad) are given intravenously. Trimetaphan is used to combat the initial increase in cerebral vascular resistance. The brain temperature has been lowered to the region of 20° C (68° F) while the rectal temperature has only fallen to about 35° C (95° F).

This work is still in the trial stage and the hazards are mainly connected with cannulation of the carotid artery.

Controlled Hypotension

For a number of years controlled hypotension using the ganglion blocking agents was used frequently in neurosurgical practice.[73–80]

Recently the greater use of controlled respiration, dehydration therapy with urea, and hypothermia, have reduced the indications for this more dangerous technique.[38] In fact some regard its use as unnecessary.[4, 5] However, used with discretion and in combination with other methods of reducing intracranial tension and bleeding, controlled hypotension still has a limited use in neurosurgical anæsthesia. It is indicated primarily when the possibility of severe hæmorrhage exists,[1] as in:

(a) Vascular abnormalities—aneurysms; angiomata.
(b) Meningiomata.

In these cases it may be combined with hypothermia.

Hypotensive anæsthesia is contraindicated if there is definite evidence of renal, hepatic or cardiac disease. It is foolhardy and unnecessary to use the method for operations in the sitting or steeply reversed Trendelenburg position. The same applies in the prone position with a foot-down tilt, as the blood pressure tends to be low in this position without ganglion blockade.

Controlled hypotension is not required for hypophysectomy and would be dangerous in those patients who have already had an adrenalectomy.

Brown[81] considers the use of induced hypotension to be unsafe in patients with a high supratentorial pressure and transtentorial displacement. The mid brain arteries are already stretched and partially occluded and a fall in arterial pressure might lead to fatal ischæmic brain stem damage. Its use in this type of case no longer seems indicated.

Technique. The drug of choice is trimetaphan camphorosulphonate (Arfonad), for with this short acting drug used in dilute solution delicate control of the blood pressure is possible. With the longer acting methonium and pendiomide there is a greater danger of initial overdosage.[1] The homatropinium derivative trophenium[82] is similar in action but liable to cause very high pulse rates.

A certain number of patients are resistant to the ganglion blocking agents. In a series combining trimetaphan with trichlorethylene the resistance rate was found to be 17%.[1] When the same drugs were combined with hypothermia this resistance increased. Since the introduction of halothane the position has changed considerably, and when this anæsthetic agent is used with the ganglion blocking drugs, the blood pressure can almost always be lowered easily. Enderby[83] suggests that this is due to the peripheral dilatation of blood vessels caused by halothane, combined with the ganglion blocking action of the hypotensive drug. He stresses that with this combination undue hypotension is less easily reversed as it must await excretion of the halothane by the lungs, and that the vasopressor drugs are less effective in the presence of halothane.

Anæsthesia is induced in the usual way and maintained with nitrous oxide, oxygen and halothane, 0·5–1%. The head end of the table is raised 5–10°, and blood pressure, pulse and respiration rate are recorded and E.C.G. tracings obtained. The hypotensive drug is not used throughout the operation but reserved for the vital stages. When required, trimetaphan is either given as a drip using a 0·2% solution in normal saline (1 G in 500 ml) or by electrically-driven syringe with a 1·25% solution (250 mg in 20 ml). An initial rate of 1 mg per minute is used while continuous blood pressure readings are taken. The systolic pressure is never allowed to fall below 60 mm of mercury unless the patient is hypothermic and then only for short vital periods of the operation. Generally a systolic pressure of 80 mm of mercury or higher is preferred, provided this is accompanied by good operating conditions. Marshall[44] considers that to lower the blood pressure to 100–120 mm of mercury is sufficient when this is combined with the other procedures already discussed. Great care is required when inducing hypotension in the hypertensive patient as the initial fall in pressure may be precipitous[1] (Fig. 23).

Severe bleeding may sometimes occur in spite of the use of a hypotensive technique and in these circumstances blood loss must be replaced very rapidly.

If trichlorethylene is used instead of halothane then the initial rate of administration required will be as high as 8 mg per minute in an effort to avoid resistance developing.[1] Whatever anæsthetic agent is chosen, the maximum dose of trimetaphan should not exceed 1G.

If controlled respiration with nitrous oxide and oxygen is combined with trimetaphan, it may be found necessary to add 0·5% halothane to the anæsthetic mixture from a vaporizer outside the circuit in order to achieve satisfactory hypotension.

The pulse rate usually rises as the ganglion blocking drug is given. This may persist, and if this is accompanied by resistance to hypotension, then the use of procaine amide has been suggested.[84] This occasionally proved useful in resistant cases, when trichlorethylene was the anæsthetic agent, but with the present use of halothane procaine amide should not be required.

The ease with which halothane and the ganglion blocking drugs combine to lower the blood pressure underline the potential danger of this combination, and the care that must be taken during their use.

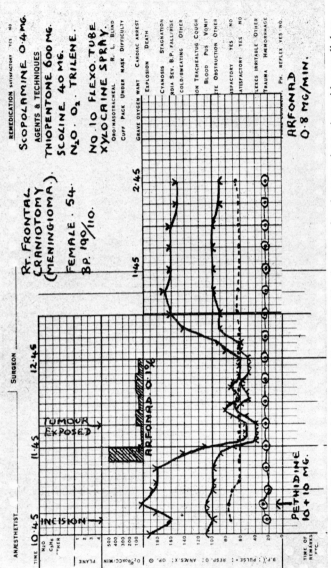

FIG. 23. Anæsthetic chart showing precipitous fall in blood pressure in a hypertensive patient with a small dose of trimetaphan.

Using 0·5% halothane with a slight head-up tilt the blood pressure may already be low and no further hypotension be required.

Posture

The position of the patient on the operating table is always of importance, and this is particularly so in the neurosurgical case where faulty position may raise the intracranial and venous pressure. Anæsthetists are aware of this and are always trying to play their part in improving operating conditions as affected by posture.

The prone position used for exploration of the spinal cord is some-

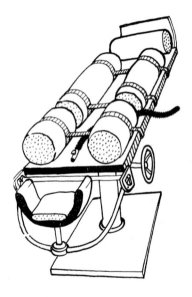

Fig. 24. Bolsters and head rest in position for the prone position.

times poorly tolerated, and if the abdomen is compressed may result in inferior vena caval obstruction and distension of the epidural veins.[85] At the same time, the tidal volume may be reduced in this position. Fig 24 shows one method of arranging bolsters along the side of the operating table which leaves the chest and abdomen free from compression. The use of controlled respiration to ensure adequate ventilation would seem to be an advantage in this position.

The use of the sitting position for exploration of the posterior fossa is now well established. The arrangement shown in Fig. 16 is convenient, as access to the posterior fossa is excellent with full head flexion. In addition the tilt of the table can be reversed without the degree of head flexion being changed. This is of value when it is desired to raise the blood pressure, either to complete hæmostasis or for resuscitation.

The patient is also sat up and may be under general anæsthesia during pneumoencephalography[86] and is in a steep reverse Trendelenburg position during section of the Vth sensory root. Anæsthetists are alert to the possibility of air embolism in these positions[1] and use a precordial or œsophageal stethoscope in case a "mill wheel" murmur gives confirmation of this complication. Whenever possible an E.C.G. apparatus is also attached. During the early stages of posterior fossa exploration regular jugular compression is applied to raise the venous pressure, and if air embolism should occur the patient is immediately turned into the left lateral head down position and the lungs vigorously inflated with oxygen. A successful outcome partly depends on the speed in recognizing and treating the complication. It should not be regarded as necessarily fatal.[1]

Head Injuries

The role of respiratory insufficiency in the mortality of severe head injuries has been discussed by Maciver and others,[52, 87, 88] and it is well established that the first line of attack in any head injury is the establishment and maintenance of a perfect airway. Anæsthetists are now playing their part in the treatment of these cases, and should be members of the team that looks after them from the roadside to the post-operative ward.

Respiratory obstruction is likely to be complicated in the head injury by respiratory depression from brain stem damage, or raised intracranial pressure. There may be associated facio-maxillary injury and the danger of aspiration of blood, C.S.F. and stomach contents. There may be simultaneous injury to the chest or pre-existing chest disease. Whatever the cause, respiratory insufficiency leads to anoxia, carbon dioxide accumulation and a rise in intracranial venous and cerebro-spinal fluid pressure, and a vicious circle of respiratory inadequacy and rising intracranial pressure is established.

Immediate treatment at the time of the accident should consist of the passage of a stomach tube[89] and if necessary the use of a cuffed endotracheal tube to maintain a clear airway, sealing off the respiratory tract.

Lewin[90] has stressed that the airway must be kept clear for 24 hours a day and that this may be possible with good nursing alone, and will be combined with the use of posture, physiotherapy, antibiotics, the control of electrolyte balance, and care of spastic limbs. If coma persists, or if there are associated injuries of the jaw or chest, and if there is pre-existing chest disease then tracheostomy may be indicated.

The value of tracheostomy in a wide variety of respiratory conditions has become recognized in recent years, not least in neurosurgical practice. It is used not only in persistent coma, but also combined with artificial ventilation in the presence of respiratory inadequacy, and following operation if there are excessive secretions or respiratory difficulty from other causes.

The benefit of tracheostomy is that not only does it relieve upper respiratory tract obstruction but also reduces the dead space and carbon dioxide retention, decreases the resistance to respiration, facilitates the removal of tracheo-bronchial secretions and results in an improved venous return and cardiac output.[1]

In addition to early tracheostomy and the essentials of good nursing Maciver[52] recommends the use of phenothiazine drugs combined with hypothermia to control rigidity and hyperthermia, and intravenous hypertonic plasma for cerebral œdema. The use of urea[48] has already been mentioned.

Radiological Investigations

Recent advances in this field have been radiological, and include improvements in contrast media, X-ray apparatus and operative technique.

The choice between local and general anæsthesia remains a controversial one for certain investigations. In some units local analgesia is used almost entirely, unless the patient is too young or too frightened to be coöperative. Others believe that general anæsthesia should be used for cerebral angiography and pneumoencephalography.

Cerebral Angiography. Often patients for this investigation have had a recent intracranial hæmorrhage and are gravely ill and suffering from the effects of either direct cerebral damage or vascular spasm and cerebral œdema.[1]

Those who favour local analgesia believe that there is less risk involved and that better pictures are obtained with the patient conscious. If during the investigation the patient's neurological or general state deteriorates, he can be returned to the ward. Using 60% Urografin subjective symptoms of flushing, heat and retro-bulbar pain are less than with other media, contrast is better, and less of the dye crosses the blood-brain barrier causing cerebral complications.

Others prefer general anæsthesia,[91] not only because it reduces emotional stress, but also because it will produce some vasodilatation which will be of value in certain intracranial vascular lesions.

The details of anæsthesia do not differ from those already described but in all neurological X-ray investigations the position of the patient is continually being changed. A cuffed flexometallic tube must be in place to maintain a clear airway in all positions of the head, and prevent aspiration of any regurgitated stomach contents. At the same time reflex response to the changing posture or dye and air injections may be controlled by intermittent suxamethonium and artificial ventilation.[2]

Brown[91] has described two patterns of hypotensive response during cerebral angiography. One was thought to be due to vascular spasm from the irritant effect of the dye on hypersensitive vessels. The other was possibly due to temporary cerebral œdema as a result of damage to vascular endothelium by Uriodone.

A hypertensive response has been found in another series of patients after subarachnoid hæmorrhage.[92]

Pneumoencephalography. During this investigation there is a danger of herniation of the medulla and air embolism.[86] The sitting position will also increase the sensitivity of the patient to hypotensive and depressant drugs and in addition postural changes may initiate reflex respiratory effects. These patients therefore require particular care and attention.

Anæsthesia and Analgesia with Patient-Coöperation

If sensory pathways are to be cut for the relief of pain and particularly accurate assessment of the extent of section is required then it is an advantage to have the patient coöperative. Similar conditions may be required for studies of cortical localization.

Segmental epidural analgesia has been used to provide complete analgesia in the operation site, the area requiring pain-relief being left unaffected for sensory testing.[93] If general anæsthesia is used and the patient allowed to regain consciousness for the moment of sensory testing then considerable time must be spent explaining the procedure to the patient before operation and arranging hand signals that he can use for communication with the anæsthetist.

One method depends on the use of endotracheal nitrous-oxide and oxygen with a suxamethonium drip.[94] The patient is allowed to wake for the period when his co-operation is required, minimal suxamethonium being used during this time. An alternative is the use of local analgesia, combined with nitrous-oxde—oxygen analgesia during the period of testing. None of the methods available is likely to be satisfactory in every case and as much will depend on the temperament of the patient as on the skill of the anæsthetist.

Normally chordotomy is performed under full general anæsthesia as the actual cord division is gross enough not to require the patient's coöperation.[2]

Local Analgesia

There have been no definite advances in the neurosurgical applications of local analgesia in recent years. Lignocaine hydrochloride (Xylocaine) 0·5–1% solution with adrenaline 1 : 250,000 is used for the majority of burr hole explorations and ventriculographies. It is also commonly used for chemothalomectomy, meningocoele operations in infants, angiography and pneumoencephalography. The use of epidural block for laminectomy[95] and particularly for prolapsed intervertebral disc operations has been recommended.[96]

Apart from these cases, the emotional and physical strain of long intracranial or spinal operations is such that general anæsthesia is essential.

Intrathecol Phenol

The use of intrathecal phenol in glycerine or "Myodil" in the treatment of intractable pain has been described by several authors[97–99] and recently a similar technique has been used to relieve spasticity and painful reflex spasms in paraplegia.[100, 101]

The illustrations, with the exception of Figs. 18 and 20 are from Ballantine, R. I. W., and Jackson, I. (1960), *A Practice of General Anæsthesia for Neurosurgery*, Churchill, London, and were originally drawn by Dr. A. M. Hall-Smith to whom I continue to be grateful.

References

1. BALLANTINE, R. I. W., and JACKSON, I. (1960). *A Practice of General Anæsthesia for Neurosurgery*. J. and A. Churchill Ltd., London.
2. WYLIE, W. D., and CHURCHILL-DAVIDSON, H. C. (1960). *A Practice of Anæsthesia*. Lloyd-Luke Ltd., London.
3. INKSTER, J. S. (1956). *Brit. J. Anæsth.*, **28**, 512.
4. FURNESS, D. H. (1957). *Brit. J. Anæsth.*, **29**, 415.
5. MORTIMER, P. L. F. (1957). *Brit. J. Anæsth.*, **29**, 528.
6. GALLOON, S. (1959). *Anæsthesia*, **14**, 223.
7. HUNTER, A. R. (1958). *Anæsthesia*, **13**, 379.
8. COPE, R. W., and GLOVER, W. T. (1959). *Lancet*, **1**, 858.
9. COURVOISIER, S., DUCROT, R., FOURNEL, J., and JULOU, L. (1958). *Arch. Int. de Pharm. et de Therapie*, 90 (May).
10. GILLETT, G. B., and KEIL, A. M. (1960). *Anæsthesia*, **15**, 158.
11. BALLANTINE, R. I. W. (1956). *Anæsthesia*, **11**, 303.
12. DODD, R. B., LIANG, H. S., and BROWN, R. J. (1957). *Anesth. et Analg.*, **36**, 52 (May-June).
13. CHURCHILL-DAVIDSON, H. C. (1954). *Brit. med. J.* **1**, 74.
14. MORRIS, D. D. B., and DUNN, C. H. (1957). *Brit. med. J.*, **1**, 383.
15. BALLANTINE, R. I. W., and JACKSON, I. (1954). *Anæsthesia*, **9**, 4.
16. BURNS, T. H. S. (1956). *Brit. med. J.*, **1**, 439.

17. RENDELL-BAKER, L. (1954). *Brit. J. Anæsth.*, **26**, 201.
18. RAVENTÓS, J. (1956). *Brit. J. Pharmacol.*, **2**, 394.
19. JOHNSTONE, M. (1956). *Brit. J. Anæsth.*, **28**, 392.
20. BRYCE-SMITH, R., and O'BRIEN, H. D. (1956). *Brit. med. J.*, **2**, 969; (1956) *Proc. R. Soc. Med.*, **50**, 193.
21. Committee on Non-explosive Anæsthetic Agents (1957). *Brit. med. J.*, **2**, 479.
22. BRENNAN, H. J., HUNTER, A. R., and JOHNSTONE, M. (1957). *Lancet*, **1**, 453.
23. MARRETT, H. R. (1957). *Brit. med. J.*, **1**, 331.
24. POPE, E. S. (1957). *Anæsthesia*, **12**, 405.
25. BROWN, T. A., and WOODS, M. A. (1958). *Brit. J. Anæsth.*, **30**, 333.
26. DELANEY, E. J. (1958). *Brit. J. Anæsth.*, **30**, 188.
27. WORINGER, E., SCHNEIDER, J., BAUMGARTER, J., and THOMALSKE, G. (1954). *Anesth. et Analg.*, **11**, 1.
28. SEDZIMIR, C. B., JACOBS, D., and DUNDEE, J. W. (1955). *Brit. J. Anæsth.*, **27**, 93.
29. HOWELL, D. A., STRATFORD, J., and POSNIKOFF, J. (1956). *Canad. med. Ass. J.*, **75**, 388.
30. BRINDLE, G. F., GILBERT, R. G. B., and MILLAR, R. A. (1957). *Canad. Anæs. soc. J.*, **4**, 265 (July).
31. GILBERT, R. G. B., MILLAR, R. A., and BRINDLE, G. F. (1960). *Canad. Anæsth. Soc. J.*, **7**, 52 (January).
32. ROSOMOFF, H. L. (1956). *Proc. R. Soc. Med.*, **49**, 353.
33. DUNDEE, J. W., and BLACK, G. W. (1960). *Anæsthesia*, **15**, 349.
34. ENDERBY, G. E. H. (1960). *Anæsthesia*, **15**, 25.
35. AYRE, T. P. (1937). *Lancet*, **1**, 561; (1937) *Anesth. et Analg.*, **16**, 330; (1956) *Brit. J. Anæsth.*, **28**, 520.
36. BALLANTINE, R. I. W. (1961). *Anæsthesia*, **16**, 502.
37. WYLIE, W. D. (1951). *G. ital. Anest.*, **17**, 305.
38. BOZZA, M. L., MASPES, P. E., and ROSSANDA, M. (1961). *Brit. J. Anæsth.*, **33**, 132.
39. BROWN, A. S. (1959). *Anæsthesia*, **14**, 207.
40. OPIE, L. H., SPALDING, J. M. K., and STOTT, F. D. (1959). *Lancet*, **1**, 545.
41. OPIE, L. H., SPALDING, J. M. K., and CRAMPTON SMITH, A. (1961). *Lancet*, **1**, 911.
42. CRAMPTON SMITH, A., and SPALDING, J. M. K. (1959). *Proc. R. Soc. Med.*, **52**, 661.
43. HUNTER, A. R. (1960). *Proc. R. Soc. Med.*, **53**, 365.
44. MARSHALL, M. (1961). *Lancet*, **1**, 745.
45. RAY, B. S. (1958). Personal communication.
46. JAVID, M. (1958). *Surg. Clin. N. Amer.*, **38**, 907.
47. STUBBS, J., and PENNYBACKER, J. (1960). *Lancet*, **1**, 1094.
48. WATKINS, E. S., STUBBS, J. D., and LEWIN, W. (1961). *Lancet*, **1**, 358.
49. SMALL, J. M. (1960). *Lancet*, **1**, 1252.
50. Annotation (1961). *Lancet*, **1**, 210.
51. HUGHES, G., MUDD, S., and STRECKER, E. A. (1938). *Arch. Neurol. Psychiat.*, **99**, 1276.
52. MACIVER, I. H., LASSMAN, L. P., THOMSON, C. W., and MACLEOD, I. (1958). *Lancet*, **2**, 544.
53. SADOVE, M. S., WYANT, G. M., and GITTELSON, L. A. (1953). *Brit. med. J.*, **2**, 255.
54. COPE, D. H. P. (1960). *Proc. R. Soc. Med.*, **53**, 678.
55. McQUISTON, W. O. (1950). *Arch. Surg.*, **61**, 892.
56. DUNDEE, J. W., GRAY, T. C., MESHAM, P. R., and SCOTT, W. E. B. (1953). *Brit. Med. J.*, **2**, 1237.
57. ROSOMOFF, H. L., and GILBERT, R. (1955). *Amer. J. Physiol.*, **183**, 19.
58. ROSOMOFF, H. L. (1956). *Proc. R. Soc. Med.*, **49**, 353.
59. COOPER, K., and ROSS, D. (1960). *Hypothermia in Surgical Practice*. Cassell and Co. Ltd., London.

60. McBurrows, M., Dundee, J. W., Francis, I. Ll., Lipton, S., and Sedzimir, C. B. (1956). *Anæsthesia*, **11**, 4.
61. Campkin, V., and Inglis, J. M. (1958). *Brit. J. Anæsth.*, **30**, 586.
62. Boba, A. (1960). *Hypothermia for the Neurosurgical Patient*. C. C. Thomas, Illinois, U.S.A.
63. Woringer, E., Shneider, J., Baumgarter, J., and Thomalske, G. (1954). *Anæsth. and Analg.*, **11**, 1.
64. Rowbotham, G. F., Bell, K., Akinhead, J., and Cairns, A. (1957). *Lancet*, **1**, 1016.
65. Sedzimir, C. B., Jacobs, D., and Dundee, J. W. (1953). *Brit. J. Anæsth.*, **27**, 93.
66. Inglis, J. M., and Turner, E. (1957). *Brit. med. J.*, **1**, 1335.
67. Swann, H., Zeavin, I., Holmes, J. H., and Montgomery, V. (1953). *Ann. Surg.*, **138**, 360.
68. Cookson, B. A., Neptune, W. B., and Bailey, C. P. (1952). *J. int. Coll. Surg.*, **18**, 685.
69. Gray, T. C. (1957). *Lancet*, **1**, 383.
70. Lougheed, W. M., and Kahn, D. S. (1955). *J. Neurosurg.*, **12**, 226.
71. Woodhall, B., and Reynolds, D. H. (1957). *Excerpta med. 1st International Congress of Neurological Surgery*, Brussels.
72. Kristiansen, K. (1961). *J. R. Coll. Surg. Edinb.*, **7**, 1.
73. Saunders, J. W. (1952). *Lancet*, **1**, 1286.
74. James, A., Coulter, R. L., and Saunders, J. W. (1953). *Lancet*, **1**, 412.
75. Aserman, D. (1953). *Brit. med. J.*, **1**, 961.
76. Sadove, M. S., Wyant, G. M., Gittelson, L. A., and Bucy, P. C. (1953). *J. Neurosurg.*, **10**, 272.
77. Saunders, J. W. (1954). *Lancet*, **1**, 1156.
78. Bozza, M. (1954). *Chirurgia*, **10**, 435.
79. Anderson, S. M. (1955). *Brit. med. J.*, **2**, 103.
80. Mazzia, V. D. B., Ray, B. S., and Artusio, J. F. (1956). *Ann. Surg.*, **143**, 81.
81. Brown, A. S. (1954). *Anæsthesia*, **9**, 17.
82. Robertson, J. D., Gillies, J., and Spencer, K. E. V. (1957). *Brit. J. Anæsth.*, **29**, 342.
83. Enderby, G. E. H. (1960). *Anæsthesia*, **15**, 25.
84. Mason, A. A., and Pelmore, J. F. (1953). *Brit. med. J.*, **1**, 250.
85. Pearce, D. J. (1957). *Proc. R. Soc. Med.*, **50**, 109.
86. Jacoby, J., Jones, J. R., Ziegler, J., Claasen, L., and Garvin, J. P. (1959). *Anesthesiology*, **20**, 336.
87. Maciver, I. N., Smith, J. B., Tomlinson, B. E., and Whitby, J. D. (1956). *Brit. J. Surg.*, **43**, 505.
88. Maciver, I. N., Frew, I. J. C., and Matheson, J. G. (1958). *Lancet*, **1**, 390.
89. Bryce-Smith, R. (1950). *Brit. med. J.*, **2**, 322.
90. Lewin, W. (1959). *Proc. R. Soc. Med.*, **52**, 403.
91. Brown, A. S. (1955). *Anæsthesia*, **10**, 346.
92. Stark, D. C. (1958). *Anæsthesia*, **13**, 391.
92. Krumperman, L. W., Murtagh, F., and Wester, M. R. (1957). *Anesthesiology*, **18**, 316.
94. Hall, K., Baldwin, M., and Norris, F. (1959). *Anesthesiology*, **20**, 65.
95. Matheson, D. (1960). *Canad. Anæsth. Soc. J.*, **7**, 149.
96. Boulton, T. B. (1959). Personal Communication.
97. Maher, R. M. (1955). *Lancet*, **1**, 18.
    Maher, R. M. (1957). *Lancet*, **1**, 16.
    Maher, R. M. (1960). *Lancet*, **1**, 895.
98. Brown, A. S. (1958). *Lancet*, **2**, 975.
99. Nathan, P. W., and Scott, T. G. (1958). *Lancet*, **1**, 76.
100. Nathan, P. W. (1959). *Lancet*, **2**, 1099.
101. Kelly, R. E., and Gautier-Smith, P. C. (1959). *Lancet*, **2**, 1102.

CHAPTER 6

ANÆSTHESIA FOR CARDIAC SURGERY

A. I. PARRY BROWN

Ventilation of the Lungs—Circulatory Hæmodynamics—Maintainance of Unconsciousness—Patent Ductus Arteriosus—Coarctation of the Aorta—Constrictive Pericarditis—Open Heart Surgery—Circulatory Arrest—Cardiac Resuscitation.

THREE notable events have contributed to the development of anæsthesia for cardiac surgery.

Over 20 years ago controlled ventilation of the lungs was found to provide a solution to the problems of the open chest. This became standard practice in British anæsthesia after an important paper by Nosworthy in 1941.[1] The introduction of the muscle relaxants in this country by Gray and Halton in 1946 allowed anæsthetists control of pulmonary ventilation without the necessity for deep general anæsthesia.[2]

Ten years ago the physiological principles of hypothermia became available to anæsthetists.[3, 4] Although this exciting advance had more limitations for cardiac than for neuro-surgery it foreshadowed the further development of profound hypothermia by Drew.[5-7]

During the last decade several types of mechanical pump-oxygenators have been used successfully for open heart surgery in man.[8-10] This technique was made possible by the discovery of heparin in 1916 by Howell and McLean.[11]

The application, modification and development of these techniques is progressing so rapidly at the present time that it may soon be possible for surgeons to offer real hope to patients with cardiac ischæmia, one of the great challenges of medicine to-day.

Ventilation of the Lungs During Cardiac Surgery

Patients with heart disease may present special problems of ventilation. They may be orthopnœic. Nursing tradition has decreed since the earliest hypotensive calamities with chloroform that patients for anæsthesia should be wheeled to the theatre lying flat. If this position is imposed on an orthopnœic patient distress is inevitable and acute heart failure may occur. Pulmonary œdema has resulted from such malpositioning before anæsthesia. In mitral stenosis the phase of the disease associated with paroxysmal nocturnal dyspnœa and in which pulmonary œdema might be expected may have passed, but the stiff and indurated lung which offers some protection against the transudation of œdema fluid through the lung capillaries makes ventilation more difficult and increases the diffusion time between the alveolus and the lung capillary. Such stiff lungs require greater than usual pressures to maintain good ventilation and when the chest is open may cause the lung to billow into the surgical field. Although this is abhorrent to the self-effacing anæsthetist adequate ventilation must be maintained and the surgical assistant urged to give more efficient retraction.

Although relatively high peak intrapulmonary pressures may be necessary for adequate ventilation, the mean pressure must be kept as low as possible. Over-enthusiastic bag squeezing may reduce the pulmonary blood flow to dangerously low levels by mechanical obstruction to the pulmonary circulation.[12] A negative phase is unnecessary, but the intrapulmonary pressure should be allowed to return to atmospheric during expiration. Vascular shunts present obvious difficulties to the maintenance of respiratory exchange. When the shunt is from right to left so that some venous blood reaches the left heart without passing through the lungs the arterial oxygen saturation is lowered by the venous admixture. Over-ventilation can correct carbon dioxide retention caused by such a shunt but the oxygen saturation can only rise to normal if the oxygen levels in the venous blood rise either by an increased rate of circulation or a reduction in the oxygen requirements of the body. When the shunt is from left to right, although there is congestion of the pulmonary vascular bed, conditions are much more favourable for anæsthesia. The high flows through the lungs ensure complete exposure of the circulating blood to the atmosphere offered by the anæsthetist. These high flows may, however, in a neglected case provoke an increased pulmonary vascular resistance with reversal of the shunt or cardiac failure.

Circulatory Hæmodynamics and Cardiac Surgery

Surgical anæsthesia is associated with loss of vasomotor control and peripheral vasodilatation. The severity of this is dependent on the depth of anæsthesia attained, but does vary with the anæsthetic agent and technique. This association is acceptable in healthy patients and may even be exploited in some circumstances, but if the heart has a low fixed output (as in a valvular stenosis or pericardial constriction), peripheral vasodilation can be disastrous. If severe falls in blood pressure result from delivering this diminished flow into a dilated vascular bed, cerebral and coronary perfusion may both become inadequate. A wise precaution is to have a syringe prepared with a vasoconstrictor drug during induction of anæsthesia in these cases. Should acute hypotension occur, no time will be wasted before the drug is in the circulation and cardiac arrest or cerebral anoxia may be averted. Mephentermine 10 mg is suitable for this purpose.

A right to left shunt is increased as the vascular resistance in the systemic circulation falls, thereby reducing the proportion of circulating blood available for gas exchange in the lungs. Because of the relative lack of circulatory disturbances, good results may be achieved by nitrous oxide and oxygen anæsthesia whilst the muscle relaxants give the conditions required for ventilation and surgery. The elimination of lung nitrogen is an essential preliminary to the management of nitrous oxide anæsthesia. If the alveolar gases contain a substantial proportion of nitrogen some hypoxia will develop before the partial pressure of nitrous oxide is sufficient to produce unconsciousness. This would be most unwelcome at the outset of cardiac surgery, so the patient is oxygenated before starting the administration of nitrous oxide. This technique introduced by Gray and his associates for patients with mitral stenosis is useful for all those in which the fall in systemic vascular resistance must be avoided.[13] In those cases of mitral valve disease in which there is right heart failure hypoxia is doubly unwelcome. Hypoxia causes an increased pulmonary vascular resistance thus demanding more work from the right ventricle. The diminished oxygen supply at a time when the cardiac muscle is overloaded may cause ventricular fibrillation.

Maintenance of Unconsciousness During Cardiac Surgery

A direct consequence of the use of muscle relaxants is the problem of how to be certain that the patient is unaware. Awareness of surgery is most likely to occur during nitrous oxide and oxygen narcosis.[14] In cardiac surgery every attempt is made to keep the anæsthetic as light as possible to avoid cardio-vascular depression, and it is therefore not surprising that occasionally patients can recall parts of the procedure. The incidence can be reduced by the inclusion of hyoscine (Scopolamine) in the premedication and the use of analgesic drugs during the procedure to reinforce the narcotic effects of nitrous oxide. Pethidine in incremental doses of 25 mg is useful and unlikely to produce cardio-vascular depression. Phenoperidine (Searle R.1406), although at present under investigation, shows promise of being a satisfactory analgesic supplement to nitrous oxide. An alternative approach is to use low concentration of halothane in oxygen to maintain narcosis. Although the associated peripheral vasodilation would seem to outweigh the advantages of a high partial pressure of oxygen in the anæsthetic mixture for procedures such as mitral valvotomy, it has been found satisfactory for use in the atmosphere to which the blood is exposed in the pump-oxygenator.[15] Here the vasodilatation may be advantageous in reducing metabolic acidosis. It is interesting to note that Trimetaphan has been used for the same purpose in profound hypothermia.[16]

Patent Ductus Arteriosus

Increased perfusion of the lungs makes anæsthesia straightforward. The correction of the lesion does not impose any increased load on any chamber of the heart, indeed, the tumultuous action of the heart is immediately quietened when the leak from the aorta into the pulmonary artery is closed. A good anæsthetic technique for thoracotomy is all that is required. Sudden hæmorrhage if the ductus should tear is a possible complication which makes an efficient intravenous drip essential. The possibility of recanalization if the ductus is ligated in continuity justifies to some surgeons the division of the ductus between clamps. This involves the closure of what are virtually lateral openings in the aorta and the pulmonary artery. A responsibility devolves on the anæsthetist to ensure that no movement of the patient can cause a clamp to slip. A more positive part can be played by the use of controlled hypotension at this stage in the operation. An intravenous drip of trimetaphan 1 mg/1 ml, started after the patient has been placed in position on the operating table and respiration has been controlled by intermittent positive pressure, will allow the blood pressure to be held at around 70 mm Hg systolic. This level of systemic pressure is well tolerated by these patients unless changes have occurred in the pulmonary vasculature in which case a reversal of the shunt would cause cyanosis. In the absence of this contra-indication the use of hypotension facilitates the dissection of the aorta, ductus and pulmonary artery and greatly reduces the risk that one or both the clamps may slip when the ductus is divided.

A problem is presented when the ductus is complicated by infective endocarditis. The high fever and septic foci in the lungs make anæsthesia more difficult. The surgery is made more hazardous by the œdema and fragility of the infected tissue, but the rewards of success are greater in that the infection becomes controllable. If a neglected case has developed increased pulmonary vascular resistance with reversal of the shunt the anæsthetic becomes difficult and dangerous, but as closure of the ductus is probably contra-indicated in these circumstances for the shunt now acts as a safety valve for the right heart, an anæsthetic is only likely to be required for some inter-current condition.

Coarctation of the Aorta

Coarctation of the aorta is related to closure of the ductus arteriosus in that a stricture of the aorta occurs at the site of origin of the obliterated ductus. This stricture produces hypertension in the upper part of the body. All or nearly all the output of the left ventricle is forced into the innominate artery and the left carotid and subclavian arteries. This may be associated with differences in blood pressure in the left and right arms. Sometimes the stenosis of the aorta distorts the left subclavian artery and reduces its blood flow. In other cases the left subclavian artery becomes virtually the direct continuation of the aorta and so takes the full force of the cardiac output. Below the stricture the aorta often shows post stenotic dilatation. The walls of the enlarged intercostal vessels which cause notching of the ribs are often degenerate and show berry aneurysms at their origin from the aorta. The operative treatment consists in applying clamps to the aorta above and below the lesion, excising the stricture and suturing the opened ends of the aorta together. If the stricture is too long or the descending aorta too degenerate, then a graft may have to be inserted. The problems to be faced are, firstly, the excessive bleeding from the chest wall because of the anastomotic channels and the hypertension; secondly, the degeneration of the walls of the intercostal arteries which may easily tear whilst the aorta is being freed for the application of the clamps, and thirdly, the clamp on the aorta above the lesion is likely to obstruct the flow of blood into the left subclavian artery. If the out-flow of the left ventricle is confined to the innominate and left carotid arteries a great rise in pressure occurs which may result in a cerebrovascular accident or left heart failure. The high pressure can be relieved by a partial left heart by-pass or by using induced hypo-tension. The latter method is preferred by the author because it is simpler and reduces bleeding from the chest wall. Organs below the clamp are adequately supplied with blood through anastomotic channels. A ganglion blocking agent is used to lower the blood pressure. Some difficulty must be expected in these cases for although

6

vaso-dilatation will occur throughout the body, it will only reduce the resistance to cardiac output in those parts above the coarctation. A fall in blood pressure does occur, but it is not so great as is met with in a normal circulation. The temptation to overdosage with the ganglion blocking drug must be resisted because when the clamps are removed after restoration of continuity to the aorta the free flow of blood into a dilated vascular bed can produce severe hypotension. The administration of these drugs whether short or long acting must be so timed that the effect is wearing off as the suturing is completed.

Constrictive Pericarditis

Decompression of the heart in constrictive pericarditis presents considerable anæsthetic difficulties. The cardiac tamponade will have produced widespread changes. The raised venous pressure results in ascites and pleural effusions. Pleural thickening limits ventilation even when the effusions have been aspirated. The myocardium is often poor and may be invaded by the tuberculous process which has caused the constrictive pericarditis. The patient requires careful preparation with digitalis and diuretics to control the water retention. Tapping the ascites and aspirating the pleural effusions before anæsthesia will make ventilation easier. Thiopentone induction is contra-indicated for besides the danger of severe hypotension from peripheral vasodilatation in this state of restricted cardiac output, dilatation of the heart occurs during the administration of thiopentone which, with a tight constriction, may cause cardiac arrest. Pre-oxygenation followed by nitrous oxide and oxygen with a muscle relaxant and controlled respiration seem suitable. These patients tend to be more difficult to anæsthetise quietly by this technique than those with mitral valve disease and it is sometimes preferable to pass through a stage of cyclopropane and oxygen. The dissection of the thickened pericardium involves some pressure on the heart and may provoke extrasystoles. Attempts used to be made to prevent these by intravenous procaine or procaine amide and by the topical application of 2% procaine to the heart by swabs during the dissection. This has fallen into disfavour because the drugs act as myocardial depressants. Cessation of the stimulus will allow normal rhythm to recur if the patient is well ventilated. Actual pressure of the heart may prevent proper filling and so embarrass the circulation. Early warning of this must be given to the surgeon. Bleeding is not a marked feature of this operation unless a down-growth of the tuberculous process into the myocardium causes a tear of heart muscle. An intravenous drip must be set up, but because of the raised venous pressure little blood should be given until the heart is decompressed. The transfusion needs to be continued slowly for 24 hours post-operatively for without it the patient may readily develop hypotension.

Open Heart Surgery Under Moderate Hypothermia

When a chamber of the heart must be laid open to give the necessary surgical access the circulation must be arrested whilst the heart is open. If tourniquets are applied to the superior and inferior venæ cavæ within the pericardium as they enter the right atrium the flow of blood into the heart can be stopped. At the same time artificial respiration should cease or all the blood in the pulmonary vascular bed will be driven on before the heart empties. If the cardiotomy is limited to 2 minutes or less and the patient is well oxygenated before the occlusion, this can be done at normal body temperature. A simple valvular pulmonary stenosis can be corrected in this way. When a slightly longer occlusion is required the survival of the cerebral cells becomes an important factor. If the brain is cooled slowly to avoid temperature gradients it will survive 10 minutes arrest at 30° C, but there is some delay in the recovery of full consciousness at the end of the operation. If the occlusion is limited to 6 minutes the recovery from the anæsthetic is as brisk as after any other thoracotomy. This limits the usefulness of moderate hypothermia to operations lasting up to from 5 to 7 minutes. The technique is suitable for the closure of atrial septal defects of the ostium secundum type and the correction of pulmonary stenosis if a greater margin of time is likely to be required than is given at normal temperatures. The myocardium becomes exhausted if it goes on beating through the period of occlusion whilst it has no coronary blood supply. The process of cooling frequently reduces its activity to a safe level, but if it is beating too vigorously Neostigmine will slow it. The dose of neostigmine is 0·005 mg/Kg, and it should be injected into the cavity of the left ventricle whilst the heart is emptying itself subsequent to caval occlusion and with a clamp across the aorta. The drug will be driven into the coronary arteries with the next ventricular contraction. In the closure of an atrial septal defect by this technique it is important to hold a reserve of oxygenated blood in the lungs. This blood can be driven into the left atrium by inflating the lungs whilst the last stitches are tightened in the repaired defect. In this way any air accidentally entering the left atrium tends to be expelled and a quantity of oxygenated blood is left ready to perfuse the coronary arteries when the tourniquets are removed and the circulation restarted. This reserve of blood is built up by a period of hyperventilation before the occlusion and the maintenance of a steady pressure of about 5 cm of water in the lungs during it. Rewarming should commence as soon as the operation begins as the temperature will continue to fall even though the surface of the body is being warmed. The occlusion should occur just as the central temperature has begun to rise, otherwise there is a risk that very cold blood from the periphery will reach the heart after the arrest of the circulation. This may precipitate ventricular fibrillation which is difficult to reverse unless the heart can be warmed. A long period of cardiac massage whilst the heart is being warmed bruises the myocardium causing a low cardiac output and hypotension post-operatively. The advantage of this technique is that no pumps are required. The patient does not need to have anticoagulants. The blood required for the operation is less and the possibility of damage to the elements of the patient's blood is reduced. It does demand certain diagnosis and speedily efficient surgery.

Open Heart Surgery Using the Pump Oxygenator

The alternative is to provide the brain with oxygenated blood from another source. It was at first hoped that the survival time of the brain could be prolonged with a low flow perfusion of oxygenated blood. Despite some successes this has not proved satisfactory because the condition of the patient steadily deteriorates due to a progressive metabolic acidosis. The aim of most workers is to perfuse at flow rates equivalent to the resting cardiac output of the patient. The required perfusion rate is calculated either as 70–80 ml/min/kg body weight or as 2,400 ml/min/sq metre body surface. The body surface area is calculated from tables based on weight and height. The oxygenator must be capable of providing efficient gas exchange at the required flow rate, and the venous and arterial cannulæ selected must be capable of carrying this blood flow. The pump is primed with sufficient heparinized blood to enable it to deliver oxygenated blood as soon as the venous blood from the patient is fed into it. A suitable thoracotomy is performed and the right atrium exposed to receive the venous cannulæ. The femoral artery is exposed to receive the arterial line. The patient is now given 3 mg of heparin per kg of body weight (or if preferred, 90 mg/sq metre surface area) and the cannulæ inserted.

Venous blood is taken from the right atrium or the superior and inferior venæ cavæ and collected in the venous reservoir of the pump oxygenator either by gravity or by maintaining a negative pressure over the reservoir. Too great an emptying pressure may collapse the veins on to the cannulæ and defeat its purpose by obstructing the flow. The venous blood must now be oxygenated. There are three main types of oxygenator: **Bubble Oxygenators** (Lillehei-de Wall) are very efficient, but the flow rate is limited because of the difficulty of preventing small bubbles entering the arterial line. **Film Oxygenators** expose the blood to an oxygen rich atmosphere either as stainless steel screens (Mayo-Gibbon), rotating discs (Melrose) or plastic rollers (Crafoord-Senning). It is feared that the exposure of the blood directly to the oxygenating atmosphere may break down some of the plasma proteins and **Membrane Oxygenators** are being developed which it is hoped may eliminate one source of damage to the blood by separating it from direct contact with the gases.

The oxygenated blood is passed through a filter into the femoral artery. The filter removes aggregations of cells and particles of fibrin which might otherwise serve as systemic emboli and also acts as a trap to prevent bubbles from reaching the femoral artery. The oxygenating atmosphere must contain some carbon dioxide or too much will be removed from the venous blood. Samples of pump arterialized blood may be examined periodically to determine the partial pressure of carbon dioxide and variations in the concentration in the ventilating atmosphere can be made in order to maintain normal figures. Alternatively, a predetermined mixture of carbon dioxide in oxygen may be used.

The balance of blood between the patient and machine must be accurately maintained. If more is coming from the venous side than is returned the patient will react as if a sudden and severe hæmorrhage had occurred. If the arterial perfusion exceeds the venous return the patient's vascular system becomes overloaded and there is danger of emptying the reservoirs and so pumping air into the arterial line. These dangers are variously countered. On the **Mayo-Gibbon** the pump lifting blood from the venous reservoir is pre-set to deliver the calculated flow of blood over the screens of the oxygenator. If the level in the venous reservoir falls because the return from the patient is insufficient, a photoelectric sensing device causes occlusion of the pipe from the venous reservoir and at the same time opens a pipe which connects the arterial reservoir to the venous side. The flow over the screens remains constant, but is made up of varying proportions from the venous and arterial reservoirs according to the level on the venous side. A second monitor keeps the level in the arterial reservoir constant by varying the speed of the arterial pump which drives the blood back into the femoral artery of the patient. If the flow of blood from the patient is sufficient to supply the venous pump, no arterial blood will be shunted over the screens, and the output of the arterial pump will equal that of the venous pump. The patient will therefore be receiving the full calculated perfusion. If there is a deficiency in the return of venous blood the shunt will open and the arterial pump will run more slowly perfusing the patient only that amount of blood which has been contributed on the venous line.

On the **Crafoord-Senning** pump the output is pneumatically controlled by the pressure in the back pads of the pump. If the pads are tightly inflated the pump output is maximal. As the pressure in the pads falls the output is reduced. The pressure in these pads is governed by the weight of blood in the arterial reservoir. There is also an electrical cut-out which would stop the pump if the level fell below the opening of the pipe carrying the blood to the pump.

In the **Melrose pump** the balance is maintained by the pump operator who varies the speed of the pump to keep the level in the reservoir of oxygenated blood steady. When the Melrose machine is used the control is, therefore, in the hands of the pump operator. The mechanical devices keep a steady balance if no large quantity of blood is being lost from the operative field, and there are no great changes in the vascular bed of the patient. They tend to exaggerate the deficiency of circulation caused by a diminution of the venous return to the heart. Any blood loss either external or due to pooling in the patient must be made good by transfusion. This can be given intravenously to the patient or into the venous reservoir of the machine.

It is usual to go on to the machine by first setting up a partial bypass. The clamps are removed from the venous lines allowing blood to flow into the machine. An equivalent amount is pumped into the femoral artery. As the flow increases up to the calculated perfusion rate ligatures can be tightened around the cannulæ in the venæ cavæ thus diverting the whole venous return to the oxygenator. It is of the utmost importance that whilst these ligatures are in position no mechanical obstruction shall occur which might cause a rise in venous pressure. Neglect which allows the maintenance of a venous pressure of over 20 cm of water severely prejudices the success of the perfusion.

Unfortunately, even the complete diversion of the caval blood from the heart does not enable the heart to be opened without loss of blood. The coronary perfusion of the heart will continue to flow mainly into the right atrium through the coronary sinus. The bronchial arterial supply to the lungs will be delivered to the left atrium through the pulmonary veins. Shunts such as from a patent ductus arteriosus can flood so much blood into the pulmonary circulation that it makes cardiotomy impracticable. Similarly the greatly increased flow through the bronchial arteries which occurs in Fallots tetralogy can cause excessive blood loss during perfusion. Incompetence of the aortic valves not only floods the heart, but does not allow the arterial perfusion to build up sufficient pressure for the circulation to the body. Special techniques are required to deal with these latter problems, but the blood flowing from the coronary and bronchial circulations must always be aspirated from the heart. It can be sucked away and discarded, but the quantities involved make this impossible except for very short periods. It can be collected in a special sucker and retransfused. A conventional sucker entrains the blood in a large volume of air. This causes frothing and injury to the red cells. A low pressure sucker of the DeBakey type may be used to diminish this hæmolysis and efforts should be made to entrain as little air as possible with the blood. Attempts have been made to reduce the frothing by blowing an atmosphere of soluble gas around the orifice of the sucker. Carbon dioxide and nitrous oxide have been tried but the least damage is done by the gentle use of a controllable low pressure. The blood from this sucker can be delivered into the venous reservoir of the oxygenator after de-bubbling.

All blood escaping into the chest aspirated in the general sucker, removed on swabs or soiling the drapes must be estimated and replaced. This estimate is made by weighing the soiled swabs and deducting the weight of the dry swabs and any irrigating lotions that have been used. The amount of blood aspirated into the suction bottle can be measured directly. Measuring cylinders placed in the suction lines at the head of the table next to the anæsthetist form a convenient way of keeping a constant check on blood loss.[16] Visual estimation must be made of blood on the drapes and spillage from the cardiotomy watched continuously. Up to a litre of blood may be concealed in the paravertebral gutters in a bilateral thoracotomy wound, so this estimate is of great importance. Failure to replace blood may become apparent whilst still pumping by a fall of venous return and by a deterioration in the E.E.G. recording if this is monitored. It becomes more obvious when the attempt is made to restore the normal circulation. Observation of the heart will show that it fails to fill properly. A pulse wave due to cardiac contraction is not superimposed on the arterial pressure created by the pump. Additional blood can be given by arterial transfusion from the pump. If the patient is under-transfused the arterial pressure will rise and quickly fall back to a level slightly higher than before. This can be repeated until a satisfactory blood pressure is maintained. The venous pressure must be watched in order to differentiate myocardial failure from hypovolæmia. Nixon[17] suggests that a careful study of the arterial pressure trace after the delivery of 80–90 ml of blood intra-arterially can be more informative. In a patient with a normal blood volume distention of the aorta with a rapid intra-arterial injection will result in a vasodilatation and a transient fall in blood pressure. In the hypovolæmic patient the constriction of the arterial bed produces a sharp rise in arterial pressure when the extra blood is delivered into the arteries. These supplements can be repeated until they cease to produce the pressor response.

Several methods have been tried to reduce the loss of blood from the open heart. The coronary circulation can be stopped by clamping the root of the aorta. After 2 or 3 minutes the ventricular muscle becomes cyanotic and then it fibrillates. A compromise solution is possible. Periods in which the clamp is removed allowing perfusion of the heart with oxygenated blood alternate with periods in which the clamp is in place and surgery can proceed unhampered by bleeding. These periods of anoxia damage the myocardium. This is shown by an inadequate cardiac output and circulatory failure when coming off the pump. At lower temperatures the myocardium survives deprivation of circulation for longer so that some workers have fitted a heat exchanger on the arterial line of the oxygenator by which the temperature of the patient may be lowered. Whilst the heart remains beating this hypothermia merely reduces the danger. Elective cardiac arrest will greatly prolong the period in which coronary perfusion can be safely stopped. Baker et al[18] made use of potassium arrest by the infusion of potassium citrate into the coronary circulation. This produces an arrest in diastole which is readily reversed when the aortic clamp is removed allowing oxygenated blood to drive the potassium from the coronary circulation. This is successful for periods of up to 20 minutes with a healthy myocardium, but damage may still be done if longer periods are required or if the myocardium is unhealthy. In aortic valvular disease the myocardium may have been damaged by involvement of the coronary orifices, but an aortic clamp must be applied before exposing the valve. One answer is to perfuse the coronaries with blood from the oxygenator by way of catheters introduced into their orifices. The other is to cool the heart to temperatures of the order of 13–15° C when cell metabolism will be so low that no anoxia will occur.

Local cooling of the heart may be achieved by coronary perfusion of cold dextran supplemented by packing a sludge of frozen sterile saline around the heart.

Much knowledge is to be gained by monitoring as completely as possible, but the consistent success of some units who record only the central venous pressure and ensure the replacement of the blood loss emphasize the value of simplicity and good clinical judgement.

E.E.G. monitoring gives a clear indication of the adequacy of the cerebral perfusion. In the post-perfusion period it gives warning of an inadequate circulation before irreversible damage is done.

E.C.G. recordings can warn of inadequate coronary flow, of abnormalities in blood chemistry and of injury to the conducting mechanism of the heart.

Arterial pressure measured by a cannula in the radial artery enables the adequacy of the perfusion to be assessed as well as giving information about the tone of the vascular bed. A record of the response to arterial transfusion when the heart has taken over the circulation after the by-pass can serve as a guide to the blood balance as described above.

A knowledge of the **venous pressure** is essential. If the drainage is by one cannula from the right atrium then a single record from a catheter passed into the inferior vena cava is sufficient. If cannulæ are placed in both cavæ through the right atrial appendage the pressures should be taken in both the superior and inferior cavæ. A rise in pressure is nearly always due to kinking or malposition of one of the venous lines. This error must be corrected immediately as organs exposed to the high venous pressure are damaged and the diminished flow to the oxygenator will soon result in inadequate perfusion. A fall in venous pressure with inadequate flow to the machine suggests concealed blood loss. Post-operatively a high venous pressure may result from over-transfusion or myocardial inadequacy, and a low venous pressure suggests hypovolæmia.

Samples of arterial blood are taken regular intervals. The oxygen saturation before going on the pump will be influenced by the cardiac lesion, but except in right to left shunts, should be normal. On the pump the blood should be fully oxygenated. There are two main causes for a low oxygen saturation. If the perfusion is inadequate severe venous desaturation may require a greater oxygen uptake than can be provided by the oxygenator. If the venous oxygen saturation is normal the low arterial saturation can be due to poor filming of the blood in the oxygenator. After perfusion a lowered arterial oxygen tension may be respiratory or circulatory in origin. The lungs may become congested and collapsed during perfusion. This makes it difficult to maintain full oxygenation of the blood. It is important to adjust the ventilation to the condition of the patient and not by previously calculated ventilatory requirements. Many authorities inflate the lungs with a mixture of 80% helium and 20% oxygen during the perfusion to prevent this deterioration of lung function. Comroe has suggested that a surface tension reducing agent normally present in the alveoli may be reduced during perfusion. The surface tension in the alveoli is, therefore, increased and this makes inflation more difficult.

The pH of the blood considered with the P_{CO_2} and the standard bicarbonate give valuable help in the anæsthetic management. The slight overventilation associated with controlled respiration during the anæsthesia before pumping lowers the P_{CO_2} below 40 mm Hg; this does not produce an equivalent rise in pH as the standard bicarbonate is also lowered. It is wise to maintain control of respiration by the use of larger doses of relaxant drugs and to restrict the alveolar ventilation to that required to balance the metabolism of the body if it is wished to transfer to the oxygenator at normal figures. The blood in the pump can be similarly tested. The blood can be freshly taken into packs or bottles containing heparin, in which case normal figures can be expected. Edglutate blood is acid with low pH and bicarbonate and raised P_{CO_2}. This blood has been drawn into bottles containing a solution of sodium ethylene diamine tetra-acetic acid with dextrose, sodium chloride and magnesium chloride and it is heparinized by adding 20 mg of heparin to each 500 ml of blood followed after mixing by 1·5 ml 10% calcium chloride. The acidity can be corrected by the addition of sodium bicarbonate and recirculating the blood through the oxygenator before connecting to the patient. There should be little change in pH during the perfusion; the early findings of a steadily increasing metabolic acidosis were presumably due to inadequate flow rates. In the post-perfusion period a metabolic acidosis due to tissue anoxia will be shown by a lowered bicarbonate, and a respiratory acidosis by a raised P_{CO_2}. Some benefit may accrue in metabolic acidosis from giving intravenous sodium bicarbonate for it is difficult to restore good cardiac action if the blood chemistry is deranged.

Circulatory Arrest with Profound Hypothermia

Great advantages accrue if complete circulatory arrest can be used for a time long enough to allow unhurried surgery. Blood loss from the coronary and bronchial circulations will cease. Hæmolysis is reduced because a sucker is unnecessary. The surgical field is unobstructed and dry. At 14° C an arrest for an hour can be survived giving ample time for most cardiac operations. Simple cooling cannot be used because the cardiac output becomes inadequate at about 28° C. There is a period of ventricular fibrillation which quietens into cardiac standstill when the temperature falls further. The use of a pump oxygenator to continue the circulation allows the fall in temperature to proceed uninterrupted by this failure. This technique has been described by Hodgson and Parkhouse[16] who emphasize the need to cool slowly thus reducing the temperature gradients between different parts of the body. They were troubled by vaso-constriction during the cooling and recommend the use of trimeta-phan ("Arfonad") 25–50 mg intravenously if the arterial line pressure rises. This helps to maintain a high perfusion rate and to avoid differences of perfusion to different parts of the body.

Drew and his collaborators have developed an alternative tech-nique which uses the lung of the patient as the oxygenator whilst two pumps take over the function of the left and right sides of the heart. First a left heart bypass is set up from the left atrium to a venous reservoir through a pump into the femoral artery. The blood passes through a heat exchanger between the pump and the patient. Cold water circulates through the heat exchanger. The aim is to perfuse the patient with blood about 6° C below body temperature. The by-pass is at first partial, but it is steadily increased until it is total. When the temperature of the heart approaches 30° C or when cardiac action is seen to be inadequate a right heart by-pass is started. A cannula in the right atrium takes venous blood to a second reservoir whence it is pumped into the pulmonary artery. The lungs are ventilated with oxygen by intermittent positive pressure. The cooling continues until an estimated brain temperature of 14° C is reached. Circulation and ventilation is then discontinued and blood from the heart is drained into the pump reservoirs. The surgeon now has a dry, still heart on which to operate. When the surgery is com-pleted the circulation is restarted and the heat exchanger is used for warming the blood. The anæsthetic management is discussed by Benazon[19] and presents no unusual problems.

Cardiac Resuscitation*

A great advance has been made in the management of acute circulatory arrest by the demonstration that cardiac massage can be carried out effectively through the closed chest.[20] Any trained

* See also Chapter 10, p. 290.

person can maintain a circulation in sudden arrest whilst further aid is fetched. Milstein has discussed the implications and outlines a model procedure.[21]

A supply of oxygenated blood to the brain must be restarted. This will require both ventilation of the lungs and cardiac massage. The patient should be placed flat on a firm surface preferably with the head low and the legs raised. This should return some venous blood to the heart. Some vigorous thumps are given to the præcordium. This has been reported as a stimulus capable of restarting the heart. The airway must be cleared and the chest inflated by mouth to mouth respiration. Inflation of the lungs may restart the heart. Success is shown by a return of the pulse, an improvement in colour and a contraction of the pupils. If there is not an immediate response external cardiac massage is started. Stand to the side of the patient. Place one hand on the end of the sternum. Press vertically down on this hand with the other using the weight of the body so that the sternum is compressed 3–4 cm towards the spine. The compression and relaxation should be repeated 60 times a minute. Ventilation of the lungs must be carried out as sternal compression does not produce an adequate gas exchange. If single-handed, the operator must interrupt the massage once a minute to give 2 or 3 mouth to mouth respirations. When assistance arrives ventilation can be continuous and if possible give oxygen by using a bag and mask. The adequacy of the restorative measures is estimated by an improvement in the colour of the patient and contraction of the pupil. A peripheral pulse may be felt in time with the massage.

A differential diagnosis between cardiac asystole and ventricular fibrillation must now be made. This can only be done by an electrocardiogram. Asystole is treated by intravenous drugs. There is no need to use the difficult and dangerous intracardiac route as an effective circulation is being kept up. 10 ml of a 1% solution of calcium chloride may be successful in restarting the heart; alternatively, 10 ml of saline containing 1 mg of adrenaline may be used. If an external pacemaker is available it may be used to stimulate the heart. Ventricular fibrillation will require electrical defibrillation, but it is useless to attempt this until the heart muscle has been well oxygenated by good massage. If cardiac massage is not producing a strong coarse fibrillation as seen in the electrocardiogram an intravenous injection of adrenaline may improve cardiac activity and prepare the heart for defibrillation.

The external defibrillator requires a greater voltage and current than those used when the electrodes are in direct contact with the heart. Large electrodes are applied to the chest at the upper and lower ends of the sternum. These electrodes must be well insulated as voltages of up to 700 volts may be required. The current is alternating and is passed for 0·1–0·2 seconds. If one shock is unsuccessful a series of 3 or more in quick succession can be tried. If an external defibrillator is not available a thoracotomy is required to permit the use of the ordinary machine. This thoractomy must be rapid because external massage must be interrupted, but there is sufficient time for sterile preparations.

There are few contra-indications to the use of external cardiac massage. After cardiac surgery it may not be successful. The heart is normally held in position by the pericardium, but should this have been widely opened the only effect of compression may be to dislocate the heart. Arrest after severe hæmorrhage may require rapid transfusion into the aorta or heart in order for massage to be successful. Cardiac tamponade is best relieved by opening the pericardium. Arrest after air embolism requires aspiration of the air and froth from the chambers that have been filled. All these cases require thoractomy.

There is a risk that ribs may be fractured by the forcible compression. This is a small price to pay if life is restored, but it emphasizes the need for confident diagnosis of arrest before employing heroic treatment.

References

1. NOSWORTHY, M. D. (1941). Anæsthesia in chest surgery, with special reference to controlled respiration and cyclopropane. *Proc. R. Soc. Med.*, **34**, 479.
2. GRAY, T. C., and HALTON, J. (1946). A milestone in anæsthesia? (d-tubocurarine chloride). *Proc. R. Soc. Med.*, **39**, 400.
3. DELORME, E. J. (1952). Experimental cooling of the blood stream. *Lancet*, **2**, 914.
4. SWAN, H., ZEAVIN, I., HOLMES, J. H., and MONTGOMERY, V. (1953). Cessation of circulation in general hypothermia. *Ann. Surg.*, **138**, 360.
5. DREW, C. E., KEEN, G., and BENAZON, D. B., (1959). Profound hypothermia. *Lancet*, **1**, 745.
6. DREW, C. E., and ANDERSON, I. M. (1959). Profound hypothermia in cardiac surgery. *Lancet*, **1**, 748.
7. DREW, C. E. (1961). Profound hypothermia in cardiac surgery. *Brit. med. Bull.*, **17**, 37.
8. MELROSE, D. G. (1953). A mechanical heart-lung for use in Man. *Brit. med. J.*, **2**, 57.
9. KIRKLIN, J. W., DESHANE, J. W., PATRICK, R. T., DONALD, D. E., HETZEL, P. S., HARSHBARGER, H. G., and WOOD, E. H. (1955). Intracardiac surgery with the aid of a mechanical pump oxygenator system (Gibbon type). Report of eight cases. *Proc. Mayo. Clin.*, **30**, 201.
10. GOTT, V. L., DEWALL, R. A., PANETH, M., ZUHDI, M. N., WEIRICH, W., VARCO, R. L., and LILLEHEI, C. W. (1957). A self-contained, disposable oxygenator of plastic sheet for cardiac surgery. *Thorax*, **12**, 1.

11. Howell, W. H., and Holt, E. (1918). Two new factors in blood coagulation—heparin and pro-antithrombin. *Amer. J. Phys.*, **47**, 328.
12. Little, D. M., Jr., and Sutton, G. C. (1955). Succinylcholine-nitrous oxide anæsthesia for mitral commissurotomy. *Canad. Anæsth. Soc. J.*, **2**, 156.
13. Gray, T. C., and Riding, J. E. (1957). Anæsthesia for mitral valvotomy: the evolution of a technique. *Anæsthesia*, **12**, 129.
14. Hutchinson, R. (1961). Awareness during surgery: a study of its incidence. *Brit. J. Anæsth.*, **23**, 463.
15. Dawson, B., Theye, R. A., and Kirklin, J. W. (1960). Halothane in open cardiac operations. *Anesth. Analg.*, **39**, 59.
16. Hodgson, D. C., and Parkhouse, J. (1961). Management of anæsthesia during profound hypothermia. *Brit. J. Anæsth.*, **23**, 303.
17. Nixon, P. G. F., Grimshaw, V. A., and Wooler, G. H. (1960). Clinical observations on vasomotor reflexes. *Lancet*, **2**, 1429.
18. Baker, J. B. E., Bentall, H. H., Dreyer, B., Melrose, D. G. (1957). Arrest of isolated heart with potassium citrate. *Lancet*, **2**, 555.
19. Benazon, D. (1960). The experimental and clinical use of profound hypothermia. *Anæsthesia*, **15**, 134.
20. Kouwenhoven, W. B., Jude, J. R., and Knickerbocker, D. G. (1960). Closed chest cardiac massage. *J. Amer. med. Ass.*, **137**, 1064.
21. Milstein, B. B. (1961). Cardiac resuscitation. *Brit. J. Anæsth.*, **33**, 498.

CHAPTER 7

ANÆSTHESIA FOR DIAGNOSTIC PROCEDURES

T. B. BOULTON

*General Considerations—Anæsthesia for Radiological Procedures
—Cardiac Catheterisation—Angiocardiography—Aortography—
Angiography—Bronchography—Tracheography—Hysterosalpin-
gography—Anæsthesia for Endoscopy—Bronchoscopy—Direct
Laryngoscopy—Bronchospirometry—Œsophagoscopy—Gastro-
scopy—Cystoscopy—Sigmoidoscopy.*

THE last decade has witnessed the increasing use of general anæsthesia as an aid to diagnostic procedures. There are several reasons
for this tendency: general anæsthesia is more comfortable for the
patient than local analgesia, it often enables the diagnostician to
"have a longer look", "get a better view", or to "take a better
picture", thus facilitating a more accurate diagnosis. Anæsthetists,
moreover, have given increasing thought to the requirements and
hazards of the various investigations.[1, 2] General anæsthesia is
indicated when the patient is uncoöperative or apprehensive, when
the procedure is uncomfortable or painful, to prevent movement of
the patient or to minimize some symptom due to the procedure
itself.[1] It is well to remember that most of these procedures have a
morbidity and perhaps a mortality of their own;[3-12] the anæsthetist
must, therefore, endeavour to ensure that the administration of an
anæsthetic neither increases the patient's symptoms nor decreases
his chance of ultimate survival. Many investigations are frightening
and uncomfortable rather than actually painful; it may well be that
the future may see an increasing use of hypnosis in this field as has
already been anticipated.[13] Before embarking on anæsthesia careful
consideration must be given both to the condition of the patient,
which may be poor because of the disease under investigation, and
to the requirements of the diagnostic technique itself.

Diagnostic procedures may be conveniently divided into Radiological procedures and Endoscopies.

Radiological Procedures

In the past the anæsthetist has often regarded the X-ray Department as a kind of medical Black Hole of Calcutta; a place where he

must perform his duties in a hot, dark room, surrounded by nightmare machines, which possibly give forth sparks and certainly emit dangerous rays, and accompanied by an assortment of physicians and technicians who all too often had scant sympathy for anæsthetic problems. The recent development of the Image Intensifier, which enables the patient to be screened on a television tube in reasonable lighting conditions and reduces the amount of radiation required, and the installation of air-conditioning have done much to reduce the environmental hazards; at the same time an appreciation of the importance of careful anæsthesia has made the anæsthetist a respected member of the diagnostic team.

Modern X-ray machines are effectively earthed and insulated and, while a non-inflammable anæsthetic is still desirable, several workers have disregarded this factor after taking suitable precautions.[14-17] Parkhouse[17] quotes the Ministry of Health Working Party 1956 "In our view the risk of an explosion in the modern X-ray room is easy to exaggerate; in particular we consider the risk of a dangerous explosion where the patient is anæsthetized with open ether in the anæsthetic room and brought in unconscious is negligible."

It has already been mentioned that the hazard from radiation has been reduced by modern radiological apparatus, in addition the use of endotracheal intubation and electronic monitoring apparatus enables the anæsthetist to keep away from the danger area. Nevertheless the radiation hazard must not be disregarded. Inglis[18] showed that, during cardiac catheterization, the anæsthetist received twice as much radiation as the radiologist and ten times as much as the radiographer, although, admittedly, the dose was well inside the permitted weekly maximum. Keen[19] has studied the radiation hazard to anæsthetists in a number of procedures; he concludes that, though the doses received are well below maximum permissible level and possibly harmless, "No radiation is safer than any radiation." The prudent anæsthetist does well to provide himself with the necessary protection, (lead apron and, when necessary, lead gloves), especially if he is frequently working in the X-ray department.

Cardiac Catheterization

Right Heart Catheterization. Right heart catheterization is of paramount importance in the assessment and selection of patients for cardiac surgery. In the last 10 or 12 years it has developed from a haphazard affair with makeshift apparatus conducted in almost total darkness to a carefully controlled and accurately monitored proceeding in reasonable lighting conditions.

Under radiological control a radio opaque catheter is inserted into the right auricle via a superficial vein (most frequently a vein of the right forearm). From the right auricle the catheter may be passed into the inferior vena cava or through the tricuspid valve into the right ventricle and on into the pulmonary vein and its branches. If there are septal defects it may be possible to pass the instrument into the left side of the heart and the pulmonary veins. Pressure tracings and oxygen saturation samples are taken from all these chambers and vessels. Assessment of this data enables the nature and extent of the malformation to be determined. The cardiologist may also require to employ certain auxiliary techniques such as the Valsalva,[20] nitrous oxide[21] and dye-dilution techniques[22] for the evaluation of intracardiac shunts and the application of the Fick principle for the assessment of cardiac output.

Cardiac catheterization is not of itself a painful procedure. It is, therefore, generally accepted that co-operative older children and adults are best handled with the aid of light sedation and distraction accompanied by local analgesia for the actual insertion of the catheter. The problem, therefore, resolves itself into that of the management of young children who cannot be expected to remain quietly at rest in the frightening conditions of the Catheterization Room.

Children submitted to anæsthesia for catheterization may be suffering from grave cardiac disabilities, they may be deeply cyanosed or in a state of incipient failure. Straining and coughing may in certain circumstances precipitate heart failure.[7] The act of catheterization itself can cause dangerous complications including cardiac arrest, gross cardiac irregularities, conduction defects, and acute anoxia due to blockage of a stenosed pulmonary valve with the catheter.[23] Blood sampling may amount to an appreciable proportion of the blood volume of a small child and give rise to hypotension and hæmorrhagic shock.[24] Ventricular tachycardia and left bundle branch block are absolute contra-indications to catheterization and serious consequences may ensue if it is attempted after recent myocardial infarct or pulmonary embolus or in the presence of subacute bacterial endocarditis or Ebstein's malformation of the tricuspid valve.[3, 25, 44]

The measurement and interpretation of oxygen tensions necessitates the inhalation of a constant concentration of oxygen which must not be greater than air. Nitrous oxide and ether[26] will interfere with the estimation of oxygen concentrations by the Van Slyke[27] method and trichlorethylene may also interfere,[28] although Keats claims that this effect is not significant.[6] Eggers[29] refers to a modification of the Van Slyke technique which takes the concentration of nitrous oxide into account.[30] The use of photo-electric analysers obviates the variation due to the use of inhaled gases and vapours.[24] Depression of respiration will decrease oxygen saturation.[31]

Manometric estimations may be invalidated by changes in the intrathoracic pressure if the patient strains, cries, or struggles. In these circumstances cardiac hæmodynamics may be seriously affected, shunts may be reversed, failure may be precipitated, and grave danger to the patient ensue.[24] Anæsthetic techniques which depress the myocardium causing hypotension may also invalidate the test.

The aim of anæsthesia is, therefore, to produce a steady basal level of sedation by a technique which does not impair respiratory or circulatory hæmodynamics and which allows the inhalation of a gas mixture which does not invalidate gas analysis. Rapid recovery is of great advantage to the patient and lessens the anxieties of post-operative care.

Inhalational anæsthesia was employed early in the development of cardiac catheterization, but soon found disfavour because of variable inhaled oxygen levels and interference with the Van Slyke estimation.[28] The majority of workers abandoned the inhalational agents and turned to heavy sedation, with or without intravenous supplementation, accompanied by local infiltration for the venotomy. Rectal paraldehyde was found to be unsatisfactory because of the exhaled vapour[28] but rectal bromethol[7, 18, 28, 32-35] and rectal thiopentone[1, 7, 18, 32, 36] were widely used for basal sedation as were oral barbiturates[35, 37] and intramuscular morphine derivatives.[37] Intravenous supplementation was carried out with thiopentone[28, 33, 34] or pethidine.[1, 7, 18]

Many workers continue to employ basal sedative techniques[37-42] and there is no doubt that good results are obtained. The use of intramuscular thiopentone and hyaluronidase has been described by Keown[7] and of intramuscular secobarbitone by Taylor.[5] The combination of phenobarbitone—$\frac{1}{4}$ grain (16 mg) per stone (6·35 kilos) body weight 3 hours pre-operatively and followed by papaveretum and scopolamine in the relatively large doses recommended by Anderson[43] 1 hour pre-operatively—has proved particularly successful;[44] local analgesia is used for the venotomy and the mixture is supplemented by intravenous pethidine when necessary. It remains true, however, that basal sedation is liable to be unpredictable in depth and duration and the danger of sudden movement is never completely eliminated. Further disadvantages are, that repeated doses of supplements, particularly thiopentone, are liable to produce cardio-respiratory depression,[8, 45] that the airway is not assured, and that heavy sedation will lead to prolonged recovery.

Recent developments have been the use of the phenothiazine derivatives and certain other newer drugs by intramuscular and intravenous injection for basal sedation, and a reappraisal of the use of inhalational agents. In the author's opinion there is much to be said for a return to inhalational methods in the light of the introduction of halothane.

The employment of mixtures containing pethidine and the phenothiazine derivatives for sedation for cardiac catheterization was pioneered by Smith, Rowe and Vlad[9] at the Hospital for Sick Children, Toronto. They use a mixture containing chlorpromazine 6·25 mg, promethazine 6·25 mg, and pethidine 25 mg, per ml in a dosage of 1 ml per 20 pounds (9·05 kilos) of body weight given intramuscularly 1 hour prior to the procedure. A reduction in dosage of up to 25% is made in the case of debilitated patients. In a series of 670 cases, 504 were well sedated, a further 122 moved on insertion of the catheter but were subsequently quiet, 26 were controlled after supplementary injections of the mixture via the catheter, and 18 cases, early in the series, were restless during the procedure but were not supplemented. There were four deaths at or shortly after catheterization, 1 of these was attributed directly to depression due to the mixture, 2 to cardiac arrest following irregularities and 1 to inadvertent injection of contrast medium into the coronary sinus at subsequent angiocardiography. The mixture did not guard against cardiac irregularities, the patients slept for a considerable time postoperatively. Other authors report favourably on techniques employing these 3 drugs.[39,46-48] Gareau, Rechere and Patoine[48] precede the mixture with 0·5–1·0 gr (32·5–65 mg) of pentobarbitone as a rectal suppository.

Ordish and Mair[49] substitute promazine (sparine) for chlorpromazine in the mixture. They argue that the former drug produces fewer side effects. The dosage employed is pethidine 1·6 mg per kilo plus 10 mg, promethazine 0·8 mg per kilo plus 5 mg, and promazine 0·8 mg per kilo, given intramuscularly 1½ hours preoperatively. Pethidine alone is given for intravenous supplementation. The reported series comprises 58 cases without mortality. Two cases required additional sedation (1 nitrous oxide and oxygen, the other rectal thiopentone). The patients slept for a considerable period postoperatively; 2 cases were given nalorphine for respiratory depression.

Lundy[8, 50] has described a complicated technique which he had used successfully at the Mayo Clinic. The sedative drugs rectal thiopentone, intramuscular dromoran, promethazine and alphaprodine are given in carefully timed and balanced dosage with the antagonists levallorphan, bemegride and amiphenazole, and vasopressors. In a series of 133 cases there were 3 deaths within 15 hours of the examination. The patients slept for 2 to 3 hours after the investigation but this was not considered to be a disadvantage.

Hydroxydione was used by intravenous injection to produce a steady state of light hypnosis by Feldman, Robbie and Monro.[31] After pre-medication with pethidine promethazine and atropine, or papaveretum promethazine and hyocine, intramuscularly, a single intravenous dose of hydroxydione 7–10 mg per pound (0·45 kilos) body weight was administered. In 25 of 60 cases nitrous oxide and oxygen was required during the venotomy, but in all but 5 cases no further sedation was necessary. Cardiac irregularities were encountered, but there were no cases of post-operative depression.

It has long been accepted as a general principle in anæsthesia that a steady state is best obtained and most easily controlled by the careful administration of inhalation agents. Anæsthetists have, however, been deterred from using volatile agents for catheterization because of the supposed effect on oxygen saturation values. Recent work has proved that satisfactory conditions can be obtained using standard gas mixtures or air.

Kepes, Livingstone and Escher[24] used a 3 : 1 nitrous oxide-oxygen mixture in 25 cases, following pre-medication with barbiturate morphia and hyocine, induction with vinesthene and ether and intubation. A photo-electric oximeter was used to determine oxygen saturations. These workers point to the advantages of a steady state, an assured airway, rapid recovery and the fact that the anæsthetist's hands can be kept away from radiation.

Keats[6] used spontaneously respired compressed air and trichlorethylene following pre-medication with pentobarbitone, chloral hydrate, pethidine and scopolamine. An ear oximeter was used to indicate that a steady state had been achieved. The Van Slyke[27] method of determining oxygen tension was employed. Experiment showed that a 2% reduction in saturation values occurred when trichlorethylene was used; this represents the anæsthetic concentration of the vapour and did not affect cardiological assessment. In a series of 225 cases there was 1 case of successfully resuscitated cardiac arrest and 4 cases died in the post-catheterization period. A technique using a carefully monitored mixture of nitrous oxide, oxygen and trichlorethylene was employed by Eggers, Stoeckle and Allen[29] in

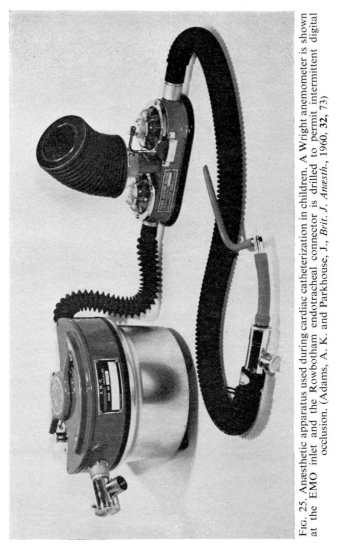

Fig. 25. Anæsthetic apparatus used during cardiac catheterization in children. A Wright anemometer is shown at the EMO inlet and the Rowbotham endotracheal connector is drilled to permit intermittent digital occlusion. (Adams, A. K. and Parkhouse, J., *Brit. J. Anæsth.*, 1960, **32**, 73)

67 cases without mortality. Norton and Kubota[51] used spontaneously respired halothane vaporized by compressed air.

An important reappraisal of the subject of anæsthesia for cardiac catheterization in children was made in a recent paper by Adams and

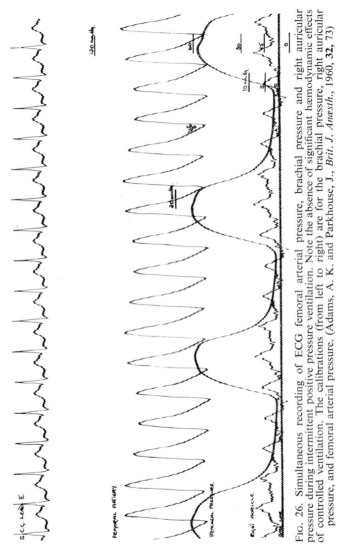

Fig. 26. Simultaneous recording of ECG femoral arterial pressure, brachial pressure and right auricular pressure during intermittent positive pressure ventilation. Note the absence of significant hæmodynamic effects of controlled ventilation. The calibrations (from left to right) are for the brachial pressure, right auricular pressure, and femoral arterial pressure. (Adams, A. K. and Parkhouse, J., *Brit. J. Anæsth.*, 1960, **32**, 73)

Parkhouse.[52] These workers have devised an inhalational method which provides a reliable steady state without interfering with the test, facilitates the use of several ancillary diagnostic techniques and allows a rapid recovery. The method employs light anæsthesia with air and ether-halothane azeotrope[53] delivered by controlled ventilation from the E.M.O. draw-over inhaler modified to deliver a known concentration of azeotrope (Fig. 25). The patients are pre-medicated with phenergan 0·5 mg and pethidine 1 mg per pound (0·45 kilos). They are then induced with azeotrope or thiopentone and intubated with the aid of succinyl choline or flaxedil. They are, thereafter, maintained on azeotrope 0·4–0·6% in air by controlled ventilation with the aid of relaxants if necessary. Arguments and evidence (Fig. 26) are presented to show that controlled ventilation, carefully used, does not affect oxygen saturation or hæmodynamics, nor does the concentration of azeotrope employed appreciably alter the oxygen saturation values obtained with the spectrophotometer. Intracardiac shunts may be demonstrated both by the nitrous oxide technique and a modified valsalva technique, the dye-dilution method could also be employed. Cardiac output can be determined by the Fick principle, minute volume being measured by a Wright Anemo-meter[54] inserted in the inlet of the E.M.O. vaporizer and expired air can easily be collected from the Ruben valve. Recovery from anæs-thesia was rapid. The only deviation in blood gas analysis was found to be that the superior vena caval saturation was often found to be higher than the inferior vena caval saturation; this is the reverse of the usual finding in the conscious state. This phenomenon had been previously described by Fieldman[35] who suggested that it might be due to reduced oxygen consumption by the brain under anæs-thesia.

A modification of the above technique has been successfully employed at St. Bartholomew's Hospital. A halothane-air mixture is delivered to the intubated patient by drawing air through a Fluotec[55] vaporizer by means of an Oxford bellows or AMBU bag fitted with a Ruben valve.[56]

There seems little doubt that carefully administered light general anæsthesia, with controlled ventilation, employing azeotrope-air or halothane-air mixtures from a draw-over vaporizer is the most logical and effective solution yet devised for this difficult pædiatric problem.

Left Heart Catheterization. Left heart catheterization is usually undertaken solely to ascertain the pressure in the left side of the heart.

The pressure in the left ventricle may be measured directly by a needle introduced through the chest wall, either posteriorly on the left or anteriorly on the right,[57] or by means of a catheter threaded through the mitral valve via a needle inserted into the left atrium at the suprasternal notch,[58] or via a catheter passed retrograde through the aortic valve;[59, 60] more recently special catheters have been passed through the interauricular septum.[44] All these procedures may be undertaken under local analgesia provided that the patient will keep still. If general anæsthesia is used (e.g. for children), any reasonable method is acceptable since the question of oxygen saturation estimation does not usually arise.

A needle may also be introduced into the left atrium through the wall of the left bronchus.[61] Wylie and Churchill-Davidson[40] recommend that bronchoscopy for this procedure is best undertaken under local analgesia supported by intravenous pethidine or chlorpromazine. They argue that intermittent inflation down the bronchoscope will be required if general anæsthesia is used and this is not practicable nor desirable under the circumstances. General anæsthesia by the insufflation technique (see p. 197) has, however, been successfully employed.[62]

Angiocardiography

The technique involves the injection of radio-opaque material into the blood stream so that, by means of successive exposures automatically controlled or by cine-angiography, the passage of the medium through the chambers of the heart may be studied. The contrast medium may be introduced, either via a cannula placed in a large superficial vein, or through the cardiac catheter directly into individual chambers of the heart (selective angiocardiography). Careful study of the sequence of filling and the dilution of medium in the various chambers will enable the radiologist to determine the nature of the cardiac malformation. This study often follows directly upon catheterization although some workers suggest a time interval of at least a week between the two investigations.[63]

The injection of the contrast medium produces unpleasant symptoms for the patient—dizziness, nausea, a sensation of warmth accompanied by throbbing in the head and faintness, and a feeling of suffocation with a desire to cough. Most adults and adolescents will, however, tolerate angiocardiography under sedation, local analgesia being administered for insertion of the cannula or catheter. Improvement in radio-opaque media has greatly contributed to the comfort of the conscious patient. If the investigation is undertaken in younger children, general anæsthesia is usually considered to be necessary and humane.

The chief hazard which confronted earlier workers was the coughing and bronchospasm with subsequent anoxia and dangerous alteration in hæmodynamics which followed the injection of the contrast medium.[33, 34, 64] In recent years three factors have contributed to increased safety—first the introduction of newer contrast media with fewer side effects, second the use of muscle relaxants, and third the use of endotracheal intubation.

The newer triodated agents—sodium diatrizoate (Hypaque, Urograffin), sodium acetrizoate (Diaginol)—produce fewer side effects and are much safer than the older drugs—diodone (Diodrast), and iodoxyl (Uroselectan, Neo-iopax)—both of which produced bronchospasm and other allergic effects, although of the two iodoxyl was considered to be the safer drug.[64] Pre-operative sensitivity testing[65, 66] of contrast media has, except in a few cases,[65] proved to be of little value. Serious reactions have followed in patients who showed no reaction to the test dose.[4, 64, 67] It is, however, often considered wise to study the effect of a small intravenous test dose at the actual time of the investigation immediately prior to the larger injection required for the actual angiocardiography.[44] The use of an anti-histamine (e.g. promethazine), either as part of the premedication or as part of the anæsthetic technique, is a wise precaution.

Complete muscle paralysis during the injection of the contrast medium has been found to eliminate bronchospasm.[68] Hay and Rees[37] draw attention to the similarity between the "bronchospasm" following the injection of contrast media and the "bronchospasm" following the inhalation of an irritant vapour; they suggest that the same receptors may be involved in both cases, and stress the fact that the paralysis of striated muscle relieves the condition. In their opinion this may indicate that anæsthetists should revise their views of the nature of the phenomenon of "bronchospasm".

The introduction of suxamethonium has greatly facilitated intubation. Cope[65] writing in 1953, and Carlsson and Wahlin[69] in a recent paper, deprecate the use of intubation in angiocardiography because of the dangers of bronchospasm and cardiac irregularities, but many anæsthetists regard intubation as an essential or useful part of their technique. Intubation ensures control of the airway, facilitates controlled ventilation and enables the anæsthetist to keep his hands away from radiation. Carlsson and Wahlin[69] investigated the possible hazards of the inflation of the stomach which frequently occurs when a tube is not used, but they conclude that the danger of altering the hæmodynamic state of the patient by this means is negligible.

The use of small doses of thiopentone to control coughing was advocated by Cope in 1953;[65] some present day workers continue to use this drug for this purpose.[46] Basal medication with promethazine-pethidine-chlorpromazine mixtures will control broncho-spasm without the use of relaxants,[70] although increments of pethidine[31] or thiopentone[71] may be necessary prior to the injection of the contrast medium. The techniques most used at the present time are intubation and the use of muscle relaxant and controlled ventila-tion throughout the procedure[37, 40] and the administration of a single dose of suxamethonium immediately prior to the injection of the contrast medium,[68] the patient being under some other form of anæsthesia or deep sedation (e.g. rectal thiopentone and intravenous pethidine,[68] trichlorethylene,[39] bromethol,[1] or hydroxydione[31].) If the air-azeotrope relaxant technique is used for cardiac catheteriza-tion, the patient is ready for angiocardiography at any time.[52] Norton and Kubota[51] find halothane-oxygen without relaxant satisfactory.

If the contrast medium is injected by means of a cannula in a peripheral vein, the anæsthetist can help to ensure maximum concen-tration in the heart by control of respiration, the intrathoracic pressure being raised by manual compression of the bag just prior to injection, and reduced, by opening the expiratory valve, as the injection is made. The medium is thus sucked into the heart as a bolus.[37] If a right to left intracardiac shunt is suspected, carotid compression may be practised in order to prevent the concentrated medium passing direct to the brain.[46]

Aortography

Visualization of the aorta and its major branches by the injection of contrast medium is of value in cardiovascular and urological surgery[72] and has more recently been used to study the aortic valves.[73] Radiologists employ two main techniques. The translumbar route[72, 74] in which an injection of contrast medium is made under pressure into the aorta as it lies on the first lumbar vertebra, via a needle inserted percutaneously from a point below the twelfth rib. The retrograde method[75] in which the medium is injected via a catheter introduced through a special cannula inserted per-cutaneously into the femoral artery. The medium may thus be injected at any desired level (e.g. the origin of the renal arteries). The aortic arch and valves may be visualized by injection via a catheter passed down the carotid artery[73] or by peripheral injection into the radial artery.[76] There is considerable controversy amongst radiologists as to the respective merits of translumbar and retro-grade methods,[72] but it would appear to the impartial outsider that the retrograde method, which is simpler and more accurate and can be easily performed under simple local infiltration, is gaining in popularity. There are, of course, occasions when the retrograde method cannot be employed, e.g. in complete aortic obstruction.

Patients submitted for anæsthesia for translumbar aortography are usually suffering from cardiovascular or renal disease or both. They may have hypertension and may well be under treatment with hypotensive agents including the recently introduced drugs bretylium and guanethidine. The combination of these drugs with anæsthetic agents which have a hypotensive action as a side effect (e.g. thiopentone), may cause sudden and dangerous falls in blood pressure. If patients are being treated with these drugs it is well to "wean" them off for 5 to 7 days before the investigation.

Stuart[10] has reviewed the hazards of translumbar aortography in relation to anæsthesia. Paraplegia has followed this investigation. In the past this unfortunate occurrence has been attributed to toxic action of the contrast agent, but it is now thought that the paralysis may be due to ischæmia following intramural injection and dissection of the intima.[77] Other complications have been extravasation of contrast medium, perithecal injection, hæmorrhage, renal failure, convulsions and pneumothorax.[78] It follows that translumbar aortography should not be undertaken lightly,[79] that intramural or periaortic injection of contrast medium is a major hazard, and that the patient must be absolutely still during the injection.

If local infiltration alone is used, the injection of the contrast medium causes various unpleasant symptoms. There is a feeling of warmth and flushing and there may be a burning pain throughout the abdomen; there may also be nausea, vomiting and faintness.[78] Even the newer contrast agents may cause these symptoms. The discomfort may compel the most controlled patient to make involuntary movements leading to intramuscular or perivascular injection.[72]

General anæsthesia for translumbar aortography has long been popular with British anæsthetists. A frequently used technique is, induction with thiopentone followed by suxamethonium and intubation, maintenance with nitrous oxide-oxygen and trichlorethylene or halothane, and a further injection of suxamethonium followed by controlled ventilation at the time of injection and radiography.

American workers are less ready to use general anæsthesia.[78] This appears to be due to unhappy experiences with thiopentone alone in the unintubated prone patient with all the dangers of consequent respiratory depression, obstruction, laryngospasm and regurgitation.[78, 80, 81]

Spinal analgesia or epidural anæsthesia are often regarded as the methods of choice in the United States.[82, 83] A block to the level of the fifth thoracic segment is necessary and this may cause hypotension and require the use of vasopressors. The main objection to these techniques is medico-legal.[10] If paraplegia should result, the syndrome may well be attributed to spinal anæsthesia rather than angiography.

Pinet[76] has described a technique of retrograde aortography through a cannula placed in the radial artery. A catheter is not used. Trimetaphan (Arfonad) 10–30 mg is administered prior to injection reducing the blood pressure and facilitating the retrograde flow of opaque medium. Pinet states that general anæsthesia is not essential, but that it is useful in lessening the subjective symptoms of hypotension and covering the insertion of the trocar.

Angiography

Other arterial and venous angiographic procedure, e.g. femoral angiography, are usually performed by direct or percutaneous puncture under local analgesia or routine general anæsthesia. A recent development has been lymphangiography. In this technique a dye (patent blue), is first injected into the webs of the fingers or toes; it is absorbed into the lymphatic vessels, one of which is then dissected out and injected with contrast medium. The anæsthetist must be prepared for the whole patient to turn blue if the investigation is prolonged. He must not, however, be led to attribute true cyanosis to the dye as has been known to happen on at least one occasion.[84]

Neurosurgical Investigations

Cerebral angiography, encephalography and ventriculography are dealt with in the chapter on neurosurgery (p. 127).

Bronchography

In this investigation contrast medium is introduced into the bronchial tree in order that its structure may be studied on the radiograph. Bronchography is at the present time less frequently necessary than in the past. This is chiefly because the antibiotic era has reduced the incidence of bronchiectasis and the number of cases requiring surgery for tuberculosis. If good pictures are to be obtained there must be careful co-operation between the anæsthetist and the surgeon or radiologist. Not only must the anæsthetist share the airway with the investigator, but he must also make himself aware of the precise conditions of timing and posturing in the particular technique employed.[85]

Patients presented for bronchography may well be poor risk cases.[85] They may be suffering from diminished pulmonary reserve and have a considerable amount of sputum. Pre-operative postural drainage for several days before the investigation must form a part of all techniques, particularly those where preliminary bronchoscopy is not routinely employed.[17, 40]

Lipiodol (iodised poppy oil), was formerly the principal contrast medium used. This agent has two main disadvantages: it tends to run rapidly from bronchi to alveoli thus confusing the picture, and it persists for several weeks as a radio-opaque substance thus preventing repeat bronchoscopy if this be required. Dinosil[86] was first introduced as a watery suspension; this has less tendency to flow into the alveoli and is absorbed in 6 to 8 hours. It is, however, more irritant to the bronchial tree than Lipiodol. Dinosil 60, an oily suspension, is less irritant than the watery suspension. The opaque medium is quickly absorbed and does not obliterate the picture with alveolar spill. The oil will, however, persist in the alveoli for some weeks.[62] The introduction of dinosil, together with a reduction in the amount of contrast medium injected, has considerably reduced the danger of iodism and other toxic reactions in present day bronchography.

Most workers use minimal local analgesia for bronchography in adults. The procedure need not be unduly uncomfortable.[40, 87] Injection through the crico-thyroid membrane[88] is now little used.[39] The contrast medium is injected over the back of the tongue blind, or with the aid of a mirror or laryngoscope,[40, 89] or by means of a catheter passed into the trachea via the mouth[90] or nose.[87] Only minimal anæsthesia is required.[87] Techniques requiring complete topical anæsthesia are neither necessary nor desirable because of the danger of toxic reaction.[12, 91, 92] Belinkoff[90] reports that the intravenous injection of nisentil depresses the pharyngeal and laryngeal reflexes facilitating laryngoscopy and tracheal catheterization for bronchography.

Some workers use general anæsthesia in adults either because they are concerned with the toxic dangers of local anæsthesia[93] or because of poor patient acceptance of local anæsthesia by certain races[85] or individuals.[16, 93] Jooste[85] reports 100 cases of successful bronchography on adult negroes with the aid of an insufflation technique similar to that described later for bronchoscopy (see p. 197). After bronchoscopy under thiopentone and succinyl choline the patient is hyperventilated with oxygen and intubated. A tube about two sizes smaller than would have been used for ordinary anæsthesia is employed in order to ensure adequate retrograde flow of insufflated oxygen. The patients are kept completely apnœic by intermittent injection of succinyl choline. An insufflated flow of $1-1\frac{1}{2}$ L of oxygen was found to secure adequate oxygenation for at least 10 minutes, but there was a gradual rise of carbon dioxide tension; this did not harm the patients in any way. The contrast medium was injected via a catheter inserted through a hole in the proximal end of the endotracheal tube. In another method[93] bronchoscopy is performed under thiopentone and succinyl choline, spontaneous respiration is then allowed to return and the medium injected through the bronchoscope by means of a catheter. Shane and Ashman[16] use a cyclopropane-nitrous oxide-oxygen mixture, injecting the contrast agent into the spontaneously respiring patient through the elbow of the endotracheal connector.

Bronchography can be carried out on children without anæsthesia or under local anæsthesia,[40, 94] but it is generally agreed that a general anæsthetic is desirable both because it is kinder and because coughing and struggling can ruin the picture.[40]

It is probably true to say that the most frequently used techniques at the present time are those based on that described by Baker.[95] The following routine is typical and satisfactory: a Cobbs adaptor is used, a gum elastic or polythene catheter is marked prior to intubation in such a way that it will just protrude beyond the end of the endotracheal tube when the mark is at the suction opening of the Cobbs adaptor. The child is premedicated with the appropriate dose of papaveretum and hyocine,[43, 96] induced with nitrous oxide-oxygen and trilene or halothane or 2·5% thiopentone and intubated after relaxation with succinyl choline. The patient is positioned on the operating table and the bronchial tree aspirated with a suction catheter; a dose of succinyl choline is given,[68, 96, 97] the lungs are inflated with oxygen, the contrast medium is injected with the measured catheter, the patient rapidly postured,[40] and the X-rays taken with the patient apnœic. Cyanosis will not occur if the patient has been well oxygenated.[40] The patient is again inflated with oxygen and then, when spontaneous respiration returns, thorough aspiration is performed. The patient is turned on the side, oxygenated, and extubated when the cough reflex returns. Some workers prefer a heavier pre-medication, e.g. with rectal thiopentone,[40, 96] but this delays recovery. Others recommend atropine alone[16] to ensure a speedy return of consciousness and this is certainly advisable in poor risk patients.[40] In some techniques the medium is injected while the patient is breathing spontaneously or controlled under deep ether,[46] although the latter will delay recovery, Shane[16] uses a nitrous oxide-oxygen-cyclopropane mixture and reports rapid recovery. Macintosh, Mushin and Lake,[98, 99] writing in 1950, objected to the method of injecting contrast medium through the endotracheal tube by means of a catheter because it was liable to obstruct a large proportion of the available airway; they recommended that the catheter alone be passed through the cords. The writer has not found obstruction of the lumen of the tube by the catheter to be a problem especially since the introduction of suxamethonium into the technique[68] means that the patient is apnœic, and therefore not respiring through the tube, at the time of injection. If obstruction of the lumen of the tube is considered to be a hazard, an endotracheal tube with a side tube for the introduction of the medium can be obtained[97, 100] or improvised[101, 102] and enables the anæsthetist to retain control of the airway.

An alternative method is the so-called "drowning technique" originally described by Jacoby and Keats[103] in 1938 and reintroduced in a modified form by Temple and Gray[104] in 1950. Parkhouse[17] has carefully analysed the results of 500 cases in which this technique was employed in an exhaustive review article on bronchography under general anæsthesia. The results obtained have been very satisfactory; there was no mortality and few complications. At least 2 weeks postural drainage precedes the investigation. Pre-medication is with atropine alone; the patient is induced with a small dose of thiopentone ethyl chloride or vinesthene and rapidly taken to the third plane of the third stage of etherization. The child is allowed to breathe air until anæsthesia just begins to lighten. The mouth is opened and 20–30 mg of oily dinosil are tipped over the back of the tongue and inhaled by the patient. As soon as inhalation has occurred an anteroposterior and right and left oblique films are exposed followed by a second anteroposterior. No posturing is required since the contrast medium is sucked into the lungs and rapidly fills the whole bronchial tree. As soon as the pictures have been taken the child is laid prone across a trolley with his head hanging down and his back is then percussed. The cough reflex returns rapidly and the bulk of the medium is expectorated.

Tracheography

This investigation consists in the injection of a small quantity of radio-opaque medium into the trachea. In infants this may be done without anæsthesia by means of a small plastic catheter passed through the cords with the aid of a laryngoscope. In older children an agent which does not depress respiration (e.g. ether) is desirable. Thorough elimination of surplus material by suction and posturing is essential at the conclusion of the procedure.[46]

Hysterosalpingography

This investigation is often performed under general anæsthesia for convenience. Measday has compared the results of a series under general anæsthesia with one without anæsthesia.[105] He comes to the conclusion that general anæsthesia should not be used, as discomfort during the test may well be a valuable warning sign.

Endoscopies

There is little doubt that endoscopy through the various orifices of the body without anæsthesia or under local analgesia alone can at times be painful, uncomfortable, frightening or embarrassing. General anæsthesia can, moreover, usually provide better operating conditions for the endoscopist. It is not surprising, therefore, that in Britain and other countries where specialist anæsthesia is readily available, there has, of late, been increasing use of general anæsthetic techniques without detriment to safety. Where expert anæsthesia is not on hand or where the endoscopist works alone for economic or other reasons local analgesia will remain the method of choice.

Bronchoscopy

This procedure presents a challenge to the anæsthetist or bronchoscopist as it necessitates actual or potential interference with oxygenation. Introduction of the bronchoscope into the lower lobe bronchus may confine gaseous exchange to a fraction of the available lung tissue. The hazard is all the greater because the patient may already have impaired pulmonary function because of the very disease for which the bronchoscopy is indicated.

Bronchoscopy can be an unpleasant or terrifying procedure for the conscious patient; patients who have undergone bronchoscopy under local anæsthesia often refuse repeat bronchoscopies and this may be a very real bar to the subsequent study of the disease.[106-108] Fairlie, in a careful study of patients who had undergone bronchoscopy under both general and local anæsthesia, revealed an overwhelming patient preference for general anæsthesia.[109]

The bronchoscopist's requirements are: first that the jaw shall be relaxed to facilitate instrumentation; this can be achieved by local analgesia and active co-operation in the conscious patient, or by the use of deep anæsthesia or light anæsthesia and muscle relaxants; and second, that the very sensitive reflexes of the bronchial tree shall be obtunded by local analgesia, deep anæsthesia, or relaxants. The bronchoscopist may also desire to observe the active or passive movements of the vocal cords, but these may be better studied at another time by simple indirect laryngoscopy with a mirror.[109]

The recent literature contains many papers devoted to anæsthesia for bronchoscopy. There is no clear-cut choice between local and general anæsthetic techniques, since many methods are a combination of both,[110] and some forms of deep sedation are almost indistinguishable from general anæsthesia. The anæsthetist must consider carefully whether or not the employment of a particular method in a particular situation is likely to assist the bronchoscopist only at the expense of increased morbidity or mortality.

Local Analgesia

The introduction of satisfactory local analgesics which have a relatively low toxicity (e.g. lignocaine), has been an important advance in topical analgesia for bronchoscopy. The application of topical analgesics to the tracheo-bronchial tree has long been associated with a disproportionate number of reactions, both cardio-respiratory and convulsive, some of which have proved fatal.[111-114] It is generally accepted that most reactions are due to overdose or rapid absorption rather than true hypersensitivity or idiosyncrasy,[115, 116] but while it is true that careful control of absolute dosage and rate of application[111, 112, 115-116] can do much to reduce this danger, it is apparent that certain drugs are particularly prone to cause reactions when absorbed from the bronchial mucosa. Amethocaine, (tetracaine, pantocaine, pontocaine), widely used, particularly in the United States, because of its profound analgesic effect, which is possibly due to its power of penetration to the deeper sub-mucous layers,[115] has been responsible for a large number of reactions.[113, 115, 116, 119, 120] Reactions due to amethocaine are usually sudden in onset and cardiorespiratory in nature, convulsions being less frequent.[115] Steinhaus[121] has reported that while the blood concentrations of amethocaine immediately following instillation into the tracheo-bronchial tree of rabbits are similar to those obtained after injection of the drug intravenously, levels obtained after the instillation of cocaine are relatively lower than those expected after intravenous injection. This difference is attributed to the vasoconstrictive action of cocaine. The addition of adrenaline to the amethocaine does not impair its rapid absorption. Clinical trial confirms the greater incidence of reactions with amethocaine as compared with cocaine.[119, 122] Amongst newer and safer local analgesics 5% cyclaine (hexylcaine) has achieved some popularity;[123-125] Orkin and Rovenstein[123] report one non-fatal reaction in 1,262 administrations and compare the drug favourably with tetracaine. Hughes used 0·5-1% dyclone with satisfactory results.[126] The antihistamine pyribenzamine (Tripelannamine), which has local analgesic properties, has been employed.[127] Kleitsch[127] using a 2% solution of tripelennamine, found that it was necessary to add an equal quantity of 0·5% amethocaine in order to prevent the symptom of retrosternal burning experienced by patients when tripelennamine alone was used.

Lignocaine (lidocaine, Xylocaine, Duncaine), is a topical analgesic which provides a satisfactory alternative to amethocaine and cocaine. Compared with the latter drugs the toxicity of lignocaine is low.[111, 128, 129] It is now widely used for bronchoscopy, particularly in Britain and Scandinavia, both with[131-135] and without[40, 136-139] general anæsthesia. The usual concentration employed is 4%. Jepsen and Kristiansen[136] report a series of 871 cases without reaction using 3-6 ml of 5% lignocaine. Intravenous pethidine was used as para-medication; the authors found that less pethidine was required when lignocaine was employed than in a similar series using cocaine. They attribute this to the central sedative effect of absorbed lignocaine. Firth[135] uses up to 25 ml in his technique.

Pre- and Para-medication for Local Analgesia. Precise control of sedation is easier by intravenous injection at the time of endoscopy rather than reliance on intramuscular or subcutaneous injection pre operatively. The intravenous administration of barbiturates for the control of established convulsions due to local analgesics is of paramount importance, but the use of drugs of this group in pre medication as a prophylactic against toxic reactions is of limited value.[113, 114, 119, 120, 122, 124]

Intravenous pethidine (Demerol, meperidine), injected slowly and intermittently in 1% solution, is a satisfactory para-medication for bronchoscopy.[110, 136, 140, 141] The drug is a good analgesic, has some sedative properties, and reduces the muscular tone of the bronchi. The dose range is from 50 mg to 200 mg in divided doses. The technique is suitable for out-patient work provided that there are facilities for a 2 or 3 hour recovery period, and may be safely used by the bronchoscopist working alone. The amount of local analgesic required is reduced.[110] Occasional cases of respiratory depression may be counteracted by the use of n-allyl-nor-morphine.[140] Nisentil (Alphaprodine), an allied drug, has also been used for bronchoscopy.[90]

The phenothiazine derivates have been used for both pre- and para-medication. The addition of promethazine (Phenergan), to pethidine as an intravenous injection undoubtedly enhances amnesia,[125] but it is doubtful whether the use of the more powerful drugs and their combinations,[112, 139, 142, 143] which are liable to render the patient semi-conscious for some hours,[139,143] has any real advantage. Hydroxydione[144, 145] (Viadril), has also been employed; not only is the recovery period liable to be prolonged with this drug but the hazard of venous thrombosis is also intro-duced.

Some workers have employed muscle relaxants on patients who have been merely sedated and not generally anæsthe-tised.[113, 142, 145, 146] The author feels that while the use of block-ing agents[115, 142] (e.g. dimethyltubocurarine), in minimal doses insufficient to cause respiratory paresis might conceivably be justified if the patient were deeply sedated, the use of suxamethonium to induce paresis on a patient pre-medicated only with morphine sulphate 10–15 mg and methantheline (Banthine) 100 mg.[146] is highly undesirable and to be deprecated.

General Anæsthesia. General anæsthesia for bronchoscopy should relax the jaw, obtund the sensitive reflexes of the tracheo-bronchial tree and permit a rapid recovery of consciousness so that the patient may cough post-operatively to clear secretions from his own airway. There are two ways of obtaining such conditions: the use of very light anæsthesia in combination with short acting muscle relaxants, and the use of light general anæsthesia combined with topical analgesia. If general anæsthesia alone is used, considerable depth is required and this will lead to an undesirably prolonged recovery period. If topical analgesia is used in combination with any form of general anæsthesia, rapid recovery of consciousness is essential in order that the voluntary cough reflex of the patient may be operative. Fairlie[109] believes that topical and general anæsthesia should not be combined, but this is an unnecessarily extreme view except possibly in the presence of copious secretions where the topical may, in any case, be ineffective.[123] Whatever the technique of general anæs-thesia, pre-medication should be relatively light to allow rapid awakening, e.g. atropine alone,[16, 147] pethidine and atropine,[180, 148] or moderate doses of an opiate combined with a belladonna derivative.[132, 134, 149]

The combination of the short acting barbiturate thiopentone and intermittent injection of the short acting muscle relaxant suxamethonium is now widely used. If satisfactory conditions are to be maintained apnœa due to paralysis of the respiratory musculature is inevitable and means must be found for maintaining oxygenation. A number of solutions to this problem have been described: (1) intermittent positive pressure either periodically by means of a

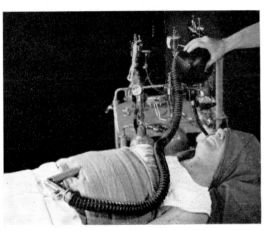

FIG. 27. Use of an inflatable cuirass in endoscopy. The illustration shows application to the chest and attachment to the Boyle's machine. (Pinkerton, H. H., *Brit. J. Anæsth.*, 1957, **29**, 422)

shortened Magill tube fitting snugly in the proximal end of the bronchoscope[150] or continuously by using a special eyepiece with a transparent window which seals the bronchoscope;[93, 151-153] the latter must, of course, be temporarily removed if sucker, or biopsy or foreign-body forceps are to be used; (2) positive pressure by means of a small endotracheal tube alongside the bronchoscope;[108, 154] many bronchoscopists would find the presence of such a tube intolerable; (3) ventilation by positive pressure or positive-negative pressure applied externally to the chest wall and/or abdomen; many workers have employed shell or wrap-round mechanical cuirass respirators for this purpose.[133, 148, 155-158] The "wrap-round" types, e.g. the Emmerson "rain-coat", are considered superior because they are easier to fit especially if the patient is obese; others use simple manual pressure[106, 109] and Pinkerton[132] has devised a useful cuirass inflated by manual compression of an ordinary rebreathing bag (Fig. 27); (4) If the insufflation method[130, 159, 160] is used, no attempt is made to ventilate the patient; oxygen is insufflated through a narrow catheter introduced prior to the bronchoscopy to the level of the carina. Oximetry shows that oxygenation is maintained at a high level, except in emphysematous patients; there is inevitably some hypercarbia but this does not appear to produce any harmful results if the procedure is limited to 10 to 15 minutes[85] although Fairley[109] believes that hypercarbia is responsible for the increased incidence of cardiac irregularities which he observed in patients under general anæsthesia.

It is inevitable that a certain number of patients anæsthetised with the thiopentone-suxamethonium technique will have a vague recollection of the procedure, particularly if they are pre-medicated with atropine alone for out-patient work.[109, 147] Fortunately the recollection is usually very hazy and rarely unpleasant. Brown and Young[147] believe that the patient should be warned of this possibility. Muscle pains following suxamethonium can also be a problem,[109] though the incidence of these can be reduced by the administration of a small dose of gallamine trethiodide with the initial dose of thiopentone.[147, 161] Some workers using the thiopentone[132, 147] suxamethonium technique spray the larynx and trachea with topical anæsthetic prior to bronchoscopy. Fairley[109] deprecates this; the author has, however, never seen this procedure cause trouble, it has the advantage that less relaxant is necessary—in fact the patient may even be permitted to respire spontaneously periodically if insufflation is being used. Topical also modifies the violence of the bouts of coughing which are liable to occur immediately post-operatively after the thiopentone-suxamethonium technique, thus preventing cyanosis and venous congestion but allowing expectoration.

General anæsthesia combined with good topical analgesia has the advantage of allowing spontaneous respiration.[149] The better the topical analgesia the lighter the general anæsthetic need be and the quicker the subsequent recovery; there may thus be some slight advantage in administering the topical analgesic before inducing general anæsthesia,[135, 162, 163] but from the point of view of the patient this is neither necessary nor desirable. Injection through the crico-thyroid membrane, or between the upper tracheal rings, gives efficient analgesia to the pharynx, larynx, and tracheo-bronchial tree with a minimal quantity of topical analgesic. The procedure need not cause the patient any discomfort and has few complications. The injection should be made immediately the patient loses consciousness after the initial dose of thiopentone.[164]

To ensure a rapid return to consciousness it is better to employ an inhalational rather than an intravenous drug[135] for maintenance of anæsthesia. Ether,[46] cyclopropane-nitrous oxide-oxygen,[16] trichlorethylene,[131] nitrous oxide-oxygen with minimal, non-paralysing doses of relaxants,[107, 162] have been used but none have the advantages of halothane.[134, 165] This powerful, non-irritant anæsthetic produces excellent relaxation of the jaw, suppresses the reflexes of the bronchial tree and has a short recovery time.

The following technique has been found to be satisfactory. The patient is pre-medicated $1\frac{1}{2}$ hours pre-operatively with pethidine 50–100 mg, levallorphan 1 mg, atropine 0·6–0·9 mg; this ensures light pre-medication without respiratory depression. On arrival in the anæsthetic room, a Mitchel[166] needle is inserted under local anæsthesia and the head is extended so that the larynx and trachea are prominent in the neck. 100–250 mg of thiopentone are then administered intravenously. As soon as the lash reflex is lost, 2 ml of 4% lignocaine are rapidly injected through the cricothyroid membrane or, more easily, between the upper two rings of the trachea; the patient gives a cough distributing the lignocaine upwards to the pharynx and downwards to the peripheral bronchi. A further small supplementary dose of thiopentone is injected to steady the patient. Oxygen (3 L), nitrous oxide (2 L) and halothane (3%) is administered by mask for 5 minutes. Laryngoscopy can then be performed with ease; the vocal cords being widely abducted, a slender polythene insufflation catheter is passed between the cords. The halothane mixture is now continued for 2 or 3 more minutes. The lungs are inflated with oxygen, the mask is removed and the

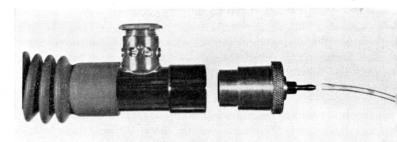

Fig. 28. Insufflation adaptor (Young, T. M., 1956, *Anæsthesia*, **11**, 252)

insufflation catheter connected to the anæsthetic machine by means of a Young's adaptor[130]; 1–3% halothane in oxygen is insufflated throughout the procedure. In robust patients 10 mg (1 ml of a 1% solution) of suxamethonium may be administered immediately prior to instrumentation and repeated as necessary during bronchoscopy; this is usually a non-paralysing dose but, should the patient be apnœic for a short period, the insufflation catheter will maintain oxygenation.

Jackson and Jackson[167] recommend bronchoscoping children without local or general anæsthesia. Although infants may be broncho-scoped without anæsthesia of any kind, the author believes older children should be saved the distress of this procedure and should always be generally anæsthetised. A technique which will allow them to breathe spontaneously should be used. Trans-laryngeal or trans-tracheal injection should not be performed on children. The technique recently described by Brown[134] is satisfactory. After pre-medication with atropine alone (under 2 years), or appropriate doses of papa-veretum and scopolamine[43] (over 2 years), the patient is induced with nitrous oxide, oxygen and halothane. Anæsthesia is continued with halothane and oxygen; laryngoscopy is then performed and the trachea thoroughly sprayed by means of a Macintosh spray[168] passed between the vocal cords. A mixture of 1·5% halothane in oxygen is blown through the side tube of the Negus bronchoscope during the investigation.

The author is of the opinion that, with the exception of the very seriously ill and moribund, the vast majority of cases can with advantage be safely and satisfactorily bronchoscoped under general anæsthesia. Techniques which involve respiratory paralysis and intermittent positive pressure ventilation are contra-indicated in patients with broncho-pleural fistula, tension cysts or superior vena caval obstruction[109, 147] and relatively contra-indicated in emphysema and in the presence of foreign bodies in the bronchial tree.[164]

Direct Laryngoscopy

Cass[169] has reviewed the anatomical abnormalities of the jaw which complicate direct laryngoscopy. These include overgrowth of the premaxilla and alveolar regions, dental overbite, and mandibles with short descending rami with obtuse angles.

All the local and general anæsthetic techniques described above for bronchoscopy have been employed for laryngoscopy. Priest and Wesolowski[172] describe the use of a relatively narrow cuffed endotracheal tube, such a tube would prove inconvenient for many endoscopists. Laryngoscopists should always be on their guard against obstructive pathology in the trachea,[11] apparatus for intubation, bronchoscopy and tracheostomy should always be available.

Bronchospirometry

This involves intubation of the left main bronchus with either a single- or double-lumen tube for the purpose of making quantitative measurements of the lungs individually.[173] The pethidine-topical lignocaine technique described under bronchoscopy is satisfactory.[136]

Oesophagoscopy and Gastroscopy

Although these procedures are frequently performed under local analgesia[127, 172] or pre-[158] or para-[140] medication alone, there is an increasing tendency to employ general anæsthesia.[40 120, 162, 174] Since the airway need not be shared with the surgeon, endotracheal intubation with a cuffed tube should be the rule. Intubation can be performed either through the nose or the mouth. If the latter route is employed, an armoured flexometallic tube should be used; the proximal end of the tube and its adaptor should be placed in the opposite corner of the mouth to that from which the surgeon introduces the œsophagoscope, (i.e. tube on the left for a right-handed surgeon, tube on the right for a left-handed surgeon). If œsophagoscopy and bronchoscopy are to be performed at the same session, œsophagoscopy should be carried out first, the endotracheal tube is then withdrawn by the anæsthetist and an insufflation catheter introduced if required.

The most satisfactory anæsthetic technique is thiopentone induction, intubation under suxamethonium followed by controlled respiration with nitrous oxide-oxygen; respiratory paralysis is maintained with intermittent doses of 1% suxamethonium. 20 mg of gallamine triethiodide should be added to the initial dose of thiopentone to minimize muscular after pains.[161] In cases of achalasial, stricture, or œsophageal bleeding, the same precautions as for a full stomach should be observed (i.e. inhalational induction with ether or foot-down tilt and rapid intubation with the thiopentone-suxamethonium technique). Sellick[176] has described a technique in which an assistant is asked to exert digital pressure on the cricoid cartilage during induction; this manœuvre obstructs the œsophagus and prevents regurgitation.

Cystoscopy and Sigmoidoscopy

Both these procedures can be performed without pre-medication as out-patient procedures. Male cystoscopy requires local anæsthesia to the urethra; lignocaine gel (Duncan Flockhart) from a specially designed disposable tube is useful for the purpose. The anti-histamine tripelennamine (pyribenzamine) has been used for its local anæsthetic effect.[140] Pethidine is a useful para-medication.[140]

General anæsthesia is increasingly used for both procedures, particularly if diathermy is to be employed or biopsies taken. Any standard technique, (e.g. thiopentone induction nitrous oxide-oxygen and trichlorethylene maintenance) may be employed. It is useful to give a small dose of a non-depolarizing relaxant (e.g. gallamine triethiodide) to reduce sphincter tone.

References

1. DUNCALF, D., and THOMPSON, P. W. (1956). *Brit. J. Anæsth.*, **28**, 450.
2. PATRICK, R. T. (1960). *Anesthesiology*, **21**, 553.
3. COURNAND, A. *et al.* (1953). *Editorial, Ann of Internal Med.*, **38**, 1081.
4. DOTTER, C. T., and JACKSON, F. S. (1950). *Radiol.*, **54**, 527.
5. TAYLOR, C., and STOETLING, V. K. (1959). *Anesth. and Analges.*, **38**, 441.
6. KEATS, A. S. *et al.* (1958). *J. Amer. med. Ass.*, **166**, 215.
7. KEOWN, K. K. *et al.* (1957). *Anesthesiology*, **18**, 271.
8. LUNDY, J. S. (1958). *J. Amer. med. Ass.*, **166**, 453.
9. SMITH, C., ROWE, R. D., and VLAD, P. (1958). *Canad. Anæsth. Soc. J.*, **5**, 35.
10. STUART, P. (1958). *Brit. J. Anæsth.*, **30**, 524.
11. HARMEL, M. H. (1956). *N.Y. State J. Med.*, **56**, 1832.
12. DIJKSTRA, C. (1958). *Bronchography*. Blackwell, Oxford.
13. MASON, A. A. (1958). *Modern Trends in Anæsthesia*, ed. Evans, F. T., and Gray, T. C., p. 255. Butterworth.
14. CARNEGIE, D. M. (1951). *Brit. med. J.*, **1**, 1230.
15. CAMPBELL, M., and HILLS, T. H. (1950). *Brit. Heart J.*, **12**, 65.
16. SHANE, S. M., and ASHMAN, H. (1956). *Internat. J. Anesth.*, **3**, 1.
17. PARKHOUSE, J. (1957). *Brit. J. Anæsth.*, **29**, 447.
18. INGLIS, J. M. (1954). *Anæsthesia*, **9**, 25.
19. KEEN, R. I. (1960). *Brit. J. Anæsth.*, **32**, 224.
20. MCILROY, M. B. (1959). *Brit. Heart J.*, **21**, 293.
21. SANDERS, R. J. *et al.* (1959). *Circulation*, **19**, 898.
22. FOX, I. J., and WOOD, E. H. (1957). *Proc. Staff Meet. Mayo Clin.*, **32**, 541.
23. COURNAND, A. (1951). *Bull. New York Acad. Med.*, **27**, 277.
24. KEPES, E. R., LIVINGSTONE, M., and ESCHER, D. J. W. (1955). *Anesth. and Analges.*, **34**, 299.
25. KISTIN, A. D. *et al.* (1955). *Amer. Heart J.*, **50**, 634.
26. COLEMAN, J. F., ZIEGLER, D., and GREEN, E. (1960). *Henry Ford Hosp. med. Bull.*, **8**, 306.
27. VAN SLYKE, D. D., and NEILL, J. M. (1924). *J. Biol. Chem.*, **61**, 523.
28. HOLLING, H. E., and ZAC, G. A. (1950). *Brit. Heart. J.* **12**, 153.
29. EGGERS, G. W. N., STOECKLE, G. E., and ALLEN, C. R. (1959). *Anesthesiology*, **20**, 817.
30. ORCUTT, F. S., and WATERS, R. M. (1937). *J. biol. Chem.*, **117**, 509.
31. FELDMAN, S. A., ROBBIE, D. S., and MONRO, J. A. (1961). *Anæsthesia*, **16**, 217.

32. SMITH, J. A. (1950). *Brit. med. J.*, **1**, 705.
33. GIBSON, J. B. (1953). *Anæsthesia*, **8**, 269.
34. ADELMAN, M. H. *et al.* (1952). *N.Y. State J. Med.*, **52**, 1866.
35. FIELDMAN, E. J. *et al.* (1955). *Anesthesiology*, **16**, 869.
36. CARNEGIE, D. M. (1953). *Proc. R. Soc. Med.*, **46**, 423.
37. HAY, J. D., and REES, G. J. (1959). *General Anæsthesia*, ed. Evans, F. T., and Gray, T. C., Ch 11, 202. Butterworth, London.
38. BLUNDELL, A. E., ANDRIELLO, R. C., and BALBONI, F. A. (1960). *Anesth and. Analges.*, **39**, 499.
39. LEE, J. A. (1959). *Synopsis of Anæsthesia*, Wright, pp. 262, 433, 502.
40. WYLIE, W. D., and CHURCHILL-DAVIDSON, H. C. (1960). *A Practice of Anæsthesia.* Lloyd-Luke, London.
41. COLEMAN, J. F., ZIEGLER, R., and GREEN, E. (1960). *Henry Ford Hosp. Bull.*, **8**, 306.
42. BLAYNEY, A. MC. (1961). *Ann. Meeting Assoc. Anæsth.*
43. ANDERSON, S. M. (1952). *Anesth. and Analges.*, **31**, 262.
44. WEITZMAN, D., and HONEY, M. (1961). *Personal communication.*
45. BEARD, A. J. W., and GOODWIN, J. F. (1956). *Brit. J. Anæsth.*, **28**, 557.
46. SMITH, R. B. (1959). *Anæsthesia for Infants and Children.* Mosby, St. Louis.
47. MITCHEL, F. N., and MINOR, G. R. (1958). *J. Pædiat.*, **52**, 16.
48. GAREAU, P. E., DECHERE, J. P., and PATOINE, J. G. (1960). *Laval Med.*, **29**, 293.
49. ORDISH, P. M., and MAIR, I. M. J. (1961). *Anæsthesia*, **16**, 188.
50. LUNDY, J. S. (1959). *J. Amer. med. Ass.*, **169**, 130.
51. NORTON, M. L., and KUBOTA, Y. (1960). *Anesthesiology*, **21**, 375.
52. ADAMS, A. K., and PARKHOUSE, J. (1960). *Brit. J. Anæsth.*, **32**, 69.
53. ADAMS, A. K., LAMBRECHTS, W. V. DE M., and PARKHOUSE, J. (1959). *Acta. Anæsth. Scand.*, **3**, 189.
54. WRIGHT, B. M. (1955). *J. Physiol.*, **127**, 25 (P).
55. MACKAY, I. M. (1957). *Canad. Anæsth. Soc. J.*, **4**, 235.
56. YOUNG, T. M. (1961). *Personal communication.*
57. BROCK, R. *et al.* (1956). *Thorax*, **11**, 163.
58. RADNER, S. (1954). *Acta. med. Scand.*, **148**, 157.
59. ZIMMERMAN, H. A., SCOTT, R. W., and BECKER, N. O. (1950). *Circulation*, **1**, 357.
60. WEITZMAN, D. (1960). *Brit. J. Clin. Pract.*, **14**, 255.
61. ALLISON, P. R., and LINDON, R. J. (1953). *Circulation*, **7**, 669.
62. HILL, I. M. (1961). *Personal communication.*
63. MEHTA, M. (1959). *Anæsthesia*, **14**, 43.
64. DOTTER, C. T., and STEINBERG, I. (1951). *Ann. of Rœntgenol.*, **20**, 39.
65. COPE, D. H. P. (1953). *Brit. J. Anæsth.*, **25**, 212.
66. TAYLOR, H. K., and MCGOVERN, T. (1943). *J. Amer. med. Ass.*, **121**, 1270.
67. COOLEY, R. N. *et al.* (1950). *Radiology*, **54**, 848.
68. INGLIS, J. M., and ASTLEY, R. (1953). *Brit. J. Radiol.*, **26**, 269.
69. CARLSSON, E., and WAHLIN, A. (1961). *Acta. Anæsth. Scand.*, **5**, 39.
70. ROWE, R. D., VLAD, P., and KEITH, J. D. (1956). *Radiology*, **66**, 344.
71. ASTLEY, R., PARSONS, C. G., and ABREU, A. L. (1959). *Proc. R. Soc. Med.*, **52**, 457.
72. STIRLING, W. B. (1957). *Aortography*, 1st Ed. Livingstone, Edinburgh.
73. SLOMAN, G. (1959). *Proc. R. Soc. Med.*, **52**, 460.
74. DOS SANTOS, R., LAMAS, C., and CALDOS, P. (1929). *Med. Contemp.*, **47**, 93.
75. SELDINGER, S. I. (1953). *Acta Radiologica*, **39**, 368.
76. PINET, F. *et al.* (1959). *J. Radiol. Electrol.*, **40**, 115.
77. GAYLIS, H., and LAWS, J. W. (1956). *Brit. med. J.*, **2**, 1141.
78. MCAFEE, J. G., and WILLSON, J. K. V. (1956). *Amer. J. Rœntgenol.*, **75**, 956.
79. LERICHE, R., BEACONSFIELD, P., and BOELY, C. (1952). *Surg. Gynæc. Obstet.*, **94**, 83.
80. DETERLING, R. A. (1952). *Surgery*, **31**, 88.

81. SMITH, P. G., RUSH, T. W., and EVANS, A. T. (1951). *J. Urol. (Baltimore)*, **65,** 911.
82. ADRIANI, J., and ROMAN, D. A. (1948). *Urol. Cutan. Rev.*, **52,** 653.
83. FELDMAN, E., GREENE, B. A., and CHINN, H. Y. H. (1954). *Anesthesiology*, **15,** 66.
84. TAYLOR, G. W. (1961). *Personal communication.*
85. JOOSTE, K. H. (1955). *Anæsthesia*, **10,** 59.
86. DON, C. (1952). *Brit. J. Radiol.*, **25,** 573.
87. BARKER, J. C. (1955). *Brit. med. J.*, **1,** 1031.
88. ARMAND-DELILLE, P. F., and LEUNDA, J. (1930). *Presse Medic.*, **38, 1,** 378.
89. SALISBURY, B. J. (1955). *Lancet*, **2,** 651.
90. BELINKOFF, S. (1956). *Anèsth and Analges.*, **35,** 246.
91. GUPTA, S. K. (1959). *Brit. med. J.*, **1,** 695.
92. HALSE, W. F., and SCHRADER, G. (1961). *Laryngoscope*, **71,** 211.
93. BERQUO, G., and FICHO, P. C. (1960). *Anesth. and Analges.*, **39,** 523.
94. HUIZINGA, E., and SMELT, G. J. (1950). *Bronchography.* Van Gorcum, Assen.
95. BAKER, A. H. L. (1939-41). *Brit. J. Anæsth.*, **17,** 112.
96. LOVE, S. H. S., and MORROW, W. F. K. (1954). *Anæsthesia*, **9,** 74.
97. MORKANE, C. J. J., and PRAYOR, W. J. (1957). *Aust. and N.Z. J. Surg.*, **27,** 155.
98. MACKINTOSH, R. R., and MUSHIN, W. W. (1950). *Brit. med. J.*, **1,** 1319.
99. MUSHIN, W. W., and LAKE, R. (1951). *Anæsthesia*, **6,** 88.
100. WAY, G. L., and JAMES, G. C. W. (1950). *Lancet*, **1,** 1073.
101. DAVISON, M. H. A. (1950). *Brit. med. J.*, **1,** 1429.
102. BERGER, H. C. (1957). *Anesthesiology*, **18,** 336.
103. JACOBY, N. M., and KEATS, G. (1938). *Lancet*, **2,** 191.
104. TEMPLE, L. J., and GRAY, T. C. (1950). *Lancet*, **2,** 116.
105. MEASDAY, B. (1960). *J. Obstet. Gynæc. Brit. Emp.*, **67,** 663.
106. CUMMINS, C. F. *et al.* (1958). *Anesth. and Analges.*, **37,** 336.
107. REITMAN, T. S. (1957). *J. Amer. med. Ass.*, **165,** 943.
108. ROGERS, F. A., and ERHARDT, K. S. (1961). *J. Thorac. Cardiovasc. Surg.*, **41,** 817.
109. FAIRLEY, H. B. (1956). *Canad. Anæs. Soc. J.*, **3,** 366.
110. KNUDSEN, E. J. *et al.* (1958). *Laryngoscope*, **68,** 133.
111. ANNOTATION (1957). *Brit. med. J.*, **1,** 276.
112. WYANT, G. M., DOBKIN, A. B., and KILDUFF, C. J. (1957). *Canad. med. Ass. J.*, **76,** 1011.
113. GUPTA, S. K. (1959). *Brit. med. J.*, **1,** 695.
114. SEEVERS, M. H. (1949). *Trans. Amer. Acad. Opth.*, **53,** 281.
115. ADRIANI, J., and CAMPBELL, D. (1956). *J. Amer. med. Ass.*, **162,** 1527.
116. HIMALSTEIN, M. R. (1956). *Arch. Otolaryng.*, **63,** 60.
117. TITCHE, L. L. (1961). *Ann. Otolaryng.*, **70,** 128.
118. McKINNEY, J. R. (1958). *Laryngoscope*, **68,** 1814.
119. WEISEL, W., and TELLA, R. A. (1951). *J. Amer. med. Ass.*, **147,** 218.
120. HEATLEY, C. A. (1956). *N.Y. State J. med.*, **56,** 367.
121. STEINHAUS, J. E. (1952). *Anesthesiology*, **13,** 577.
122. TELLA, R. A., and WEISEL, W. (1956). *Arch. Otolaryng.*, **63,** 115.
123. ORKIN, L. R., and ROVENSTEIN, E. A. (1956). *J. Amer. med. Ass.*, **160,** 1465.
124. HULSE, W. E., and SCHRADER, G. (1961). *Laryngoscope*, **71,** 211.
125. PINO, D. M., and VAN HOUTEN, R. J. (1958). *J. thorac. Surg.*, **35,** 825.
126. HUGHES, F. A., BURWELL, J. R., and PATE, J. W. (1956). *J. thorac. Surg.*, **32,** 135.
127. KLEITSCH, W. P. (1959). *Arch. Otolaryng.*, **69,** 45.
128. MULLER, O. V. (1952). *Farmakologi Nyt Nordisk Forlag.* Arnold Busck, Copenhagen.
129. CRAWFORD, O. *et al.* (1951). *South M.J.*, **44,** 1073.
130. YOUNG, T. M. (1956). *Anæsthesia*, **11,** 252.
131. ROBINSON, C. L. N., and MUSHIN, W. W. (1956). *Brit. med. J.*, **2,** 324.

132. PINKERTON, H. H. (1957). *Brit. J. Anæsth.*, **29**, 421.
133. SLEATH, G. E., and GRAVES, H. B. (1958). *Canad. Anæs. Soc. J.*, **5**, 330.
134. BROWN, D. (1959). *Anæsthesia*, **14**, 135.
135. FIRTH, J. D. A. (1960). *Anesth. and Analges.*, **39**, 175.
136. JEPSEN, O., and KRISTIANSEN, F. (1959). *Danish med. Bull.*, **6**, 228.
137. BOUCHER, H., and ROUMAGNAC, H. (1951). *Bronchoscopie, Oesophagoscopie et Gastroscopie*, **2**, 137
138. POWER, D. J. (1957). *Canad. Anæsth. Soc. J.*, **4**, 89.
139. BIENIAS, G. B. (1959). *Arch. Otolaryng.*, **70**, 758.
140. JOHANSEN, S. H. *et al.* (1957). *Danish med. Bull.*, **4**, 16.
141. ALTMAN, M. M., and FIALKOV, G. (1957). *Arch. Otolaryng.*, **65**, 221.
142. WYANT, G. M. (1958). *Canad. Anæsth. Soc. J.*, **5**, 363.
143. GONZALO, P. H. (1957). *Arch. Otolaryng.*, **65**, 13.
144. BOLSTAD, D. S., and DITZLER, J. W. (1958). *Ann. Otolaryng. Rhinol.*, **67**, 1154.
145. BENDA, R. *et al.* (1958). *Dis. Chest.*, **33**, 488.
146. ALVER, E. C., and LEEK, H. (1955). *Arch. Otolaryng.*, **62**, 399.
147. BROWN, D., and YOUNG, J. U. I. (1959). *Brit. med. J.*, **1**, 693.
148. TOKER, P. (1955). *S.A. med. J.*, **29**, 40.
149. MACINTOSH, R. R. (1954). *Anæsthesia*, **9**, 77.
150. CHURCHILL-DAVIDSON, H. L. (1953). *Anæsthesia*, **8**, 128.
151. HERRON, R. A. C. (1950). *Anæsthesia*, **5**, 40.
152. MATHEWSON, H. S. (1956). *Anesthesiology*, **17**, 623.
153. KOVACS, S. (1957). *Anesthesiology*, **18**, 335.
154. LAMMERT, T. K. (1961). *J. Amer. med. Ass.*, **175**, 49.
155. POLISHAR, I. A. *et al.* (1958). *Trans. Amer. Acad. Ophthal. Oto-laryng.*, **62**, 178.
156. BAYUK, A. J. (1957). *Anesthesiology*, **18**, 135.
157. HELPERIN, S. W., and WASKOW, W. H. (1959). *Anes. and Analg.*, **38**, 444.
158. BUCHANAN, D. P. (1960). *Amer. J. Dig. Dis.*, **5**, 121.
159. CHEATLE, C. A., and CHAMBERS, K. B. (1955). *Anæsthesia*, **10**, 171.
160. BUCK, H. A. (1955). *Anæsthesia*, **10**, 313.
161. MORRIS, D. D. B., and DUNN, C. H. (1957). *Brit. med. J.*, **1**, 383.
162. SCHOEMPERLEN, C. B. (1958). *Dis. Chest*, **33**, 617.
163. EVERSOLE, U. H. (1956). *Surg. Clin. of North Amer.*, **32**, 135.
164. ALLEN, H. A. *et al.* (1956). *Anesth. and Analges.*, **35**, 386.
165. MARRETT, H. R. (1957). *Brit. med. J.*, **2**, 331.
166. MITCHEL, J. V. (1962). *Anæsthesia*, **24**, 258.
167. JACKSON, C., and JACKSON, C. L. (1950). *Bronchoesaphagology*. Saunders, Philadelphia and London.
168. MACINTOSH, R. R. (1947). *Lancet*, **2**, 54.
169. CASS, M., JAMES, N. R., and LINES, V. (1956). *Brit. med. J.*, **1**, 488.
170. YOUNG, T. M. (1958). *Anæsthesia*, **13**, 419.
171. SCHWEIZER, O., and HOWLAND, W. S. (1959). *N.Y. State med. J.*, **59**, 3955.
172. PRIEST, R. E., and WESOLOWSKI, S. (1960). *Trans. Amer. Acad. Ophthal. Oto-laryng.*, **64**, 639.
173. CARLENS, E. (1949). *J. thorac. Surg.*, **18**, 742.
174. SPELLBERG, A. (1959). *Gastroenterology*, **36**, 120.
175. SHANE, S. M. *et al.* (1958). *Laryngoscope*, **68**, 25.
176. SELLICK, B. A. (1961). *Lancet*, **2**, 404.

CHAPTER 8

OBSTETRIC ANÆSTHESIA AND ANALGESIA: RESUSCITATION OF THE NEWBORN

The late R. J. HAMER HODGES and M. E. TUNSTALL

Obstetric Anæsthetic Services—Maternal Mortality and Morbidity due to Anæsthesia—Fœtal Mortality and Morbidity due to Anæsthesia—Regional Analgesia for Cæsarean Section—General Anæsthesia for Cæsarean Section—Special Requirements in Emergencies—Anæsthesia for various Obstetric Manœuvres and Instrumental Delivery—Hypoæsthesia or Ataralgesia—Hypnosis—Heart Disease—Eclampsia—The Flying Squad—Relief of Pain in Childbirth—Resuscitation of the Newborn.

ENCOURAGING results have been obtained in this field and the standard of obstetric anæsthesia has been generally raised. Obstetricians and anæsthetists have worked together to ensure that obstetric units obtain specialized anæsthetic services in keeping with modern requirements.

All maternal and fœtal risks associated with obstetric anæsthesia can be reduced by an improved anæsthetic technique and obstetric anæsthetic inter-departmental liaison.[1] As both specialties realize their obligation in this respect avoidable maternal and fœtal deaths will diminish. But there are little grounds for complacency and at the present time an obstetric-anæsthetic service equal to that provided in many general and specialized operating theatres is uncommon in this country.[1] Avoidable maternal deaths still occur and the maternal risk involved when anæsthesia is casually administered to the mother has long been appreciated but also there is now a greater awareness among anæsthetists of the particular hazards to the fœtus of all forms of anæsthesia. Effects on the fœtus of inexpert anæsthesia which can be lethal[2] often go unrecognized.[3] In some centres active neonatal resuscitative procedures are either non-existent[4] or ineffectual,[5] and the responsibility for the organization and institution of such therapy is vague.[6] Much remains to be done, but much has been and is being achieved.

Obstetric Anæsthetic Services

General Principles. The organization of round-the-clock staffing in a modern obstetric unit has been pioneered and fully analysed in the

United States of America by Hingson and his colleagues.[7, 8] Essential requirements are the procurement and maintenance of competent staff, the institution of safe standard procedures, the provision of the right equipment, and an adequate and efficient record system. Facilities for education and research are necessary in order to improve upon anæsthetic and resuscitative techniques.[8] Such services have been associated with a marked reduction in maternal mortality related to anæsthesia.[7-10]

Many practical advantages are to be gained from the participation of anæsthetists in the obstetric team[11] and the obstetrician has enough to do without acting simultaneously as accoucheur, anæsthetist and pædiatrician. Anæsthetists should be available to give advice and assistance in obstetric emergencies and to evaluate and administer supportive therapy in hæmorrhagic and hypotensive states which are important factors in the production of fœtal hypoxia as well as maternal morbidity and mortality.[11] Anæsthetists also are often in the best position to care for the infant after delivery especially during operative obstetrics[6, 11-13] and to keep an adequate clinical record of drug administration and resuscitative procedures in the immediate perinatal period. These records are essential to all forms of research associated with perinatal mortality.[14]

The results associated with the establishment of a complete twenty-four hour anæsthetic and neonatal resuscitative service in one unit have been analysed.[1, 3, 15] The introduction of this service facilitated an extension of the current obstetric policies of greater active intervention in difficult and complicated labours because firstly, any decision to operate was immediately implemented, and secondly, the task of the surgeon was rendered less onerous by the use of a modern anæsthetic technique which was safe for both mother and child. Over a five year period the Cæsarean section rate for the whole district served by the unit was increased threefold and the perinatal death rate was lowered from 39 to 29 per thousand total births. Now that maternal mortality has fallen so low the perinatal mortality rate remains the only figure by which the efficiency of any service associated with overall maternal and fœtal care can be properly assessed. Without exaggerating the significance of anæsthesia in maternal and fœtal welfare, and recognizing that expert and safe obstetric management is obviously the overriding consideration, it can be concluded that a readily available and specialized obstetric-anæsthetic and neonatal resuscitative service is an essential requirement of a modern obstetric department.[1] Such services should become commonplace and must eventually be universally available.[1] These services should be extended through the obstetric flying squad to domiciliary practice and should provide training facilities not only for anæsthetic registrars but for junior obstetric staff also. For those intending to practice domiciliary midwifery instruction in active resuscitation of the newborn and some basic anæsthetic training might well be regarded as essential requirements.

Personnel. Not only must anæsthetic and resuscitative techniques fulfil ideal requirements as regards the mother and child but they must be safe and suitable for handling by "residents" after 3–6 months practical experience of general anæsthesia. Some obstetric emergencies require the initiation of treatment within a few minutes in order to prevent loss of life of the mother or child. This means that resident doctors are essential to a comprehensive maternity service and therefore the techniques taught to and used by these residents must be applicable to all the emergencies they might encounter.

Anæsthetic Equipment. A modern maternity department should be equipped no differently from a general operating theatre, yet many delivery rooms are totally obsolete for operative obstetric deliveries.[16] The obstetric anæsthetist is still called upon to anæs-thetize patients on beds often immobilized in positions incompatible with the safe induction of anæsthesia. The recurring invention of specially designed maternity beds, underlines their deficiencies. If all the essential refinements advocated by discerning anæsthetists in the interests of safety[17] were embodied in one unit then the resultant "bed" would differ little from a standard operating table. The sooner this metamorphosis is completed the better.

All operative deliveries should and can be conducted on a standard operating table in a maternity operating theatre and all minor proce-dures involving anæsthesia similarly. Some obstetricians have had no difficulties in meeting the wishes of the anæsthetist in this respect and the added safety has been appreciated by all.[1, 3, 18] The use of maternity beds should be restricted to normal deliveries and used as a compromise for emergency operative delivery only when absolutely necessary. For these emergencies specially designed beds should always be available and instant control of a tilting mechanism which operates either way is an essential feature[17] (Fig. 29). Cramped and ill-equipped labour rooms do not conform with modern standards for operative deliveries yet in the United Kingdom some maternity units do not contain their own operating theatre, Cæsarean sections being delivered in a general surgical theatre. This may be at some distance removed, and possibly preoccupied, and it still happens that an urgent

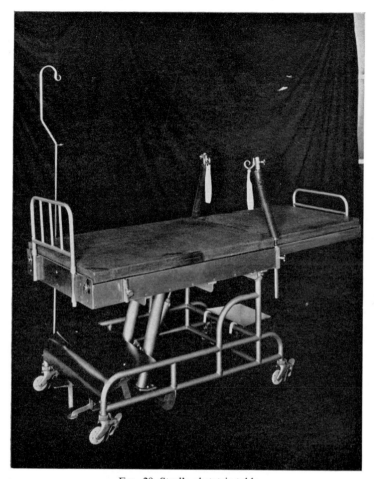

FIG. 29. Steel's obstetric table

Cæsarean section has to wait its turn on a list of surgical acute cases.[19] Most obstetric anæsthetists look forward with impatience to the time when all units have laid their own theatre and the "forceps delivery in bed" will be as dead as the "kitchen table tonsillectomy".

Records. The importance of completing full accurate records has frequently been denied but objections are not valid when records are simplified, systematically completed and methodically planned for a preconceived investigation.[14] The specifically designed punch record card used in the Portsmouth Group of Hospitals has proved invaluable.[14] A thin recording sheet is used loosely attached along the lower edge of the card, separated from it by a carbon so that reduplicated observations can be recorded with the minimum of inconvenience. Subsequently the sheet can be detached and incorporated into the clinical notes of both mother and child. A simple and quick reference to the maternal perinatal state and the first few minutes of the infant's life provides invaluable data for the anæsthetists, the obstetricians and the pædiatricians.[14]

Maternal Mortality and Morbidity due to Obstetric Anæsthesia

Mortality and Morbidity. In spite of some reduction in maternal deaths almost three quarters can still be regarded as primarily due to the anæsthesia.[20] Probably 20–40 maternal deaths due to anæsthesia occur each year in England and Wales.[18, 21] These disasters occur during both major and minor procedures as well as postoperatively after their successful conclusion. All anæsthetics administered to pregnant women especially during labour carry additional hazards, and none is trivial or should be undertaken lightly. Inhalation of vomitus, primary cardiac failure, cardiovascular collapse and convulsions have all been responsible for maternal mortality, and deaths still occur with all the recognized anæsthetic techniques employed, inhalational, intravenous, spinal, epidural, and local infiltration. Most deaths directly attributable to anæsthesia follow inhalation of vomited or regurgitated stomach contents and most avoidable deaths following major obstetric operations are associated with either hæmorrhage or shock.[20] The lack of some obvious precaution such as planned endotracheal intubation[20] or the pre-operative institution of intravenous therapy in emergencies,[22] or the absence of some supportive therapy[23] is often a contributory factor. Anæsthetic deaths still occur as the responsibility of the single-handed obstetrician[20] and it is sometimes difficult or impossible to obtain an experienced anæsthetist at short notice.[19]

Anæsthesia in an obstetric department should be under the control of a consultant anæsthetist responsible for the anæsthesia and the instruction of his juniors and available for consultation by them in case of difficulties.[20] Special attention should be paid to the problems of vomiting and regurgitation.

Prevention and Treatment of Vomiting and Regurgitation. In pregnant women emptying of the stomach is delayed, and hiatus herniation often unsuspected, is an added risk,[24] and many patients present as emergencies. With inhalational anæsthesia active vomiting may occur during induction or post-operatively. Vomiting during induction leads to delay and the risk of fœtal death from maternal hypoxia, if not maternal death. Endotracheal intubation with a cuffed tube is not yet routinely practised[20] and some anæsthetists feel that anæsthesia should be so light that even pharyngeal stimulation with an oral airway would be contra-indicated as likely to provoke reflex vomiting.[16] But operative manipulations or fundal pressure may precipitate the eruption of stomach contents during general anæsthesia and without endotracheal intubation the risk of aspiration is very great.[25]

Spinal anæsthesia may promote vomiting,[26] and passive regurgitation may occur during operation under conduction anæsthesia as with inhalational techniques. Vomiting may be induced under epidural or spinal anæsthesia by a rapid fall of blood pressure, or a rapid rise due to administration of vasopressors particularly in conjunction with ergot derivatives.[27]

Often the central nervous depression, which results when a conduction block is supplemented with other agents[28] increases the risk of inhalational asphyxia.

The oral intake of women in labour should be restricted. When labour is prolonged only fluids and isotonic glucose by mouth supplemented if necessary by intravenous therapy should be the aim.[16] Aspiration of small quantities of acid gastric contents can prove fatal[29] and administration of antacids to reduce gastric acidity has been suggested.[21] Gastric aspiration through anything less than a size 10 œsophageal tube is likely to be ineffectual[16] and in any event can never be a certain means of emptying the stomach. But the reduction of intra-gastric pressure is of course helpful. In one series 19 deaths due to inhalational asphyxia occurred after the "stomach had been emptied pre-operatively" by stomach tube.[25] The initiation of active vomiting by apomorphine has been recommended[30] and has advocates[31] but others regard the safety of this measure as suspect and the procedure unjustified.[3]

The use of conduction anæsthesia decreases but does not nullify the risk of inhalation of gastric contents due to vomiting[7, 26, 23] and this form of anæsthesia is not applicable to all obstetric procedures. The maintenance of light general anæsthesia has in the past been advocated in the sanguine expectation that the patient's own active reflexes protect her in these planes but this is not substantiated by the facts.[32] Various methods of blocking the cardia, œsophagus, and pharynx have been suggested but are unproven in practice. Induction of anæsthesia in the lateral or head-down position has been used in order to minimize the effect of vomiting or regurgitation should it occur, but it would seem more practical to attempt to reduce the incidence of such complications rather than merely try to render them innocuous.

Endotracheal intubation of the mother therefore is inevitably the answer to the problem of vomiting and regurgitation. Intubation protects the mother during the entire operative procedure and if the endotracheal tube remains *in situ* until the patient is almost awake safe emptying of the stomach may be provoked or, if vomiting occurs shortly after extubation, the patient's reflexes and the presence of the anæsthetist should help to ensure the prevention of inhalation.

The problem is now resolved into the avoidance of vomiting or regurgitation in the interval between the commencement of production of unconsciousness and the safe positioning of the endotracheal tube.

With an inhalational induction the risk of vomiting remains until the equivalent of stage II anæsthesia is passed and is only reduced by the smoothness and speed of the technique. With the production of light sleep by a minimal dose of intravenous barbiturate the risk of vomiting is diminished by the extreme rapidity of the induction but the risk is always there and it requires the nearly simultaneous onset of immediate paralysis by a relaxant drug to eliminate this risk.

The risk of regurgitation is minimized by intubating under deep inhalational anæsthesia without relaxants, but this introduces the factor of delay and of drug depression of the fœtus.

While the risk of vomiting prior to intubation is eliminated by induction of sleep with an intravenous barbiturate injection followed immediately by an injection of a rapidly acting paralysing drug such as suxamethonium, the problem of regurgitation remains. This problem can be solved. Recently, for patients paralysed prior to endotracheal intubation, a method of manual cricoid pressure, performed by an assistant, has been advocated to prevent fluid regurgitating into the pharynx.[33] This method shows great promise and it remains to be seen whether it will supersede the convenience and safety of a method which has already been shown to have solved the problem of regurgitation, the steep head-up position.

The Head-up Position. The use of the head-up position during the induction of anæsthesia was first suggested by Morton and Wylie.[34]

The practical safety of the technique has been tested[18, 35] and recently 2,000 such obstetric anæsthetic inductions[3] have been reported without maternal death or serious morbidity and with few technical difficulties. A sleep dose of thiopentone followed immediately by suxamethonium[3] was used and rapid endotracheal intubation carried out, and the interval between the production of unconsciousness and the onset of paralysis was minimal.

No routine attempts were made to empty the stomach nor induce vomiting before anæsthesia in this series. Gastric aspiration in particular instances was only considered necessary in less than 1 per cent of patients and the deliberate induction of vomiting by means of drugs[30] was considered an unjustifiable assault on the mother.

It has been suggested that rapid induction and intubation in the head-up position is a method only for the experienced expert and that its success depends on a degree of sleight of hand.[36] This has not only been disproved by current experiences[1, 3, 18, 37] but in any event major obstetric anæsthesia, conduction or general, should no longer be in the hands of anæsthetists who cannot perform endotracheal intubation, speedily, dexterously and without fail. Patients exist who cannot easily be intubated but are very rare and this possibility is no contra-indication to the technique. In these circumstances the passage of a wide bore stomach tube can be simply performed[38] and as in the single instance in the series of 2,000 patients reported[3] the anæsthetic can be continued with a light inhalational technique without a relaxant. Alternatively Sellick's cricoid pressure manœuvre[33] performed by an assistant could be used while inhalational anæsthesia beyond stage II is established by controlled respiration before the return of any neuromuscular conduction is allowed. No reminder should be necessary of the possible vagal effects of the sudden introduction of an inhalational agent in high concentration to a paralysed patient. A prior check on all equipment particularly laryngoscope and sucker must be carried out routinely and laryngoscopy must never be attempted before full neuromuscular block is established, to avoid stimulation of vomiting before paralysis is complete.[3] This technique of induction of anæsthesia in the head-up position appears to have been reasonably tested in practice and found to protect the mother from the dangers of vomiting and regurgitation.

Treatment of Inhalational Asphyxia and Aspiration Pneumonitis. Should active vomiting occur during induction of inhalational anæsthesia the mask should be removed, the patient turned on her side and a steep head-down position adopted. The jaw should be opened if necessary using force and solid material rapidly scooped away. Suction should be used to clear the pharynx of fluid and oxygen administered. If cyanosis persists the larynx should be visualized, sucked out and endotracheal intubation performed when the trachea is cleared. Oxygen by positive pressure may be needed and the danger of disseminating inhaled solids and fluids must be appreciated, though this may be less than the danger of hypoxia. Should cardiac arrest occur, immediate oxygenation and cardiac massage is imperative. When the immediate emergency is past bronchoscopy and bronchial suction may be performed. If inhalation of gastric contents has occurred the bronchi may be washed out with 10–20 ml of normal saline. Hydrocortisone 100 mg or prednisolone 21-phosphate 20 mg is given at once intravenously and post-operatively a careful clinical watch should be kept for pulmonary œdema associated with cyanosis, dyspnœa and bronchospasm over the next few hours. If very severe bronchospasm and cyanosis occurs it will be necessary to paralyse the patient and institute intermittent positive pressure oxygenation therapy as well as administering further intravenous steroids. The treatment of the subsequent pneumonitis is aided by the administration of antibiotics.

The implication of recent experimental work[39] is that, in all cases where aspiration of acid gastric contents, even in small quantities, is suspected, hydrocortisone 100 mg should be given at once. This should reduce the severity of the subsequent pneumonitis and it is particularly useful in the treatment of severe bronchospasm should it occur.

Fœtal Mortality and Morbidity due to Obstetric Anæsthesia

Over recent years perinatal mortality has remained disappointingly stable. Approximately two-thirds of this apparently irreducible mortality is associated with hypoxia.[4] Factors associated with fœtal hypoxia during anæsthesia have been analysed[40] and recently reviewed and re-assessed.[3] Maternal respiratory depression and hypoxia, maternal hypotension, depression of the fœtal respiratory centre and delay in delivery of the hypoxic fœtus from its intolerable environment all reduce the chances of survival of the infant, particularly in cases of prematurity and frequently in cases of postmaturity, and are all factors which may be produced by analgesia or anæsthesia. The decreased vital capacity of the full term pregnant woman may be aggravated by previous sedation and with inhalational anæsthesia maternal oxygenation may be further decreased as respiratory depression occurs. Loss of vaso-motor control and depression of cardiac output in deep anæsthesia may result in maternal hypotension and decreased placental circulation. In these circumstances even in the presence of high oxygen administration fœtal hypoxia can follow. With cyclopropane there is a depression of oxygen saturation of the fœtal blood.[41] This agent may also have some invidious effects on the fœtal myocardium in the presence of the hypoxia and hypercarbia of fœtal distress.[42] Inhalational anæsthetics, ether, chloroform, trichlorethylene, cyclopropane, and halothane all carry an inevitable risk of drug depression to the fœtal respiratory centre.

The dangers of fœtal hypoxia due to maternal hypotension have been further investigated and assessed.

Hon[43] stresses that while as yet the role of maternal arterial blood pressure in maintaining intervillous blood flow (and hence adequate fœtal oxygenation) has not been fully clarified there is an increasing body of evidence suggesting that it is of paramount importance. The possibility of conduction anæsthesia increasing uterine tone and so further reducing placental flow must also be considered. Maternal hypotension under conduction anæsthesia can be dramatically aggravated by adoption of the supine position[7, 44, 45] which together with the maternal respiratory embarrassment which may follow intercostal paralysis[16] may further aggravate fœtal hypoxia. The prevention and treatment of maternal hypotension and special considerations of fœtal oxygenation are discussed later.

Special Fœtal Dangers in Emergencies. Recently many obstetricians have advocated more active treatment of the obstetric emergencies associated with hypoxia, ante-partum hæmorrhage and fœtal distress, for theoretically the majority of fœtal loss in these circumstances is avoidable. In practice also there is evidence that a higher standard of obstetric care could reduce the mortality in areas where it is high[46] and in ideal circumstances early active intervention in emergencies appears to lead to greater fœtal salvage.[1, 3] To implement this policy safely without increasing the risks of maternal or fœtal death, anæsthetists must co-operate fully in the obstetric team. The special danger to the fœtus in emergencies is delay. The passage of time is, in itself, lethal but this is not the only aspect of emergency deliveries which can concern the anæsthetist.

In many instances urgent operative deliveries are associated with the birth of depressed, often premature infants and immediate resuscitative procedures are imperative. Anæsthetists therefore must provide anæsthetic services and anæsthetic techniques compatible with immediate and safe operative conditions for any emergency operative delivery at all times. Anæsthesia should be induced with the minimum of delay and facilities should be provided for immediate neonatal resuscitation on delivery when necessary. The special considerations of as short an "induction-delivery interval" as is compatible with maternal safety are discussed later.

Regional Analgesia for Cæsarean Section

(*a*) **Local Infiltration.** In the past many women must have suffered the "Cæsarean under local" not as an elective technique but as a direct result either of the obstetrician's mistrust of all forms of anæsthesia or of the complete absence of all forms of specialized anæsthetic aid.

Nowadays if specialized anæsthetic aid is readily available such a procedure is less often justified.

(*b*) **Epidural Analgesia.** Epidural analgesia is the choice of many authorities[16, 47, 48, 49] but the technique requires considerable manual skill and strict attention to numerous details and does not lend itself to occasional use.[49] Lignocaine 22–24 ml of a 1·75% solution with 1 : 250,000 adrenaline is advocated[47] the injection being made through the twelfth thoracid interspace. The use of an indwelling catheter reduces the dangers of inadvertent dural puncture and Foldes uses a mean dose of 24 ml of 3% 2-chloroprocaine with added adrenaline injected through a catheter inserted in the third or fourth lumbar interspace.[49] Others report favourably on the low toxicity, rapidity of action, and high diffusibility of 2-chloroprocaine[50, 51] Supplementation is needed commonly to allay excitement and anxiety, when retching occurs in transperitoneal operations, or to cover inadequate analgesia and is needed in 58·8 per cent of patients.[49] Mackay[28] states that almost all need some form of general anæsthesia during the course of their operation. Light general anæsthesia or the intravenous administration of small doses of promethazine, pethidine, or other agents may be used, but the great advantage of the technique claimed (the lack of drug intoxication of the fœtus) is thereby lost. The risks following vomiting and regurgitation should it occur are also increased. The need to supplement epidural analgesia is an important and disturbing factor.[16]

In the hands of the experienced epidural analgesia is satisfactory for Cæsarean section but there is a definite incidence of failure variously stated from 2·5[47] to 10 per cent.[52]

Anæsthetists undertaking subarachnoid or epidural blocks must not only be experienced and competent in the management of patients under total sympathetic blockade[7, 53, 54] but must be able, and prepared, to give continuous oxygen, if necessary by endotracheal controlled ventilation[7] and the dangers to the mother and fœtus of hypotension must be realized. The prevention and treatment of maternal hypotension is discussed with spinal analgesia.

(c) **Spinal Subarachnoid Block.** Recently there has been a swing away from subarachnoid techniques to the relatively safer epidural blocks. In part this has been due to overpublished litigation which has followed instances of neurological sequelæ attributed to subarachnoid injection. Some authorities, however, still use spinal analgesia for from 44[55] to 95 per cent[10] of Cæsarean sections, and in many areas spinal anæsthesia has been traditionally and safely used for many years. Over a period of twelve years Thorne[55] has seen no major neurological sequelæ. With the patient in the lateral position, 10° head down, subarachnoid puncture is conveniently made in the third or fourth lumbar interspace and "heavy" nupercaine (1/200 in 6% glucose) 1·2–1·4 ml is injected. In North America 6·0–8·0 mg of "pontocaine" in 2·0–2·5 ml of 10% glucose is popular.

Makepeace[56] found that 10·8 per cent of Cæsarean sections conducted under spinal analgesia suffered from post-spinal headaches but the use of a 25 gauge spinal needle has helped to reduce the incidence of this complication to 1 per cent.[57] It is also suggested that dehydration and blood loss during labour are etiological factors in post-spinal headaches and adequate hydration of the obstetric patient is important in this respect.[57, 58]

Conduction techniques sometimes fail, frequently need supplementation, and are contra-indicated in emergencies, maternal hypotensive states, and acute and chronic anæmias.[7, 11, 16, 21, 42, 48, 59, 60] This reduces the validity of the arguments in their favour. When there is good reason for the patient to remain awake or when some positive contra-indication to general anæsthesia exists conduction analgesia is indicated. When there is urgency or the anæsthetist is unfamiliar with epidural blocks spinal analgesia is the technique of choice.

(d) **The Dangers of Maternal Hypotension.** Forthman and Adriani[61] in a series of 391 sections conducted under spinal analgesia noted a degree of hypotension in 82 per cent, with an average systolic blood pressure fall for the whole series of 30 mm Hg and Kennedy[45] noted hypotension in 17·7 per cent of 600 patients under spinal anæsthesia prior to delivery. Lund shows that 10–13 per cent of epidural anæsthesia is associated with falls in blood pressure of up to 50 mm Hg.[62] Fœtal bradycardia occurs after 4 minutes when maternal pressure falls to 80 mm Hg.[53] Tensions of 100 mm Hg may be associated with fœtal bradycardia of a definite hypoxic type within a few minutes.[43] There is little doubt however that if maternal hypotension is sufficiently severe and prolonged the fœtus will die but the significance of moderate degrees of maternal hypotension may not be reflected in the perinatal mortality rates since lesser degrees of fœtal damage may be manifest only by various nervous system lesions which appear later in life.[43] Some authorities feel that maternal hypotension poses no great problem and can be easily corrected[53] but continuous readings of the maternal blood pressure and the prompt correction of hypotension are mandatory if the fœtus is to have the best chance of surviving labour and delivery with an intact nervous system.[43] This is particularly true if the mother has received conduction anæsthesia and labour is being stimulated with an oxytoxic drug.[43] Vasopressors are commonly advised prophylactically, before the block or during injection but if this is done the use of ergot drugs, which may be required as uterine stimulants during the procedure may lead to severe hypertension and headaches,[45] and cerebro-vascular disasters.[63] Foldes[64] therefore uses a continuous intravenous infusion of vasopressor drugs during all conduction analgesia during obstetric procedures and titrates the administration against the maternal blood pressure. This latter procedure would appear to be the most reasonable method of dealing with this particular hazard. The possibility of large doses of vasopressor drugs crossing the placental barrier and adversely affecting the fœtus has to be noted.[16]

(e) **Maintenance of Blood Pressure.** Ephedrine sulphate intramuscularly 25 mg can be administered 10 minutes prior to subarachnoid block for Cæsarean section and has been found to reduce the incidence of hypotension from one in four to one in eight,[63] while 20 mg at the completion of a caudal block almost completely prevented the occurrence of profound and rapid hypotension.[65] This should not be given in the presence of hypertension or toxæmia.[65] Should hypotension still occur it may respond to intravenous ephedrine but this leads to compensatory tachycardia in 25 per cent of patients. With ephedrine or adrenaline; trichlorethylene, cyclopropane or halothane cannot safely be used and cardiac arrhythmias may occur. Methoxamine hydrochloride is free from this danger[65] and 8 mg intramuscularly may be used as a prophylactic dose during conduction block.

The use of a continuous infusion of intravenous vasopressor[64] already mentioned, provides the greatest safety and allows closer control of the danger of severe hypotension or hypertension. Drugs suitable for use in this manner are mephentermine sulphate and particularly metaraminol bitartrate (aramine). This latter vasopressor has replaced a 1-noradrenaline "drip" in many clinical situations and there is a lesser likelihood of local tissue necrosis due to extra-venous injection, or precipitous falls of blood pressure on with-drawal.[22]

Maternal hypotensive states call not only for intravenous suppor-tive therapy but oxygen should be given continuously by mask.

General Anæsthesia for Cæsarean Section

The ideal anæsthetic for Cæsarean section should be applicable to all cases. It has been held that conduction anæsthesia though contra-indicated in emergencies provides, in elective cases, better oxygena-tion and less respiratory depression of the fœtus than general anæsthesia.[42, 66, 67] This view can now be challenged for using light general anæsthetic techniques with complete neuromuscular block full oxygenation of mother and child can be ensured.[3, 15, 18]

"Balanced" anæsthetic techniques[52, 68-72] have been in use since the first reports of Gray,[73] Davenport and Prime[74] but as yet there seems to be no agreement as to the optimum balance and there remains a reluctance to abandon completely the traditional agents for anæsthetic maintenance.[75] Even in minimal quantities ether,[76] trichlorethylene,[64] cyclopropane[42, 72] and halothane[77] have all been shown to be dangerously depressant to the fœtus and the advantages to be gained by excluding these agents from the maternal and fœtal circulation should be self evident. A comprehensive series of obstetric anæsthetics excluding all such depressant drugs and using an anæsthetic technique based on minimal thiopentone, suxameth-onium and nitrous oxide-oxygen only has recently been carefully evaluated.[1, 3, 15, 18]

The head up tilt is used during induction of anæsthesia to obviate the danger of regurgitation, and endotracheal intubation is routinely employed. This technique gave promise[18] of having a higher degree of maternal and fœtal safety than any general anæsthetic technique previously described for obstetrics and latterly over 2,000 obstetric anæsthetics including 1,500 operative deliveries have been analysed.[3] The technique used is as follows:

All patients are pre-medicated with atropine 0·6 mg and when pre-operative fœtal distress or ante-partum hæmorrhage is present the mother is pre-oxygenated. On an operating table in a steep head-up position a sleep dose of thiopentone (usually 200–250 mg) is admini-stered followed immediately by 50 mg of suxamethonium. Uncon-sciousness and neuromuscular block occur almost simultaneously and as soon as muscle fasiculations cease endotracheal intubation with a cuffed tube is performed, and the table is immediately lowered into a slight head-down position. Anæsthesia is maintained with nitrous oxide 6 L/min and oxygen 4 L/min only until delivery and suxamethonium is used to maintain full neuromuscular block, to control reflex movements, and to facilitate controlled respiration. Immediately prior to delivery the patient is inflated with 100% oxygen. After the umbilical cord is clamped anæsthesia may be maintained in any manner convenient to the anæsthetist but is maintained at a light level, however, suxamethonium being used for abdominal closure. All patients have active pharyngeal reflexes before extubation.

Hodges and Tunstall[3] reviewing over 2,000 obstetric anæsthetics conducted under this technique, state that evaluations and comparisons of maternal and fœtal mortality associated with previously used general anæsthetic and conduction techniques are no longer valid. They feel a complete re-assessment is necessary in the light of advances in general anæsthetic techniques. They give their reasons for choice of agents for Cæsarean section as follows:

Atropine. Reduction in vagal tone is essential in operations conducted under light anæsthesia and all general anæsthetics should be preceded by atropine 0·6 mg.

All sedative pre-medication is absolutely contra-indicated. Opiates administered to the mother pre-operatively decrease the incidence of fully active infants delivered and enhances the respiratory depressant effects of prematurity and pre-operative fœtal distress. It is not always possible to minimize pre-operative sedation but deliberate operative pre-medication can and should be avoided.

Thiopentone. Thiopentone should be used neither to produce nor maintain surgical anæsthesia but to ensure smooth and rapid induction to the level of unconsciousness only.

An anæsthetic induction using nitrous oxide-oxygen alone has a theoretical appeal but the likelihood of maternal vomiting and regurgitation with all its associated dangers is increased. Thiopentone ensures a smoother, safer and more rapid induction than is possible with any other technique which completely offsets the minimal effects on the infant which can be disregarded in practice.[6]

Using minimal sleep doses of thiopentone the theoretical danger of hypotension following induction in the head-up position[36] has been of no practical significance in the series of patients reported.

Suxamethonium. Suxamethonium is used because it provides conditions compatible with immediate endotracheal intubation, controls reflex responses in the lightest plane of anæsthesia and provides the shortest possible interval between the production of unconsciousness and the occurrence of total paralysis. Furthermore a large mass of clinical and experimental evidence now confirms the previous observation[18] that the fœtus is completely unaffected. Suxamethonium does not cross the placental barrier except in many times the paralysis dose[78] and in any event the neonate is particularly resistant to the effects of this drug.

D-tubocurarine and gallamine triethiodide are not considered ideal because conditions compatible with immediate smooth endotracheal intubation are not obtainable without high dosage, time factors preclude test doses, significant amounts may cross the placental barrier[79-81] and the neonate is suceptible to these agents particularly. In the mother there has been a tendency to produce a change in response to suxamethonium following prolonged oxytocin administration[82] but further observations[83] suggest that this action is likely to be of practical significance only in prolonged administrations of oxytocin and any residual paralysis responds immediately to the administration of neostigmine.

Nitrous Oxide. Nitrous oxide of all the inhalational agents affects the fœtus and the mother's vital centres least. Nitrous oxide (6 L/min) and oxygen (4 L/min) administered by controlled respiration in a fully paralysed patient is all that is required to maintain analgesia and amnesia once full saturation has been achieved. The induction dose of thiopentone is sufficient to cover the stimulus of intubation and skin incision which immediately follows. It must be remembered that the use of low gas flows, particularly in a circle system, considerably delays the achievement of nitrous oxide "saturation" for any given percentage. The positive advantages of the controlled administration of an oxygen-rich mixture to a fully paralysed patient cannot be too strongly emphasized and such administration prior to delivery leads to a significant increase in available oxygen in the fœtus.[84] The authors do not consider that the administration of any other inhalational agent prior to delivery is justified.

This technique of anæsthesia for Cæsarean section has been used by one author in St. Mary's Hospital, Portsmouth since 1952, and in this unit is considered the anæsthetic of choice at the present time. In the series of 2,000 obstetric anæsthetics reported[3] 654 infants were delivered by section with no maternal or fœtal anæsthetic mortality. In 226 infants when neither pre-operative fœtal distress nor antepartum hæmorrhage was a complicating factor no infant was lost from any cause whatever and the overall perinatal mortality in mature infants in both complicated and elective cases was 1·7 per cent. In all the 654 infants the neonatal morbidity was extremely low and 83·6 per cent of infants established spontaneous respirations within 5 minutes of delivery, more than three-quarters of these within 60 seconds.

Special Requirements in Emergencies, Prematurity and Fœtal Hypoxia

Induction Delivery Intervals. By induction delivery interval is meant the time from the commencement of the thiopentone injection to when no part of the baby (excluding the cord) is within the mother.

The thiopentone suxamethonium sequence described allows a more rapid induction delivery interval than any other technique.

A short induction delivery interval, especially in association with a short decision delivery interval which is affected by such factors as the proximity of an immediately available operating theatre, competent resident staff, and an obstetric anæsthetic service, undoubtedly saves life. In a consecutive series of 23 instances of prolapse of the cord in the first stage of labour[3] only one infant was lost and that from avoidable non-anæsthetic factors.

It has also been shown[3] that an induction delivery interval over seven minutes significantly depresses the respiratory activity of babies where there is fœtal distress, ante-partum hæmorrhage or prematurity, and is due to prolonged examination, and other technical complications rather than to anæsthesia per se.

In some centres up to 60 per cent of Cæsarean sections may be urgent or emergencies, and in these circumstances the time factor alone renders conduction techniques incompatible with fœtal welfare.[3] With epidural techniques the operation cannot be commenced within 20 minutes of the "test dose" apart from the time taken to prepare and perform epidural puncture.[7] Even if preliminary "scrubbing up" is omitted, 15–18 minutes is the shortest possible time before operation can be started.[64, 27] With spinal anæsthesia an induction delivery of 16·7 minutes can be achieved[67] excluding preparation and puncture time.

Using the general anæsthetic technique described[3] an induction delivery of less than 7 minutes can be achieved in 53 per cent of patients. In this series infants with pre-operative fœtal distress were delivered more rapidly and with the more experienced anæsthetists and surgeon in dire emergencies an I.D.I. of 2 minutes and less was achieved. Furthermore the corrected perinatal mortality among 236 infants with pre-operative fœtal distress was 5·0 per cent and among 200 patients with ante-partum hæmorrhage the perinatal mortality was 5·1 per cent. There can be little doubt that speed in itself was life saving in many of these cases. Altogether, there are obvious advantages to be derived from as short an induction delivery interval as is compatible with maternal safety, particularly in emergencies.

Fœtal Oxygen Saturation. Fœtal bradycardia indicative of distress almost invariably responds to the administration of oxygen to the mother. In the absence of previous maternal respiratory depression or decreased oxygen intake this improvement is due both to increased oxygen carriage in the plasma and to an increased maternal hæmoglobin saturation. Replacement of nitrogen in the maternal circulation with oxygen represents an additional 10% of available oxygen per 100 ml of blood for the fœtus.[84] The slope of the newborn oxygen dissociation curve also ensures that even a small increase in oxyhæmoglobin is beneficial to the fœtus.[84]

McClure[84] shows that babies born of mothers who receive oxygen for more than 10 minutes prior to delivery have a considerable increase in available oxygen compared to babies of mothers who receive no oxygen. With 11 to 15 minutes and more than 15 minutes administration the figures were 21% and 40% above that of the control study.

Cooperman[85] studying the oxygen saturation of newborn infants by means of ear oximetry has recently made an interesting observation. In a mother sedated heavily or late in labour the oxygen saturation in the newborn infant is higher in infants delivered vaginally under inhalational anæsthesia with adequate oxygen content than those delivered vaginally under pudendal block probably because the depressed maternal respirations are stimulated in the former instance. Further, Henderson et al.[12] state that the oxygen saturation of the newborn is slightly lower under spinal than general anæsthesia probably due to blood pressure instability in the former case. This has probably always been so but this "advantage" of general over conduction anæsthesia has been masked and far overweighed in the past by the concurrent central depression of the fœtal respiratory centre inherent in the inhalational technique. An initial high oxygen saturation at birth avails little if followed by a long period of apnœa or respiratory depression. This objection no longer holds good for fœtal respiratory depression and can and should be avoided in modern general anæsthesia.

Initial oxygen saturation of the newborn infant, therefore, is improved considerably by an oxygen rich maternal intake and an increased maternal respiratory action before delivery. The certain way of ensuring this is by deliberate positive pressure respiration with an oxygen enriched mixture as described in the general anæsthetic technique advocated.[3, 15]

ANÆSTHESIA FOR VARIOUS OBSTETRIC MANŒUVRES AND INSTRUMENTAL DELIVERY

Of the above procedures four are such that their complications could result in the necessity for immediate abdominal section, and for three of the procedures uterine relaxation could be said to be essential. General anæsthesia of the type described for Cæsarean section offers every advantage. Combined with safety, the anæsthetist possesses complete control of the situation whatever development takes place and the patient's vasomotor system is virtually unimpaired. Uterine relaxation is provided by the ready addition of ether, or for short procedures, amyl nitrite, and is independent of anæsthetic requirements.

Endotracheal intubation and the possibility of suxamethonium muscle pains could be considered unnecessary for examination under anæsthesia or external version. But it is not possible to forecast the immediate consequences of these procedures. Recently a mother collapsed during attempted external version under general anæsthesia. Immediate laparotomy revealed an extra-uterine pregnancy and free blood in the peritoneal cavity. The mother lived, and the fact that she was already intubated, on controlled respiration and without impairment of vasomotor control, played no small part in her survival.

Assisted Breech Delivery

The anæsthetic problems of assisted breech delivery have not changed and have been described by Law and Ransom.[86] In order to avoid delay or early operative intervention it is important that until the baby is delivered to the level of the inferior angles of the scapulæ the mother should be conscious and have minimal impairment of the perineal reflexes.

Extradural analgæsia, especially when administered by means of a catheter placed *in situ* prior to the second stage of labour, has obvious advantages, but the routine use of pudendal block shortly before episiotomy prior to delivery of the buttocks has the most advocates, and is adequate for forceps delivery of the after-coming head. At any moment, however, the obstetrician may require the mother to be unconscious.

With general anæsthesia even though intra-abdominal pressure has been reduced by the part delivery of the baby the danger of vomiting and regurgitation is aggravated by the patient being immobilized in the lithotomy position. Fortunately the effects of general anæsthesia on the fœtus at this stage are minimized by the virtual occlusion of the umbilical cord.

There are three approaches to the problem of providing a short anæsthetic to a patient in the lithotomy position at the end of the second stage. Firstly there is intravenous anæsthesia. It is likely that a short acting barbiturate is used by very many anæsthetists for assisted breech delivery and the reduction of intra-abdominal pressure already mentioned is probably no mean factor in diminishing the potential hazards of this technique. Secondly, Sellick's cricoid pressure manœuvre[33] which is yet to be proved over a large series of cases would enable safe intubation of the mother to be performed and the use of a standard technique such as that recommended for Cæsarean section would then be truly of universal application for all obstetric procedures. Thirdly, there is the rapid induction of inhalational anæsthesia. The cyclopropane "Vinesthene" induction used by Ransom deserves to be described in greater detail. Unconsciousness is produced with extreme rapidity thereby reducing the chance of stage II vomiting and, according to duration and method of maintenance, recovery of consciousness is also very rapid. The technique is as follows: with an oxygen flow rate of 1 L/min and a cyclopropane flow rate of 750 ml/min, following application of the facepiece, the lever of the Boyle's bottle containing 10–20 ml di-vinyl ether is rapidly advanced followed by rapid depression of the plunger. The mixture is delivered into a Waters re-breathing system with the absorber removed. Intravenous atropine is necessary and with a Didcott diaphragm[87] the needle may be left *in situ*, an advantage during any anæsthetic procedure.

Anæsthesia for Instrumental Vaginal Delivery

Pudendal Block. In simple procedures pudenal block is often the technique of choice, and is already well documented. Pudendal block by itself is applicable to only 60 per cent of all forceps deliveries, but it is claimed that if preceded by 100 mg. of pethidine and 12·5 mg of chlorpromazine it is then applicable to 94 per cent of such deliveries using Keilland's forceps.[88] Others[75] suggest that the block should be combined with techniques of inhalational analgesia or of ataralgesia. Such supplementation, however, unless it is nitrous oxide and oxygen only, may destroy the advantage of the "local" technique, the avoidance of circulating toxic or depressant agents to the foetus. Even light anæsthesia reintroduces the dangers of vomiting and the pethidine chlorpromazine sequence can cause maternal respiratory depression or hypotension[89] and marked foetal respiratory depression.[90]

Idiosyncrasy to local agents is rare but fatal convulsions have been reported following 70 ml of 1·5% lignocaine used for pudendal block,[20] a seemingly inexcusable overdose.

Spinal Subarachnoid Block. The "saddle-block" technique is suitable and "nupercaine hyperbaric" solution 0·4 to 0·8 ml is recommended. The injection should not be given during uterine contractions.[64] The lateral position can be used with 15–20 degrees head-up during the injection[16] but some prefer a slight head-down tilt[55] or sit the patient up for 2–3 minutes after injection.[91] Perineal reflexes are lost with subarachnoid "saddle-block" therefore it should not be used in the early stages of breech deliveries to avoid unnecessary extractions.[91] Recently it has been shown that lignocaine is more effective than nupercaine and requires less supplementation.[92] The upward spread of any subarachnoid block may be unpredictable in pregnancy and a high block may decrease uterine contractions, but recent work suggests[93] that this is more likely due to concurrent hypotension rather than interference with motor innervation. In 5 per cent of such "low blocks" serious hypotension requiring treatment occurs[7] and treatment should follow the lines already outlined. Very large series of forceps deliveries have been safely conducted under subarachnoid block but Sears,[91] however, reporting a 20-year series without major complication, reports a 3 per cent failure rate and an 8·9 per cent incidence of retention of urine and 14·1 per cent incidence of persistent post-spinal headaches. Thorne,[55] however, in a 13 year period found 11 per cent of mild headaches only.

Epidural Analgesia. This technique is of less confirmed value especially in emergencies owing to the time factor and the relatively high failure rate[16] but is applicable if labour has been conducted under the continuous lumbar or caudal technique for planned elective low forceps and assisted delivery. Some prefer the technique to subarachnoid block as the spread is more predictable.[94] Lignocaine by caudal injection 1·5% in the lateral position[55] (25–30 ml with adrenaline) or 2% (14–16 ml) by lumbar epidural injection with the patient sitting may be used.[94]

General Anæsthetic Techniques. With the ready availability of a safe and rapidly induced general anæsthetic obstetricians will tend to favour general anæsthesia even for low forceps deliveries. However, some believe general anæsthesia to be unjustified because local blocks are satisfactory in most instances.[95] But local blocks sometimes fail to provide adequate pain relief, complications do sometimes arise, and general anæsthesia may suddenly be necessary for some unexpected intra-uterine manipulation. In these circumstances the conversion of a "local" into a general anæsthetic may be hazardous particularly if the patient is already immobilized in a position incompatible with safe induction of anæsthesia. Therefore others[3, 83, 15] argue that general anæsthesia is justifiable even for these procedures, especially as a modern technique[3, 18] can be rendered safe for the mother and perhaps even safer for the child, leading to less fœtal depression than does the narcotic supplementation often necessary with regional analgesia. However, in the hands of the inexperienced, general anæsthesia for these minor procedures can be the most hazardous in all obstetrics. The same regard for detail and danger is necessary as with major obstetrical operations. If the patient is to be anæsthetized on an operating table an experienced anæsthetist may use the technique recommended for Cæsarean section described previously.[3, 18]

In the last six years at St. Mary's Hospital, Portsmouth, the great majority of such procedures has been so managed without any anæsthetic maternal or fœtal mortality or morbidity.[83] Endotracheal intubation protects the mother from the dangers of vomiting and regurgitation (particularly hazardous if the patient is to be later immobilized in the lithotomy position) and controlled ventilation with a high proportion of oxygen leads to improved oxygen saturation of mother and child. When previous sedation has been given to the mother, infants delivered under general anæsthesia have a higher oxygen saturation (as determined by ear-oximetry) than those delivered under pudendal block.[85]

If the facilities for this type of general anæsthesia are not present, or if the patient is already immobilized in some position incompatible with its safe induction, then alternative techniques must be adopted in the interest of maternal safety.

Nitrous oxide and oxygen may not provide adequate general anæsthesia without hypoxia and in such a situation is very likely to cause vomiting. Trichlorethylene with nitrous oxide and oxygen is a useful light anæsthetic. Nitrous oxide-oxygen-ether or cyclopropane-nitrous-oxide-oxygen sequences are commonly employed using an 80 : 20 nitrous-oxide-oxygen mixture in a semiclosed circuit at 10 to 12 L/min flow with 5% carbon dioxide and gradually introducing ether, or cyclopropane-nitrous-oxide-oxygen

(750 ml: 1,500 ml: 1,500 ml) in a closed circuit with assisted respirations, the flow being reduced (300 ml : 1,000 ml : 1,000 ml) after stabilization. No airways are used to avoid pharyngeal stimulation and anæsthesia is kept on a light plane.[16] Another alternative is the cycloproprane "Vinesthene" induction described under assisted breech delivery.

The Occasional Anæsthetist

To recommend a general anæsthetic to the occasional anæsthetist is not easy. Open ether is perhaps the safest way of maintaining anæsthesia but the problem is the induction. Here di-vinyl ether (Vinesthene) would seem to offer advantages[96] as it provides a smooth and rapid induction, it is probably safer than ethyl chloride and it is certainly preferable to the stormy open ether or potentially dangerous chloroform techniques often used. Di-vinyl ether is marketed in 25 ml bottles and this is sufficient for an open drop induction with overlap and transference to open ether. The quantity is such that with an open drop technique overdose would be almost impossible. Intravenous atropine and a reasonably clear nasal airway beforehand is essential. The left lateral head down position is advised.

With all these latter inhalational techniques the anæsthetist must not delude himself as to the possible anæsthetic origin of any resultant neonatal depression and, should it occur, should not dismiss it as obstetric in origin.

Hypoæsthesia or Ataralgesia

This method[97, 98] leads not to anæsthesia but to a condition in which freedom from apprehension, discomfort, and pain is produced with loss of sensible awareness of environment.[16] The technique is to employ a phenothiazine derivative (chlorpromazine or promethazine) a narcotic (pethidine or alphaprodine) with or without a narcotic antagonist (levallorphan or nalorphine) in various combinations and by slow intravenous injection.[16] The fine endpoint is not easy to achieve, however, and the mental indifference, uncoöperation and sometimes confusion which occurs can be a great disadvantage. Mepazine has been used[98, 99] and is said to disturb the mental state less. Other disadvantages of this method apart from mental disorientation are that there can be no attempt to hurry the onset of hypoæsthesia and that supplementation with light inhalational anæsthesia or local infiltration or block is often necessary.[16] The danger of the technique appears to be the unpredictable potentiation of narcotics which occurs with phenothiazine derivatives[90] and the sudden and severe hypotension which can follow particularly when chlorpromazine is used.[16] These factors are probably responsible for the unpleasantly large incidence of gross neonatal depression which has been noted.[16, 90]

The incidence of hypotension with chlorpromazine is stated to be 33 per cent and although less when promazine is used, the use of such mixtures can be dangerous especially in association with conduction anæsthesia or analgesia especially if chlorpromazine is used.[100] At the present time other methods of anæsthesia appear to provide as good results to the mother and less dangers to the fœtus and the use of ataralgesic mixtures in obstetrics is not yet established[75] and their routine use is not advocated.[16, 75, 90]

Hydroxydione ("Viadril", "Presuren"). Hydroxydione has been used successfully in Cæsarean sections and favourable impressions in small series have been reported.[95, 101–104] Some degree of neonatal depression has been noted, however,[105, 106] and no properly controlled study as to the effect of this drug on the neonate has yet been carried out. Induction following 0·5–1·0 G intravenously usually takes 3–7 minutes[104] and is normally vomit free. Anæsthesia can be supplemented by nitrous oxide–oxygen or ether, intubation is possible without relaxants and an analgesic may be administered if necessary, but thiopentone should not be used.[104]

The high incidence of local venous thrombosis related to chemical damage of the intima at the injection site is a serious disadvantage which has not been reduced by any of the modifications of administration advocated.[107]

Because of the severe disadvantages of local thrombosis, the slowness of anæsthetic induction, and the need for supplementation together with the unproven effects of the drug on neonatal activity, the use of hydroxydione in obstetrics is not advised at the present time.

Hypnosis

Many major procedures such as Cæsarean section can be successfully carried out under hypnotic trance[108] and August claims success in 16 out of 29 such procedures. Also determinations of acid base status of the neonate after birth have shown[109] a significantly greater ability of a "hypnotized" group to readjust and recover from the effects of asphyxia as compared to even non-medicated groups delivered under regional analgesia. Furthermore it is an undoubted fact that hypnosis alone, among the methods of pain relief, is not listed among the causes of maternal or fœtal death. Hypnosis therefore should not be lightly dismissed and all should remember that the achievement of a pain free labour depends to some extent on the personality of the doctor and the practice of some degree of hypnotic suggestion with success is "certainly not outside the capacity of anyone prepared to spend the necessary time with the patient".[75]

Many of the claims of hypnosis however, are based on unsubstantiated nubulous impressions[110] and it is quite apparent that the method is too unpredictable and unreliable to form a satisfactory routine alternative to chemical analgesia and anæsthesia.[111, 75] Some patients refuse hypnosis, some only accept with reluctance[110] and the hypnotic state is easily disturbed by many extraneous factors particularly in ward patients. The failure to maintain trance may lead to increased duration and severity of labour and to aggravate postpartum depression.[111] The best results appear to be obtained in selected patients by selected hypnotists,[75] but only 40 to 50 per cent of patients can be regarded as satisfactory even in experienced hands.[111, 110] August[110] claims that no conditioning is necessary and that hypnosis is successful in a large number of patients if combined with intravenous analgesics. Some would regard the dosage of the supplementation suggested (50–100 mg of intravenous pethidine repeated 2 to 4 hourly) as firstly sufficient in itself and secondly destroying the object of the technique.

Heart Disease

During pregnancy the cardiac output increases together with the blood and plasma volumes. Some state the danger of cardiac failure is greatest at the 32nd week[100] or between 32nd–36th week[104] and that failure seldom occurs thereafter but an analysis of maternal deaths shows[20] that although 50 per cent of deaths take place during pregnancy, acute failure can occur at any time and not during any particular month. The risk of failure increases with maternal age and successive pregnancies and labour.[77] At term the uterus contains $\frac{1}{6}$th of the total blood volume. Labour increases the cardiac work load and anything likely to accentuate this load should be avoided. Anxiety, sudden changes in posture, or unnecessary physical strain should be avoided. The lateral and not the lithotomy position should be used during delivery. Opinions as to the advisability of Cæsarean section have been divided. The opinion that section "spares" the mother the strain of labour and delivery is not entirely acceptable and recently it has been shown that the hæmodynamic changes associated with emptying the uterus are largely unavoidable and the increased cardiac work load is inevitable regardless of manner or method of emptying be it by Cæsarean section or vaginal delivery.[112] This increased load is due to 500–600 ml of blood being suddenly returned to the systemic circulation from the uterine sinuses. This would appear to confirm that Cæsarean section should be reserved for circumstances in those patients where there is an obstetric indication apart from heart disease.[112]

Anæsthesia may be required in such a patient for assisted or operative delivery. Local block or infiltration might be regarded as indicated for vaginal delivery but anxiety must be avoided and it must be remembered that an "inadequate 'local' is worse than a good 'general' ".[75]

Caudal or lumbar epidural or continuous spinal techniques are considered the method of choice by some[100] who nevertheless stress the dangers which may follow the associated sympathetic denervation. With sympathetic block and the alteration in hæmodynamics fœtal oxygenation may be severely jeopardized especially during uterine contractions.[100] In some patients however, the bloodless phlebotomy which may be achieved by conduction analgesia and sympathetic block may be indicated and beneficial.[104] When necessary hypotension should be combated by posture and oxygen rather than by vasopressors which should be used as a last resort only.[100]

General anæsthesia is regarded as best especially for major procedures by many anæsthetists. The reduction in work it ensures when delivery is imminent is beneficial and outweighs all possible disadvantages.[75] Ergot administration should be avoided as it may precipitate pulmonary œdema.[75, 104]

Eclampsia

This condition may be controlled by heavy sedation or by reduction of blood pressure. Where specialized techniques are called for by the obstetricians such as an infusion of trimetaphan or lumbar epidural blockade[27] the advice of anæsthetists may be sought. Also, in the treatment of eclamptic fits, an intravenous barbiturate, the administration of 100% oxygen, and possibly paralysis and controlled respiration may be required.

It should be remembered that as a result of the depression of liver function that occurs in pre-eclamptic toxæmia and eclampsia that in some cases prolongation of the effects of suxamethonium, due to its delayed hydrolysis, may be expected. This is no contra-indication to the use of this drug in operative cases under general anæsthesia provided the rules of relaxant technique are understood. Any results of mishandling the consequences of repeat injections of suxamethonium without proper regard for the effects of the first and possibly second injection cannot be ascribed to some special deleterious relationship between pre-eclamptic toxæmia and suxamethonium.

Halothane

Halothane depresses uterine contractility and therefore predisposes to post-partum hæmorrhage[77, 113–117] and Vasicka and Kretchmer[93] with continuous intra-amniotic pressure recordings have shown that halothane rapidly affects the uterus. The intensity of the uterine contractions is markedly diminished with first plane halothane anæsthesia and practically abolished with second plane.

Its effect on the fœtal respiratory centre will vary with the concentration administered to the mother but is unlikely to differ much from that of ether of trichlorethylene.

Hypotension, an important factor with halothane, adversely affects the placental circulation, and constitutes another contraindication to its use in obstetrics.

Halothane therefore may have a place during induction of anæsthesia or during intended uterine relaxation but it cannot be recommended for routine use in obstetric anæsthesia at the present time.

The Flying Squad

Modern obstetric anæsthetic techniques have been taken into the home[118] and all the equipment necessary to provide maximum safety, with the exception of an operating table, can be conveniently carried by a flying squad. The thiopentone suxamethonium intubation nitrous-oxide oxygen sequence used on a patient lying across a low divan bed in a small room may well be viewed askance but remedies for the two main hazards, failed intubation and or regurgitation, have already been suggested earlier in this chapter. Different centres will continue to have differing views on flying squad anæsthesia but the safety of an endotracheal tube cannot be over-estimated.

Relief of Pain in Childbirth

While modern alchemists pursue their golden quest for the pain-relieving drug which does not depress respiration, there has been no fundamental change in the techniques of pain relief in childbirth.

Pethidine combined with a narcotic antagonist[119] is used in many centres to reduce its respiratory depressant effect and is still the principal drug used in this country for raising the threshold of pain in labour.[120]

There is a growing suspicion that there are deleterious effects of nitrous oxide-air on the fœtus and research is being undertaken to decide on a suitable mixture of nitrous oxide and oxygen for use by midwives in this country. Whether ultimately district midwives will administer nitrous oxide-oxygen mixtures in their patients' homes remains to be seen. There will be a choice of either using a smaller version of the Lucy Baldwin Apparatus for Obstetric Analgesia which is already on the market or, since the discovery that nitrous oxide and oxygen mixtures remain in a single gas phase, up to 2,000 lbs. per sq. in. on the gauge,[121] a fixed percentage nitrous oxide and oxygen mixture from one cylinder. In either case the much increased cylinder usage will involve transport problems that will have to be either the responsibility of local health authorities or supplying retail chemists.

Techniques of pain relief during labour by means of continuous extradural analgesia are well known and are extremely effective and previously held beliefs as to the effect of segmental anæsthesia on uterine contractions have been questioned.[93, 122] Segmental block of T11, T12 and L1 will completely relieve the pain of uterine first stage contractions. Pelvic pain in the later stages of labour is relieved by sacral extradural analgesia but owing to the resultant loss of the perineal reflex, delivery by forceps is the rule.

Mention must be made of psychoprophylactic methods of pain relief.[123, 124] The experience of pain with contractions of the uterine muscle is attributed largely to a conditioned reflex of expectation of pain and this reflex may be replaced by another in which uterine contraction is felt to be painless. The many effective means of relief of pain in childbirth which singly may not be of universal application, may be considered as a patchwork quilt in which psychoprophylaxis, hypnosis, and Dr. Grantly Dick Read's method are adjacent.

Another approach to the relief of pain in labour is by abdominal decompression which is also claimed to considerably shorten the first stage.[125] The technique is based on the physical and physiological advantages of allowing freedom of the uterus to assume a spherical shape during contractions. This is effected by subjecting the abdomen to a negative pressure by a device similar to that of a cuirass respirator. The technique appears to be very effective and justice to it cannot be done in such a short summary.

Finally, trials are taking place with the use of morphia and its partial antagonist tetrahydroaminacrine (Tacrine Hydrochloride) in obstetrics. This appears to be worthy of further investigation but no results have been published at the time of writing. It should be noted that tacrine potentiates and prolongs neuromuscular block produced by suxamethonium.

Summary

1. There is an increasing awareness of the necessity for an obstetric anæsthetic service and inter-departmental liaison with the incorporation of the anæsthetist in the obstetric team.
2. While maternal safety remains a prime consideration, increased attention is being paid to the effects, on the fœtus, of anæsthetic and analgesic agents and, of the physiological changes induced in the mother by these agents. The importance of delay in peri-natal mortality and morbidity is apparent and anæsthetic techniques have been designed to facilitate minimum decision-delivery intervals when necessary, to provide maximum certainty, and to be safe for the mother and the child.
3. Endotracheal intubation of every woman past the 28th week of pregnancy requiring a general anæsthetic is being recognized as a normal procedure in obstetrics.
4. The use of nitrous oxide–oxygen mixtures by midwives is being contemplated.

RESUSCITATION OF THE NEWBORN

Early oxygenation and expansion of the lungs after clearance of the airway are paramount in the treatment of asphyxia neonatorum. They are important factors in the establishment of the changes in circulatory hæmodynamics which should take place in the first few minutes of life.[138]

When respiratory depression is due to hypoxia direct oxygenation is a more logical way of achieving the onset of respiratory activity than by attempting to stimulate the respiratory centre by means of drugs or violent mechanical stimulation. In view of the safety of modern methods of artificial respiration it seems hardly justifiable to wait in hope for the terminal gasps which might break the vicious circle of hypoxia and respiratory depression.

According to the severity and duration of the asphyxial process, physiological and biochemical changes have been induced which may ultimately cause death in circulatory failure in spite of the initiation of respiration.[126]

Figures quoted from the Perinatal Mortality Survey of the National Birthday Trust Fund have shown that more than half the intra-partum deaths that occurred in March 1958 in this country showed only signs at post mortem of asphyxia during labour and that 40 per cent of all babies dying from the results of intrapartum asphyxia were alive at the moment of birth. This gives an idea of the magnitude of this problem.

Clearly, prevention of asphyxia is the goal which all would seek and anæsthetists are playing their part in developing techniques without adverse effect on the fœtus which facilitate rapid delivery where speed is essential.[3]

In the absence of any or adequate respiratory movement resuscitation is most rapidly and effectively achieved by the introduction of oxygen into the lungs and there is evidence that this is best achieved by intermittent positive pressure respiration (I.P.P.R.). Techniques of resuscitation of the newborn are notoriously difficult to evaluate statistically because of the virtual impossibility of applying controls with so many variables related to childbirth. However, "Airway clearance, intubation and positive pressure inflation alone have stood a reasonable test of time."[131] Therefore it is convenient to make the assumption that oxygenation is the first and foremost method of treatment for the asphyxiated or apnœic baby, then to select the most effective method of oxygenation, and then to show that this method does no harm. Intermittent positive pressure respiration has been assessed.

A consecutive series of 342 babies following operative delivery between January 1957 and July 1961 who were intubated at birth for the purposes of endotracheal aspiration or oxygenation have recently been carefully studied.[6, 127] Each record of the procedure on the obstetric anæsthetic record card and each case record was closely scrutinized. This was combined with direct questioning of medical and nursing pædiatric staff and examination of perinatal post mortem reports. Not one of these 342 intubated babies had any complication due to endotracheal intubation and the use of I.P.P.R. Shock, infection, laryngeal trauma, emphysema or pneumothorax due to these procedures were never encountered.

While there are differences between the physiological, biochemical and anatomical state of the newborn and that of the baby several hours old, there is no reason to suppose that intermittent positive pressure oxygenation at birth, using the principles, technique and apparatus of neonatal anæsthesia, is much more dangerous than at a time several hours later when major surgery for congenital defect, perhaps lasting several hours, may be undergone.

I.P.P.R. is of course possible without an endotracheal tube, but in the newborn, to be certain of not forcing pharyngeal debris down the trachea, direct laryngoscopy is necessary and then the stomach is liable to be inflated necessitating further interference to prevent splinting of the diaphragm.

Resuscitation of the newborn as in obstetrics and obstetric anæsthesia requires resident medical staff. Therefore in large and busy units there is as much to be said in favour of standardization of resuscitation procedure as there is for anæsthetic procedure, particularly when what is done is subjected to research scrutiny and is intended to provide a constant safe and ready service for the community.

Indications for Active Resuscitation

Hypoxia is never beneficial and there can be no justification for withholding remedies which have been shown to be without harm. The school of thought which allows nature to take its course follows one or two lines of argument. Firstly it is not obvious that early artificial oxygenation influences the subsequent intelligence of the newborn that survive. Secondly, active resuscitation of a severely asphyxiated baby may help to save the life of a child already doomed to severe mental or physical handicaps.

The former is no strong argument and in the latter case many babies known to have been severely asphyxiated at birth have subsequently rated high in intelligence.[128] The statistical follow up into childhood of these babies is fraught with pitfalls, but while the incidence of gross neurological abnormality (as opposed to intelligence) is greater in severely asphyxiated babies than normal controls, the figure is small.[128]

Any baby born flaccid, apnœic, with a bradycardia or with a barely perceptible heart beat should be intubated at once. The heart rate is the most important single guide to the need for oxygenation. In the presence of a satisfactory heart beat, colour and muscle tone the treatment of apnœa, primary or secondary, may be expectant and after pharyngeal aspiration an oxygen funnel poised over the baby's face will be of good effect at the next gasp. Should there be any deterioration, intubation and I.P.P.R. should be proceeded with at once.

With expansion of the lungs the resistance to blood flow through the pulmonary circulation is lowered which enables the right ventricular outflow to be directed along its proper course. Delay in expansion of the lungs at birth can serve no useful purpose and where this does not occur immediately, assistance is required. The work of Karlberg and his associates[129] suggests that if the child does not breathe at birth then immediate efforts should be made to expand its lungs by positive pressure ventilation possibly even before the cord is divided. The respiratory distress syndrome has been related to failure of early and adequate lung expansion in the presence of asphyxia at birth and it has been proposed that early intervention could lower the incidence of this condition.[126]

Endotracheal Aspiration

The indications used for endotracheal intubation of the newborn for the purposes of aspiration vary according to current attitudes toward the procedure. Debris obstructing the larynx or trachea may be heard, seen, manifested by paradoxical respiratory movement, or intelligently anticipated. It is known from the figures quoted from the Perinatal Mortality Survey that the combination of postmaturity in the baby and toxæmia in the mother is likely to result in asphyxia during labour with meconium aspiration and while newborn lungs must be capable of coping with a certain amount of thin liquor, a large quantity, or material that is thick is not tolerated.

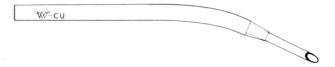

FIG. 30. Neonatal tube. Sterilized disposable "Riplex" non-toxic plastic catheter. (Two-thirds actual size) (Mfr: Wm. Warne & Co. Ltd.)

The trachea may be aspirated direct or via an endotracheal tube. In the latter instance a special sterile disposable plastic catheter is ideal. This is designed for a dual purpose and provided with an end and side hole in close proximity.[130] The catheter must be cleared frequently as blockage occurs after about two inches of material have been withdrawn. If material to be aspirated is very thick, suction must be applied directly to the endotracheal tube. The tube is removed while maintaining suction and is then re-inserted for repeat suction or oxygenation. It is a sound principle of pædiatric anæsthesia that final extubation should always be under positive pressure.

It is relevant at this stage to point out that the majority of apparatus for delivering oxygen by nasal catheter delivers at an obstructed pressure of 5 lb per sq in. gauge or more. No matter how slowly the oxygen is bubbled through a Wolffs bottle or humidifier its pressure is that of the reducing valve. One is able to visualize the possible consequences of misplacing such a nasal catheter.

Intragastric Oxygen

This technique was still in use in major obstetric units in this country in 1961, but is useless and dangerous and has been authoritatively and finally condemned.[131-133]

Endotracheal Intubation

Complications. Intubation of the newborn is not difficult. It merely requires adequate initial supervision, with perhaps prior practice on stillbirths. No medical man or woman likely to be presented with an asphyxiated baby should be without this skill. Complications are due to inability to visualize the larynx, to recognize what is visualized or to the use of force, but are unnecessary and none were seen in a recent large series.[127] Inexperienced operators may cause trauma due to initial laryngoscopy or to intubation. Barotrauma is another entirely preventable complication.

Infection is an overrated danger as thousands of babies every year escape infection following the blind pharyngeal proddings with the standard suction catheter operated by midwives. Similarly in the first half of a recent large series of intubations,[127] sterile equipment was not used and no infection was attributable to the manœuvre. However, with the advent of a sterile disposable neonatal tube,[130] there is now no justification for running the hazard of introducing a virulent organism into the pharynx or trachea of a newborn baby. The incidence of intra-partum pneumonia is raised where the membranes have been ruptured more than 24 hours and it may be necessary to resuscitate babies already possessing a respiratory infection and lowered resistance. The Perinatal Mortality Survey has shown, to be hoped for the last time, that the majority of cases of pneumothorax encountered at post mortem in March 1958 had had no mechanical resuscitation applied to the lungs at all. This condition is probably due to stop valvular or check valvular bronchial obstruction and the high pressure swings the infant is capable of producing. A possible interpretation of these findings would be that early intubation, aspiration and careful inflation would reduce the incidence of these complications.

Apparatus and Technique. A sterile disposable Cole plastic endotracheal tube has been marketed[130] specifically for resuscitation of the newborn. It is easy to insert and requires no stylet. Connection devices from oxygen apparatus are easily applied and removed which allows convenient performance of endotracheal suction procedures. The shoulder which rests at laryngeal level prevents endobronchial intubation by the relatively inexperienced. An internal ledge is present but is surmounted by the suction catheter if it is rotated and pushed, particularly if the head of the infant is extended (Fig. 30).

A plastic "intravenous" tube with a Luer mount is conveniently used for endotracheal suction.[130] An end hole and side hole are in close proximity and it reduces the chances of suction biopsy (Fig. 31).

The Jackson Rees modified Ayres T-piece system is one of the most effective devices for controlled respiration in neonates. No mano-meter is required and as Jackson Rees states,[132] it would require a very strong hand to achieve the pressures equivalent to the pressure

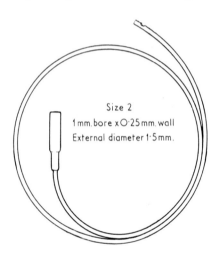

Size 2
1 mm. bore x 0·25 mm. wall
External diameter 1·5 mm.

Fig. 31. "Riplex" Portsmouth pattern IV/R catheter, sterile and disposable
(Mfr: Wm. Warne & Co. Ltd.)

swings up to 70 cm achieved by the newborn establishing respiration. It is important to remember that a newborn baby's lung can with-stand a momentary high pressure better than a sustained lower pressure.

For resuscitation procedures, where usually artificial respiration is not prolonged, an alternative is available to the T-piece system. This is a pressure controlled oxygen supply delivered by a nozzle with a side hole which can be intermittently occluded by the operator's finger. The endotracheal tube remains held in place by one hand and the nozzle is conveniently detached and replaced, if suction is required, by the other.

Incidence of Intubation. In a recent large series after Cæsarean section the incidence of intubation was 26 per cent which is related to criteria adopted for intubation.[127] It seems reasonable to suggest also that at least 50 per cent of all babies delivered by Cæsarean section should have pharyngeal toilet under direct vision.

Fifty per cent of the intubated babies quoted in the series established effective respiratory movement in under six minutes.[127] 12 per cent were intubated for the purposes of endotracheal aspiration only.

Metabolic Exhaustion

Not all babies born with a beating heart survive the effects of severe asphyxia even if receiving adequate oxygenation. Changes due to asphyxia, including the prolonged fœtal hypoxia of toxæmic placental insufficiency, render the newborn liable to die of cardiovascular failure. Glycogen depletion of the heart and liver is known to occur.[134] Acid-base and electrolyte imbalance[135, 136] may take several hours to restore. If asphyxia has been severe the resultant acid-base disturbance impairs both cardiac and renal function and also affects the immature enzyme systems which only work within very restricted ranges of pH.[126] Early pulmonary oxygenation is paramount, but here specialized methods of resuscitation such as hypothermia,[137] transfusion of oxygenated blood,[137] and the correction of biochemical and electrolytic disturbances play their role.

Responsibility for Resuscitation

"Whether it is Obstetrician, Anæsthetist or Pædiatrician, whoever is there and whoever is competent must be ready to take immediate responsibility. The Obstetrician cannot divest himself of concern and responsibility in this respect and must be adequately trained in resuscitation drill. For one thing he is more likely to be present at delivery."[131]

However, in many units, when an anæsthetist is present he is often asked by the obstetrician to undertake resuscitation of the newborn. The obstetrician is frequently fully occupied and the anæsthetist using modern anæsthetic techniques with endotracheal intubation may safely direct his attention to the baby while remaining at the mother's head. Therefore anæsthetists should be prepared to resuscitate the newborn and play their part in teaching the principles and techniques of I.P.P.R. to all junior staff.

Summary

"There is no longer any doubt as to how asphyxiated infants should be resuscitated, it should be by some sort of positive pressure ventilation."[132]

References

1. HODGES, R. J. H., and FOLEY, J. J. (1962). To be published.
2. BUTLER, N. R. (1960). *Brit. J. Anæsth.*, **32**, 102.
3. HODGES, R. J. H., and TUNSTALL, M. E. (1961). *Ibid.*, **33**, 572.
4. BUTLER, N. R. (1961). Personal communications.
5. Editorial (1960). *Brit. med. J.*, **1**, 483.
6. HODGES, R. J. H., TUNSTALL, M. E., KNIGHT, R. F., and WILSON, E. J. (1960). *Brit. J. Anæsth.*, **32**, 9.
7. HINGSON, R. A., and HELLMAN, L. M. (1956). *Anæsthesia for Obstetrics.* Lippincott, Philadelphia.
8. CULL, W. A., and HINGSON, R. A. (1957). *Bull. Maternal Welfare*, **2**, 11, American Committee on Maternal Welfare, Inc., Chicago.
9. CULL, W. A. (1960). *J. Amer. med. Ass.*, **172**, 416.
10. PILSBURY, S. G. (1960). *Ibid.*, **174**, 2151.
11. ABRAMSON, H. (1960). *Resuscitation of the Newborn Infant.* Mosby, St. Louis.
12. HENDERSON, H., MOSHER, R., and BITTRICH, N. M. (1957). *Amer. J. Obstet. Gynec.*, **73**, 664.
13. KINCH, R. A. H. (1959). *Canad. Anæsth. Soc. J.*, **6**, 90.
14. HODGES, R. J. H. (1959). *Brit. J. Anæsth.*, **31**, 32.
15. HODGES, R. J. H. (1961). *Proc. S.W. Obstet. Gynæc. Soc.* Pergamon Press, Oxford.
16. CRAWFORD, J. S. (1959). *The Principles and Practice of Obstetric Anæsthesia.* Blackwell, Oxford.
17. STEEL, G. C. (1961). *Brit. med. J.*, **1**, 963.
18. HODGES, R. J. H., BENNETT, J. R., TUNSTALL, M. E., and KNIGHT, R. F. (1959). *Brit. J. Anæsth.*, **31**, 152.
19. CLAYE, A. (1961). *J. Obstet. Gynæc. Brit. Commw.*, **68**, 577.
20. WALKER, A. L., WRIGLEY, A. J., ORGANE, G. S. W., CHAMBERLAIN, R. N., and MARTIN, W. J. (1960). *Reports on Public Health and Medical Subjects, No. 103.* H.M. Stationery Office, London.
21. DINNICK, O. P. (1957). *Proc. R. Soc. Med.*, **50**, 547.
22. CAVANAGH, D. (1961). *Obstetrical Emergencies.* Thomas, Springfield, Illinois.
23. KLEIN, M. D., CLAHR, J., TAMIS, A. B., and SOLKOW, M. (1953). *New York State J. Med.*, **53**, 2861.
24. DINNICK, O. P. (1961). *Lancet*, **1**, 470.
25. EDWARDS, G., MORTON, H. J. V., PASK, E. A., and WYLIE, W. D. (1956). *Anæsthesia*, **2**, 194.
26. STEARNS, A. B., and FREDRICKSON, G. C. (1957). *Illinois med. J.*, **112**, 267.
27. EISEN, S. M., ROSEN, N., WINESANKER, H., HELLMAN, K., AXELROD, H. I., ROTENBURG, M., RELLE, A., and SHEFFMAN, E. (1960). *Canad. Anæsth. Soc. J.*, 7. 280.
28. MACKAY, I. M. (1957). *Ibid.*, **4**, 112.
29. MENDELSON, C. L. (1946). *Amer. J. Obstet. Gynec.*, **79**, 224.
30. HOLMES, J. M. (1956). *J. Obstet. Gynæc. Brit. Emp.*, **63**, 239.
31. Editorial (1958). *Obstet. Gynec. Surg.*, **13**, 333.
32. HODGES, R. J. H. (1959). *Brit. med. J.*, **1**, 1528.
33. SELLICK, B. A. (1961). *Lancet*, **2**, 404.
34. MORTON, H. J. V., and WYLIE, W. D. (1951). *Anæsthesia*, **6**, 202.
35. SNOW, R. G., and NUNN, J. F. (1959). *Brit. J. Anæsth.*, **31**, 493.
36. SYKES, M. K. (1960). *Ibid.*, **32**, 199.
37. HODGES, R. J. H., TUNSTALL, M. E., and BENNETT, J. R. (1960). *Ibid.*, **32**, 619.
38. AINLEY-WALKER, J. C. (1961). *Ibid.*, **33**, 171.
39. BANNISTER, W. K., SATTILARO, A. J., and OTIS, R. D. (1961). *Anesthesiology*, **22**, 440.

40. HODGES, R. J. H., WILSON, E. J., KNIGHT, R. F., and TUNSTALL, M. E. (1960). *Brit. J. Anæsth.*, **32**, 16.
41. SJOSTEDT, S. and ROOTH, G. (1958). *Acta. anæsth. Scand.*, **2**, 99.
42. APGAR, V., HOLADAY, D. A., JAMES, L. S., PRINCE, C. E., and WEISBROT, I. M. (1957). *J. Amer. med. Ass.*, **165**, 2155.
43. HON, E. H., REID, B. L., and HEHRE, F. W. (1960). *Amer. J. Obstet. Gynec.*, **79**, 209
44. HOLMES, F. (1957). *J. Obstet. Gynæc. Brit. Emp.*, **64**, 229.
45. KENNEDY, R. L., FRIEDMAN, D. L., KATCHKA, D. M., SELMANTS, S., and SMITH, R. N. (1959). *Anesthesiology*, **20**, 153.
46. BAIRD, D. (1960). *Lancet*, **2**, 557.
47. DAWKINS, C. J. M. (1956). *Postgrad. med. J.*, **32**, 544.
48. EBBLI, C., and BARRICALLA, A. (1959). *Acta. anæsth. Scand.*, **Supp. 2.**, 9.
49. FOLDES, F. F., and CRAWFORD, J. S. (1959). *Ibid.*, **Supp. 2.**, 15.
50. NELLERMORE, C. W., MOORE, D. C., BRIDENBAUGH, L. D., CASADY, G. N., and BRALY, B. (1960). *Anesthesiology*, **21**, 269.
51. ANSBRO, F. P., PILLION, J. W., BLUNDELL, A. E., and BODELL, B. (1958). *New York State J. Med.*, **58**, 3447.
52. KOLSTAD, P., and SCHYE, K. F. (1957). *Acta. obstet. gynæc. Scand.*, **36**, 233.
53. EBNER, H., BARCOHANA, J., and BARTOSHUK, A. K. (1960). *Amer. J. Obstet. Gynec.*, **80**, 569.
54. GREENE, N. M. (1958). *Physiology of Spinal Anæsthesia.* Baillière, Tindall and Cox, London.
55. THORNE, T. C. (1961). *Personal Communication.*
56. MAKEPEACE, A. W. (1958). *Obstet. and Gynec.*, **11**, 438.
57. EBNER, H. (1959). *Curr. Res. Anesth.*, **38**, 378.
58. SWEENEY, T. R., CASEY, E. S., RAHEB, E. B., and WELNA, J. A. (1959). *Amer. J. Obstet. Gynec.*, **78**, 415.
59. BONICA, J. J. (1957). *J. Amer. med. Ass.*, **165**, 2146.
60. MOYA, F. (1960). *Bull. Sloane. Hosp. Women*, **6**, 41.
61. FORTHMAN, H. J., and ADRIANI, J. (1957). *Curr. Res. Anesth.*, **36**, 63.
62. LUND, P. C., CWIK, J. C., and QUINN, J. R. (1961). *Ibid.*, **40**, 153.
63. CASSIDY, G. N. (1960). *J. Amer. med. Ass.*, **172**, 1011.
64. FOLDES, F. F. (1961). *Personal Communication.*
65. DE JONG, R. H. (1961). *Curr. Res. Anesth.*, **40**, 384.
66. APGAR, V. (1953). *Ibid.*, **32**, 260.
67. MINTZ, N. (1960). *Amer. J. Obstet. Gynec.*, **79**, 224.
68. MCKECHNIE, F. B., and CONVERSE, J. G. (1955). *Ibid.*, **70**, 639.
69. CRAWFORD, J. S., and KANE, P. O. (1956). *Brit. J. Anæsth.*, **28**, 146.
70. BINGHAM, W. (1957). *Anæsthesia*, **12**, 435.
71. DUFFIELD, J. R., WAYBURNE, H., FABERLAN, H., HILLMAN, L., ABRAMS, M. W., FREINKEL, A., ZWICK, N., COHEN, D., DICKSON, D. N., FAIN, H. R., MARCUS, E., RAUTENBACH, L., and ROSENZWEIG, O. M. (1958). *Med. Proc.*, **4**, 306.
72. DANCE, C., jr., and WARD, R. (1958). *Curr. Res. Anesth.*, **37**, 249.
73. GRAY, T. C. (1947). *Brit. med. J.*, **1**, 444.
74. DAVENPORT, H. T., and PRIME, F. J. (1950). *Ibid.*, **1**, 1347.
75. WYLIE, W. D., and CHURCHILL DAVIDSON, H. C. (1960). *A Practice of Anæsthesia.* Lloyd-Luke, London.
76. PHILLIPS, K. G. (1959). *Amer. J. Obstet. Gynec.*, **77**, 133.
77. MONTGOMERY, J. B. (1961). *Brit. J. Anæsth.*, **33**, 156.
78. KVISSELGAARD, N., and MOYA, F. (1961). *Anesthesiology*, **22**, 7.
79. CRAWFORD, B. S., and GARDINER, J. E. (1956). *Brit. J. Anæsth.*, **28**, 154.
80. BECK, VON H., and NOLD, B. (1957). *Der Anæsthetist.*, **6**, 93.
81. SCHWARZ, H. (1958). *Ibid.*, **7**, 299.
82. HODGES, R. J. H., BENNETT, R., TUNSTALL, M. E., and SHANKS, R. O. F. (1959). *Brit. med J.*, **1**, 413.
83. HODGES, R. J. H. *Unpublished data.*

84. McClure, J. H. (1960). *Amer. J. Obstet. Gynec.*, **80**, 554.
85. Cooperman, N. R., Rubovits, F. E., and Hesser, F. (1961). *Ibid.*, **81**, 385.
86. Law, R. G., and Ransom, S. (1954). *Brit. med. J.*, **1**, 562.
87. Didcott, C. C. (1961). *Anæsthesia*, **16**, 503.
88. Scott, J. S., and Gadd, R. L. (1957). *Brit. med. J.*, **1**, 971.
89. Holmes, J. M. (1960). *J. Obstet. Gynec. Brit. Emp.*, **67**, 115.
90. Hodges, R. J. H., and Bennett, J. R. (1959). *Ibid.*, **66**, 91.
91. Sears, R. T. (1959). *Brit. med. J.*, **1**, 755.
92. Peterson, W. F. (1961). *Amer. J. Obstet. Gynec.*, **81**, 1249.
93. Vasicka, A., and Kretchmer, H. (1961). *Ibid.*, **82**, 600.
94. Rodriguez, R. L. (1959). *Acta. anæsth. Scand.*, **Supp. 2.**, 59.
95. Donald, I. (1960). *Brit. J. Anæsth.*, **32**, 106.
96. Dawkins, C. J. M. (1959). *Acta anæsth. Scand.*, **Supp. 2.**, 5.
97. Hayward-Butt, J. T. (1957). *Lancet*, **2**, 972.
98. Hayward-Butt, J. T. (1958). *Ibid.*, **1**, 379.
99. Purkis, I. E. (1958). *Canad. med. Ass. J.*, **78**, 245.
100. Cull, W. A., and Hingson, R. A. (1960). *Clin Obstet. and Gynec.*, **3**, 14.
101. Harbort, C. (1957). *Zentralbl. f. Gynäk.*, **79**, 1172.
102. Zinser, H. K., and Bachmann, F. F. (1958). *Ibid.*, **80**, 1831.
103. Galley, A. H., and Lerman, L. H. (1959). *Lancet*, **1**, 332.
104. Evans, F. T., and Gray, T. C. (1959). *General Anæsthesia, Vol. II.* Butterworth, London.
105. Kivalo, I., and Tammisto, T. (1959). *Acta. anæsth. Scand.*, **Supp. 2.**, 35.
106. John, H. (1958). *Zentralbl. f. Gynäk.*, **80**, 1791.
107. Robertson, J. D., and Williams, A. W. (1961). *Anæsthesia*, **16**, 389.
108. Winkelstein, L. B., and Levinson, J. (1959). *Amer. J. Obstet. Gynec.*, **78**, 420.
109. Moya, F., and James, L. S. (1960). *J. Amer. med. Ass.*, **174**, 2026.
110. August, R. V. (1961). *Hypnosis in Obstetrics.* McGraw Hill Co., London.
111. Winkelstein, L. B. (1958). *Amer. J. Obstet. Gynec.*, **76**, 152.
112. Adams, J. Q. (1961). *Ibid.*, **82**, 673.
113. Dixon, G. D., and Matheson, D. I. (1958). *Canad. med. Ass. J.*, **79**, 365.
114. Embrey, M. P., Garrett, W. J., and Pryer, D. L. (1958). *Lancet*, **2**, 1093.
115. Mackay, I. M. (1957). *Canad. Anæsth. Soc. J.*, **4**, 235.
116. Russell, J. T. (1958). *Anæsthesia*, **13**, 241.
117. Kay, H. T. (1958). *Ibid.*, **13**, 192.
118. Argent, D. E., and Evans, M. D. (1961). *Lancet*, **1**, 994.
119. Bullough, J. (1957). *Brit. med. J.*, **2**, 1051.
120. Seward, E. H., and Bryce-Smith, R. (1957). *Inhalation Analgesia in Childbirth.* Blackwell, Oxford.
121. Tunstall, M. E. (1961). *Lancet*, **2**, 964.
122. Tunstall, M. E. (1960). *Brit. J. Anæsth.*, **32**, 292.
123. Chertok, L. (1958). *Les Methods Psychosomatiques d'Accouchement sans Douleur.* L'Expansion Scientifique Française, Paris.
124. Lamaze, R. (1958). *Painless Childbirth.* Burke, London.
125. Heyns, O. S. (1959). *Med. Proc.*, **5**, 121.
126. James, L. S. (1959). *Pediatrics*, **24**, 1069.
127. Tunstall, M. E. (1961). *Proc. S.W. Obstet. Gynæc. Soc.* Pergamon Press, Oxford.
128. Benaron, H. B. W., Tucker, B. E., Andrews, J. P., Boshes, B., Cohen, J., Fromm, E., and Yacorzynski, G. K. (1960). *Amer. J. Obstet. Gynec.*, **80**, 1129.
129. Karlberg, P. (1960). *J. Pediat.*, **56**, 585.
130. Tunstall, M. E., and Hodges, R. J. H. (1961). *Lancet*, **1**, 146.
131. Donald, I. (1961). *Proc. S.W. Obstet. Gynæc. Soc.* Pergamon Press, Oxford.
132. Rees, G. J. (1961). *Ibid.*
133. Cooper, E. A., Hylton Smith, and Pask, E. A. (1960). *Anæsthesia*, **15**, 211.
134. Dawes, G. S., Mott, J. C., and Shelley, H. S. (1959). *J. Physiol.*, **146**, 516.

135. USHER, R. (1961). *The Metabolic Changes in Respiratory Distress Syndrome of Prematurity*. Ciba Foundation Publication.
136. USHER, R. (1959). *Pediatrics*, **24,** 562.
137. WESTIN, B., MILLER, J. A., NYBERG, R., and WEDENBERG, E. (1959). *Surgery*, **45,** 868.
138. DAWES, G. S. (1961). *Brit. med. Bull.*, **17,** 148.

Chapter 9

MECHANICAL VENTILATION OF THE LUNGS

A. R. Hunter

Manually-operated Ventilators — Methods — Principles — Circulatory Effects—Design of Respirators—Classification of Respirators—Cycling—Patient-triggered Ventilators—Determining the Extent of Mechanical Ventilation—Monitoring the Ventilator.

One of the most striking developments in anæsthesia in the last few years has been the transfer of emphasis in matters involving the artificial ventilation of the lungs from controlled respiration as it is conducted in the operating theatre to the performance of artificial respiration as a therapeutic measure in the treatment of disease. The immediate stimulus for this development came from an appreciation of the need for an effective method of treating poliomyelitis affecting the respiratory mechanism.[1] It was however quickly found that other states of respiratory insufficiency could be satisfactorily treated by means of mechanical ventilation of the lungs and where special units for the purpose are available they are used to the full. Just how worthwhile their work is can be seen from the reports which have been published.[2-10]

The result of this has been that the physiological and clinical problems of mechanical ventilation of the lungs have become of more importance than the machines used for the purpose. For this reason this chapter is concerned essentially with such basic matters. Those who seek specific information concerning the structure and properties of individual respirators are referred to the exhaustive Cardiff monograph on the subject.[30]

MANUALLY OPERATED VENTILATORS

The simplest contrivances for mechanical ventilation of the lungs are operated by intermittent manual pressure. The commonest of these are the time honoured bag and expiratory valve, with or without a soda lime canister, and the Oxford bellows. Two interesting machines have however come to the fore in the course of the last few years. The first of these is the Cardiff ventilator.[11] This requires

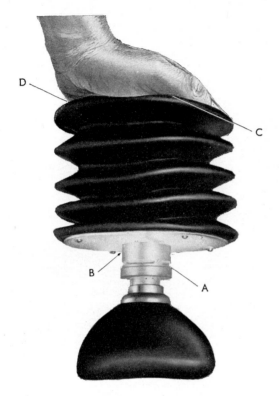

FIG. 32. The Cardiff Ventilator (M.I.E. Ltd.).

atmospheric air for its operation. This is drawn into a spring loaded bellows through a one way valve and discharged through yet another valve to the patient. This valve also provides an open passage to the exterior in expiration.

Another similar apparatus is the Ambu[12]. This consists essentially of a bag whose walls are rendered semi-rigid by a lining of sponge rubber. Air is drawn into the bag through a valve, is pushed into the patient's lungs through a Ruben valve,[13] and escapes to the exterior through the same valve. The Ruben valve which is used in this apparatus is that specially designed for use during controlled respiration. In this the expiratory disc, which in the more orthodox version prevents the entry of external air in inspiration, is removed. (Fig. 34.)

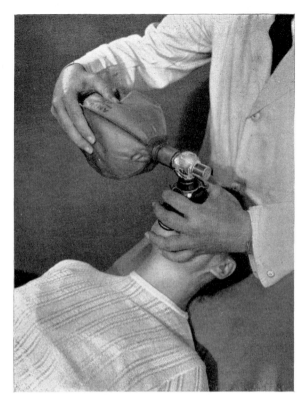

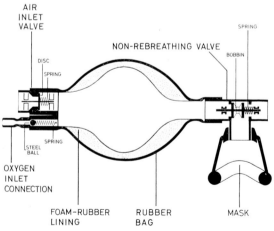

AIR
INLET
VALVE

SPRING

DISC

NON-REBREATHING VALVE

BOBBIN

SPRING

SPRING

STEEL
BALL

OXYGEN
INLET
CONNECTION

FOAM–RUBBER
LINING

RUBBER
BAG

MASK

FIG. 33. The Ambu Resuscitator (B.O.C.).

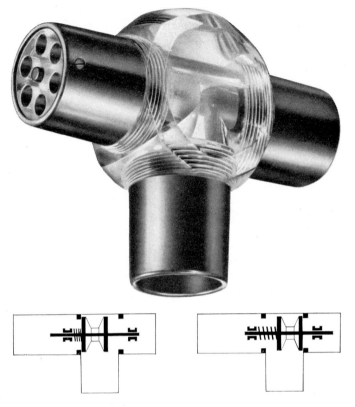

(a) Inspiratory position.   (b) Expiratory position.
FIG. 34. Ruben Valve (B.O.C.). Diagrammatic.

MEANS OF MECHANICAL VENTILATION

Automatic machines for ventilation of the lungs operate in two ways. Some apply intermittently changing pressures to the thorax and abdomen from without, and thus reproduce the respiratory movements. In consequence air is displaced in and out of the lungs. Others apply alternating pressures to the airway and thus achieve respiratory exchange.

Respirators Acting by External Pressure

Tank Respirators. The tank respirator is the most elaborate of the machines used for artificial respiration. It consists essentially of a coffin-like container which encloses the trunk and limbs of the patient but not his head and neck. The latter passes through a sponge rubber collar which fits so tightly that leakage of air in and out of the main container cannot occur. Respiratory movements are produced by the intermittent application of negative pressure to the enclosed space surrounding the trunk. The details of what happens in terms of pressure and volume changes in the airway and lungs are discussed at length by Spencer.[14] In essence they are identical with those produced by the intermittent application of positive pressure to the airway (*vide* p. 255) save that the sign of many of the pressure changes, relative to that of the atmosphere is reversed.[15] For example the return of blood to the heart still fails during the inspiratory stroke but the cause is not positive pressure applied to the mediastinum but negative pressure applied to the abdomen.[35, 36]

The classical example of this type of machine is the Drinker-Both respirator which has been known for many years. Recently this machine has been re-designed so that the container opens for nursing purposes like an alligator's jaws, on a hinge at the foot, the patient meantime being ventilated by some other method. The problems of having the patient always on his back, a considerable drawback to the earlier models, have been overcome by Kelleher[16] whose apparatus is so designed with two mattresses that it is possible to rotate the patient into the prone position without removing him from the respirator. These machines, like their predecessor the original Drinker-Both apparatus, have their tank mounted on a central spindle so that it is possible to tip the patient head-down or foot-down, as may be necessary. Kelleher's apparatus can also rotate on its long axis.

Most workers have found it difficult to combine tracheostomy with treatment in a tank respirator. A few, however, have succeeded in this too, and in their units tank respirators are used for the treatment of spinal poliomyelitis and all other forms of acute respiratory insufficiency not associated with laryngeal paralysis.

Cuirass Respirators differ from tank machines in that only the abdomen and chest are enclosed for the production of respiratory movements. The limbs are free. For the latter reason a cuirass apparatus is often used in the mobilization of a patient with long standing respiratory insufficiency—usually not amounting to complete paralysis. The first such machine, the Bragg Paul, was in fact built for this very purpose.[17]

The earliest cuirass respirators, and some which are of more recent design, operate by the rhythmic inflation and release of a rubber bag confined between an inexpansible cuirass and the patient's chest and abdomen. The rise in pressure in the bag compresses the trunk and air is driven out of the lungs. Inspiration occurs as a result of the elastic recoil of the thoracic cage to the resting position. Such an apparatus has been found useful for maintaining oxygenation during endoscopic procedures.[18] It is, however, generally accepted that such positive pressure cuirass respirators are unlikely to main-

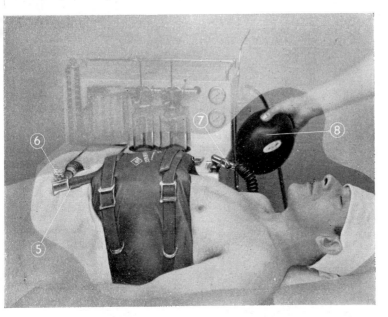

FIG. 35. Pinkerton's Cuirass Respirator (M.I.E.).

tain a completely adequate tidal exchange for a long period[19, 20] and they should be regarded as assistants of respiration rather than a complete substitute for it.

Another group of cuirass respirators operate by negative pressure. These consist essentially of a rigid shell which is fitted over and secured to the front and sides of the patient's chest and abdomen. A pneumatic or sponge rubber cushion round the edge of the shell ensures that its fit is airtight. Intermittent negative pressure is applied to the space under the shell and respiratory movements are produced in exactly the same way as with a tank respirator. When the shell covers the entire chest and abdomen these machines are more effective than positive pressure cuirass ventilators. Further they produce "normal" ventilation rather than an intermittent reduction of functional residual capacity. The Rotaventilator is such a machine and versions of the Monaghan[21] and Emerson[22] ventilator can be used with a shell cuirass during bronchoscopy.

The most elaborate cuirass ventilator is the recent version of the Emerson. In this there is a perforated metal cuirass, as in the other types of machine, but the cuirass, the patient's trunk and proximal

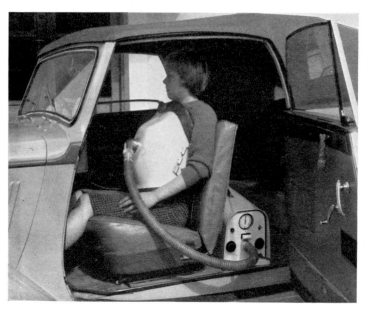

FIG. 36. The Rotaventilator. (Cape Eng. Co., Warwick).

limbs are enclosed in a light pliable plastic garment like a plain night-dress with a loose collar and short sleeves. These and the skirt of the garment are wrapped loosely round the patient and an intermittent negative pressure is applied to the space under the cuirass. The clinging properties of the garment are such that it automatically forms an airtight seal at the openings and the patient is to all intents and purposes in a tank respirator, though the only rigid portion of the machine is the cuirass and in some instances a back plate. It is claimed that this apparatus will produce an adequate tidal volume with the application of pressures as small as -20 cm H_2O (Fig. 37).

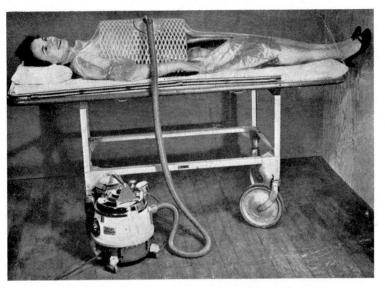

Fig. 37. The Emerson Cuirass. (Garthur Ltd., Buckingham).

The vast majority of the machines for mechanical ventilation of the lungs are of the intermittent positive pressure variety and the remainder of this chapter will concern itself primarily with these.

PRINCIPLES UNDERLYING MECHANICAL VENTILATION OF THE LUNGS

The basic principle underlying intermittent positive pressure ventilation of the lungs is that pressure applied to the airway increases the capacity of the chest; when the pressure is withdrawn the lungs return to their original size. The tidal exchange obtained depends on the resistance which the patient opposes to inflation. This opposing resistance consists of two moieties, the elastic recoil of the lungs and thoracic cage on the one hand and the frictional resistance to the flow of gas through the respiratory passages on the other. Both these quantities can be measured.

Compliance. The elasticity of the lungs and chest wall is measured as its reciprocal, the compliance, i.e. the number of ml of gas pushed into the chest by an increase in intra-alveolar pressure of 1 cm of water. Compliance is normally measured by raising the pressure in the respiratory tract by some mechanical means and maintaining the pressure at a constant level until no further air enters the lungs, a state which is achieved only after some seconds of inflation. The lungs are then allowed to empty themselves, and the amount of gas blown into them divided by the inflation pressure gives the compliance.[23, 24, 25] Compliance measured in this way is the total compliance of the patient's respiratory mechanism. It is possible

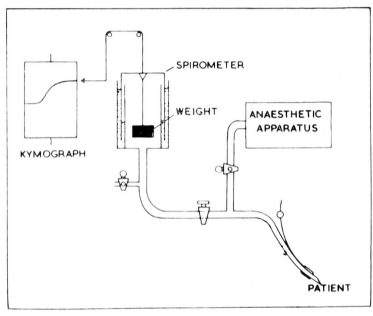

Fig. 38. Apparatus for determining the Compliance in Anæsthetized Patients. The Kymograph records the amount of anæsthetic mixture taken from the spirometer which is weighted to act as a source of constant pressure. (Newman *et al.*, 1959, *Brit. J. Anæsth.*)

to measure independently the compliance of the lungs and that of the thoracic cage. The portion of the pressure applied used in expanding the lungs alone is obtained by measuring the pressure difference between the airway and the œsophagus. The remainder of the pressure which moves the viscera and chest wall is the pressure swing in the œsophagus relative to external pressure.

The following figures for compliance are given.[26] The compliance of the isolated lung is said to be 130–220 ml/cm H_2O. The total compliance, i.e. the combined compliance of the lungs and of the chest wall, is 120 ml/cm H_2O and that of the anæsthetized subject 62 ml/cm H_2O.[27, 28] The compliance of the patient on artificial ventilation of the lungs is also considerably less than that of the normal conscious subject. It may be as little as 28 ml/cm H_2O.[29]

Airway Resistance. The frictional resistance to the passage of gases along the airways will vary with their flow rate. Mushin and others[30] quoting from Comroe[31] gave a figure for normal subject of 2 cm of water resistance per litre per second of flow rate. As the peak respiratory flow rate during normal quiet breathing need not be much more than 60 L/min, i.e. 1 L/sec, it is obvious that at rest this quantity cannot be of great importance. They point out however that much higher values for airway resistance may be present in asthma and in emphysema. These higher resistances are partly due to bronchial narrowing which converts the laminar flow, in which resistance varies

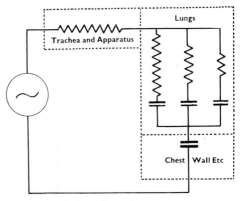

FIG. 39. Electrical analogy of respiratory mechanism.

directly with the flow rate, to turbulent flow in which resistance increases as the square of the flow rate. Because of this change in the resistance as airway diameter is reduced, a comparatively small reduction can have a relatively enormous effect in increasing resistance at the point at which turbulence develops. To avoid unnecessary increases in airway resistance every possible care should be taken during the conduct of mechanical ventilation to remove secretion which might narrow the trachea and bronchi, or water which might condense in the tubes connecting the respirator to the patient. The special importance of this can be seen from the fact that a rind of secretion no thicker than about 1 mm within a tracheostomy tube doubles the resistance to the passage of gases through it.[32]

The resistance opposed by the lungs to pressure applied to the airway has the dual character of resistance and elasticity. This gives to them properties analogous to those of an electrical circuit in which a number of condensers are charged through resistances.[23, 33] In such a circuit the amount of electricity which enters any individual condenser varies not only with the resistance and the capacity of the condenser. It is also influenced by the time for which an applied voltage acts. (There is a considerable local variation in the lungs, both in frictional resistance to air entry and in compliance.) The result is that the distribution and the amount of expansion of the entering air produced by a given inflation pressure depend not only on the size of

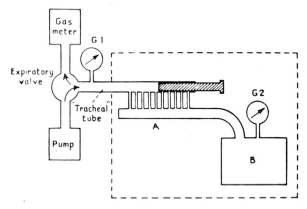

Fig. 40. Mechanical Model for Testing Respirators. The frictional resistance to the passage of gases along the fine tubes in parallel represents the airway resistance. (A). The elastic resistance of the gas in the reservoir (B) to compression represents compliance. (*Lancet*, 1955).

the inflation pressure but on the time interval over which it is applied.[102] A mechanical arrangement of frictional and elastic resistance to gas pressure in a model lung has been made for the testing of respirators (Fig. 40).

Though the compliance of the lungs and the airway resistance form the theoretical background to the clinical problem of artificial ventilation it is important to realise that the duration of the inspiratory stroke of a machine is never long enough to take up all the compliance. Further the reading shown on the pressure gauge of the ventilator is by no means that applied to the lung alveoli.[34] In consequence forecasts of the necessary pressure to produce a given tidal volume in a patient which are based directly on the compliance and airway resistance will be most misleading; they are invariably too small. Further the overall compliance and the patency of the airway of the patient on mechanical ventilation vary quite considerably from hour to hour, if not from minute to minute. The use of a respirator with a preset inflation pressure is therefore regarded by many workers as a too uncertain means of producing a constant tidal volume to be clinically acceptable.

CIRCULATORY EFFECTS

There is an extensive literature on the subject of the circulatory changes produced by IPPR and on those in patients in tank respirators.[35,36] Little attention seems to have been given to the principles underlying the design of cuirass respirators or to the disturbances of the circulation which might be expected to follow their employment. There is no reason however to assume that there is any basic difference in the three groups.

The circulatory disturbance produced by mechanical ventilation of the lungs falls into two distinct parts. First there are effects within the thorax. Secondly, there is an upset of the pressure gradient, apparent mainly in the veins, between the thorax and the adjacent parts of the body. The changes within the thorax depend on whether the chest wall has been breached by operation or by injury, or is intact. In the latter case the mediastinum can be regarded as fluid-containing space through which pressure is transmitted freely and evenly. During the inflation stroke of IPPR the pressure in this space becomes relatively more positive by an amount roughly equal to half the pressure applied to the airway. This pressure is applied equally to all the chambers of the heart and therefore cannot directly affect the pressure differences generated by cardiac contraction. However, since the absolute pressure in, for example, the left ventricle, is raised during the entire contraction by an amount equal to the pressure transmitted to the mediastinum, there will be a similar rise in the systolic blood pressure in the peripheral vessels during the inflation stroke,[37] an observation which has been made by every anæsthetist who has taken the blood pressure of a patient during mechanical ventilation of the lungs. Likewise, though the pressure difference generated by the right ventricle will, as long as the venous return remains the same, be unaffected by IPPR while the chest is closed, the absolute pressure in the pulmonary vessels will also be raised by an amount equal to the pressure transmitted through the mediastinum.[38] This increase in pressure is sufficient to overcome any tendency on the part of these vessels to collapse as a result of the pressure applied to them from the airway.

When the thorax is open the position is quite different. The heart and the mediastinal structures are now exposed to the atmosphere and both lungs are largely free from the constraining effects of the elasticity of the chest wall; the pressure of the atmosphere has ready access to the mediastinum. In the circumstances the whole of the pressure difference between the airway and the mediastinum is taken up in the lungs—which are in fact now easier to inflate. There is however a larger pressure difference between the alveoli and the heart whose chambers are now all at atmospheric pressure. In this situation inflation pressures approximating to the normal pulmonary arterial pressure can appreciably compress the vessels in the lung and thus cause fall in blood pressure. Since an upset of the venous return is not implicated a negative phase in expiration does not improve matters.[37]

The most obvious effect of IPPR however is on the venous return. Normally the mean venous pressure in the thorax is subatmospheric while that in the great veins at the root of the neck and in the upper abdomen is slightly positive. Further the act of spontaneous inspiration in which the capacity of the thorax is increased by active contraction of muscles, makes this pressure even more negative. During the inflationary stroke of IPPR however the pressure in the thorax may thus become more positive than that in the abdomen. The immediate result of starting mechanical ventilation of the lungs must therefore be a reversal of the pressure gradient on which the venous return depends. Cardiac output in consequence falls.[40] In clinical practice however compensation for this change occurs quite readily[41] even in such unlikely subjects as those who have just undergone a cardiac operation.[42] The basis of the compensation appears to be a vasoconstriction since it is aided by vasoconstrictor drugs[43] and abolished by ganglion blockers[44] and spinal anæsthesia[45] in experimental animals and in man by diseases which interrupt the sympathetic outflow e.g. acute polyneuritis and upper spinal cord transections.[103, 104, 105] On the other hand it is also prevented by exsanguination and barbiturate overdosage[45] which do not necessarily make vasoconstriction impossible; so the point cannot be regarded as fully proved.

It is the mean intrathoracic pressure which determines the degree of circulatory upset in a susceptible subject.[41] This pressure was found by Opie and others to be raised by $+ 3\cdot5$ to $+ 5\cdot9$ cm H_2O during IPPR with some ventilators.[46] The latter of these pressures was such that it would within half an hour produce syncope in a minority of healthy subjects. It was therefore obviously to be regarded seriously.

The mean intrathoracic pressure depends on the mean pressure in the patient's airway. This can be reduced in two ways.[46] First the employment of a negative phase in expiration of –5 to –10 cm H_2O keeps the airway pressure down to levels comparable to those in normal spontaneous breathing. It has however recently been shown that a negative phase increases physiological dead space and this reduces efficiency of ventilation.[106] Where no apparatus with a negative phase is available shortening the duration of inspiration will allow more time for expiration and thus lower the mean intrathoracic pressure. Shortening duration of inspiration will be liable to reduce the overall minute volume output of the machine.[64]

If the peak inspiratory flow rate of the output of the ventilator is only of the order of 30 L/min underventilation will result from this. Where, however, the peak flow rate is of the order of 50–90 L/min it is possible to reduce inspiration to one-third or less of the total respiratory cycle without undue reduction in minute volume. Under such circumstances the rise in mean intrathoracic pressure is of the order of 3·5 to 4·0 cm H_2O and this is much less serious.[46]

Some have said however that the inspiration : expiration ratio is important also in its own right. According to them, increasing the number of heart beats in the expiratory phase minimises the blood pressure fall due to IPPR.[47] Decreasing their relative number exaggerates it even when there is sufficient additional negative pressure in expiration to keep the mean intrathoracic pressure constant.[37]

THE DESIGN OF RESPIRATORS

The basic desiderata in the design of a respirator for IPPR were summarized in 1955 as follows.[48] First, the apparatus must be capable of producing correct pulmonary ventilation. Secondly, a low mean intrathoracic pressure must be maintained. In order that this should be so the apparatus must be capable of an instantaneous output of 40 to 80 L/min at all rates. The pressure produced by the respirator must collapse immediately the inspiratory phase is complete; negative pressure during expiration is an additional aid to a mean low intrathoracic pressure. It is desirable that where the patient is making spontaneous but inadequate attempts to breathe, the machine should be able to match them. It should be possible to add oxygen to the air with which the lungs are inflated. Humidification of the inspired gases should be feasible. Arrangements for the use of the apparatus either with air in the ward or in the operating theatre with anæsthetic gases will add to its value. If an apparatus is to be used in anæsthesia, closed circuit operation is desirable as an alternative.

The usefulness of a respirator is governed by the type of energy used to drive it. If it is electrically operated there is inevitably a risk of explosion with inflammable anæsthetic agents. This difficulty is avoided when the driving force is the energy of compressed gas. If this gas is provided by a cylinder however the consumption is to some extent a limiting factor on usefulness. When this is high and even a large cylinder runs out within an hour or two, the apparatus is obviously unsuitable for long term artificial respiration therapy. An entraining device goes some way to reduce consumption and offset this drawback. The difficulty is eliminated completely where the source of the driving gas is the air from a compressor. Very few compressors are spark-proof and unless they are remote from the respirator itself the explosion risk once more appears. An even cheaper yet satisfactory substitute for a compressor is the blower unit of an ordinary domestic vacuum cleaner. This has been successfully employed to provide the energy for the Newcastle respirators.[49, 50] An arrangement for using the driving gases of a respirator to ventilate the patient is a useful economy.

A large number of workers have had a wide experience of therapeutic artificial ventilation since the criteria in the first paragraph were laid down. Nonetheless, though there has been occasion to amplify them, these desiderata remain basically unchanged. Thus it is now stated that a respirator should be so constructed that it can deliver a tidal volume varying from 80 to 1,000 ml in one second[51] against the frictional resistance to the passage of gases along the airways and the elasticity of the lungs and thorax. Machines are now available with even higher peak flow rates than 80 L/min.[52, 53] There has too been something of a change of heart concerning the maximum safe inflation pressure.[54] The limiting factor is the tolerance of the lung tissue to applied pressure. It is probable that even abnormal lungs will withstand inflation pressures of 25[55] to 30 cm[56] of water. In a normal individual as much as 37 cm of water can be used with safety.[57] High pressures, however, will be required only when there is partial obstruction of the airway and there is not under these circumstances the same likelihood of their reaching the delicate alveoli to damage them nor of their transmission to the mediastinum.

THE WAVE-FORM

Of all the features of respirators, perhaps the wave-form shows the greatest variation. There are however certain rules, all of which are aimed at the employment of a wave-form which will give the lowest mean airway pressure for a given tidal volume and therefore the lowest possible overall pressure in the mediastinum.

Inflationary Stroke. It was originally calculated that an inflationary stroke in which the pressure rose rapidly to a maximum level and stayed there throughout the entire inspiratory stroke was that which gave the most satisfactory ventilation of the lungs.[4] With such an inflationary stroke the flow of gases into the patient is maximal

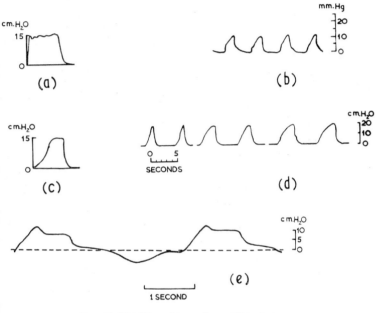

FIG. 41. The Wave-form of some Respirators.

(a) Radcliffe.	(d) Blease.
(b) Smith-Clarke.	(e) Engstrom.
(c) Beaver.	

immediately after full inflation pressure is developed and tails off to negligible values as the pressure is maintained.[58, 59] It has been shown that with this type of apparatus prolongation of the inflationary stroke much beyond one second gives very little increase in the amount of air which passes into the lungs.[59] The Radcliffe respirator is the classical example of such a machine.[60, 61] It, with other similar ventilators,[53] undoubtedly produces a useful tidal volume with a shorter inflationary period than any other type of apparatus and in consequence the inspiration : expiration ratio can be reduced to as little as 1 : 3. The only drawback is that this sudden building up of pressure in the chest is sometimes uncomfortable for the patient and frankly painful for one who has had a recent thoracotomy or chest injury. It is also believed by some that the frictional resistance in the airway generated by the high initial flow rate[55] makes such machines unsatisfactory in patients with bronchial narrowing.[62] Some believe too[63, 64] that patients find it difficult to synchronize their own respiratory efforts with such machines. Smith-Clarke and Galpine concluded that wave-form mattered less than mean airway pressure[65] and the respirator designed by them also has a sharp initial build-up of pressure, which will under most circumstances be followed by a continuing climb.[65]

The respirators employed by many anæsthetists in operating theatres have a different design. In them the pressure-wave is approximately triangular and the inflation pressure goes on increasing steadily throughout the entire inspiratory phase.[66] Such machines include the Aintree, Fazakerley, Blease and Newcastle respirators. It has been shown that for one such respirator, the Blease P6 apparatus, the volume of gas pushed into the lungs increases quite considerably with increasing duration of inspiration.[64] No work seems to have been done in relation to other respirators of this kind in clinical use but it is very probable that the Beaver, which has an intermediate type of pressure wave, will also have properties in relation to duration of inflation which will be intermediate between those of the Blease and the Smith-Clarke. Since in the Beaver and Smith-Clarke machines duration of inflation cannot be directly altered the matter is more of theoretical than of practical importance. The Oxford workers however believe that wave-form does not greatly modify the effects of changing duration of inflation.[106]

The Expiratory Phase. There is universal agreement that in every respirator in clinical use the pressure in the patient's lungs should fall as quickly as possible immediately after the end of inspiration.[58] It is also generally agreed that if the pressure during this phase of respiration is sub-atmospheric the negative pressure will be transmitted to the mediastinal contents, with the result that the mean pressure throughout the entire respiratory cycle will be more nearly atmospheric.[46] There is however some argument as to whether the negative pressure should exist only in the early stages of expiration[65] or whether it should persist throughout the entire cycle, or whether it should be present only during the latter part of expiration. Those who believe that it should be present during the whole expiratory period point to its transmission to the mediastinum and argue that it must result in an improved venous return. Others however believe that the sudden application of suction to the respiratory tree can lead to collapse of bronchi in patients with a tendency to respiratory trapping,[67] as occurs in emphysema, and that in such patients a more gradual decline in pressure is more satisfactory.[68] This latter type of pressure wave is produced by the Barnet and Engström respirators.[52] (The latter apparatus also combines the characteristics of the two previously described wave-forms in its inspiratory stroke in which the first part of the wave is triangular like those of the other respirators used in anæsthesia but this period is followed by a plateau during which the pressure is maintained at a constant level until the start of expiration.) The American literature contains descriptions of respirators working almost entirely at sub-atmospheric pressures, e.g. with a pressure swing of 0 to —10 cm of water.[44] In fact, however, such respirators have not found acceptance possibly because of the marked increase in physiological dead space produced by the application of negative pressure to the airway. There is a widespread, though probably groundless,[45] fear that expiratory pressures of less than —5 cm of water may lead to the development of pulmonary œdema.

Expiratory Valves. In order that a satisfactory wave-form for mechanical ventilation of the lungs should be obtained the pressure in the apparatus must collapse at once as soon as inspiration is at an end. There must therefore be minimal resistance to expiration. To this end it is desirable that an expiratory valve should open freely to the atmosphere. Some expiratory valves operate near to the patient. Such are the Ruben valve,[69] which is incorporated with the Ambu resuscitator,[12] the Fink valve[70] and the Beaver valve. The first of these exists in two forms. One of these is designed for use with the patient breathing spontaneously. When it is used for artificial ventilation of the lungs however with a flow which exceeds the patient's minute volume it is very common for the little bobbin to jam in the inspiratory position with the result that the gases from the machine continue to pass into the patient's lungs and cannot escape in expiration. This difficulty is readily overcome when the standard Magill attachment is in use by placing a Heidbrink expiratory valve somewhere between the bag and the Ruben valve.[71] If the Heidbrink valve is left slightly open excess gases can be pushed out through it with the result that the bag never becomes "tight" and the little bobbin in the Ruben valve is free to return to the expiratory position at the end of each inflationary stroke. A pattern of Ruben valve without the expiratory disc is available for use during controlled respiration[13] (*vide* p. 245). It cannot be used with the patient breathing spontaneously.

The Beaver valve consists essentially of a rubber diaphragm which is readily displaced in its casing. It bulges slightly toward the patient in inspiration and toward the machine during the expiratory phase.

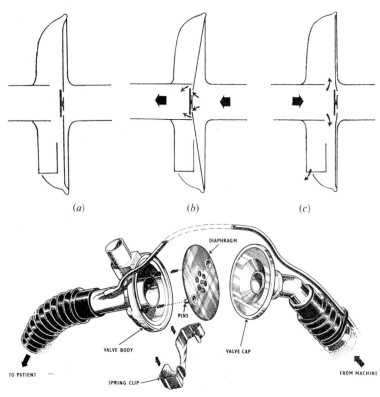

(a)   (b)   (c)

FIG. 42. The Beaver Valve.[73]

(*a*) Neutral position.   (*c*) Expiration.
(*b*) Inspiration.   (*d*) Sprung diagram.

In inspiration the diaphragm impinges on the collar-like open end of the metal tube leading to the patient. Gases pass through holes in its centre to the patient. These cannot however leak out into the expiratory port. During expiration the diaphragm is pushed toward the machine end of the valve and the small rounded metal plate mounted on it occludes the holes and prevents any back-flow, though gases are free to escape to the exterior. This arrangement makes it impossible for any negative pressure generated in the machine to be transmitted to the patient.

The Beaver valve has undoubted advantages. It has a far lower resistance to expiration than any other expiratory mechanism built into a respirator without a negative phase. Further, the machine to which it is fitted "fails safe", i.e. if the respirator stops accidentally it leaves the patient with an open and unobstructed tube through which he can breathe air if he has some residual spontaneous respiratory activity. The dead space of the Beaver valve is small. Further, the respirator to which it is fitted does not require a heavy double hose which may by its weight pull on the tracheostomy tube and cause pain, or even drag out a tube which has been insecurely fixed.

The Beaver valve has two quite serious drawbacks. First, it ceases to function satisfactorily if the diaphragm becomes wet, as it must inevitably do if a humidifier is in use. It is therefore necessary to change the diaphragm for a dry one at least every 4 hours. Secondly, the diaphragm is likely to chatter in a patient who is to some extent breathing with the respirator. When this happens it is possible for some of the gases pushed out by the machine to pass directly to the exterior without reaching the patient. For this reason metering of the expired minute volume, an essential part of the control of artificial respiration, must be carried out with the Beaver valve, not at the expiratory port, but in the tube connecting the valve to the tracheostomy. Only a Wright anemometer is small enough to do this without at the same time adding intolerably to the dead space and even this meter can only be used for a few minutes before water condenses in it and upsets its accuracy.

Mechanically Operated Expiratory Valves. The vast majority of respirators in current use are fitted with mechanically operated expiratory valves. There are no special problems in the design of these. They all however impose a certain amount of resistance to the passage of the expired gases.[63] In the vast majority of respirators too, there is an appreciable length of hose connecting the patient to the valve. Very often this hose is interrupted by a trap in which water vaporized from the humidifier or from the patient may condense. In addition the expired gases are passed through a measuring device before they reach the exterior. All these contrivances add their quota to the resistance to expiration and though the pressure immediately outside the expiratory valve may be atmospheric, the pressure at the tracheostomy or, worse still, at the bifurcation of the trachea, is unlikely to fall to this level during expiration unless negative pressure is applied at some stage during this phase of respiration. On the other hand it is a comparatively simple matter to arrange for the application of negative pressure during inspiration where a mechanically-operated expiratory valve is built into the machine itself. It is very much more difficult to do this where the expiratory valve opens to the atmosphere close to the patient.

THE CLASSIFICATION OF RESPIRATORS

It is possible to classify the many different types of intermittent positive pressure respirators available in a multitude of ways; thus it would be proper to speak of electrically driven respirators, compressed-air driven respirators or of square-wave respirators and triangular-wave respirators, pressure, volume and time cycled respirators, pressure generators and flow generators, and so on. It is, however, most satisfactory to classify respirators firstly according to their characteristics in use.

Therapeutic artificial ventilation of the lungs is now carried out almost exclusively under the immediate supervision of nurses. Reliability, therefore, is an over-riding consideration. To this end it has been suggested that respirators should primarily be classified into two groups, viz. those in which the pressure exerted by the machine has been fixed beforehand and those in which the volume which the machine will deliver has been set—in simpler terms, pressure pre-set and volume pre-set machines.[66] This is no new idea. It is in fact contained in a paper by Mushin and Rendell Baker published in 1954[73] and the words "volume limited" and pressure limited" are largely used to describe respirators in the transatlantic literature.[74] Alternatively, the converse description of "pressure variable respirator" is applied to the volume pre-set machine for reasons which will become apparent presently, while the pressure pre-set machine is described as "volume variable". In many papers the terms "pressure cycled" and "volume cycled" are used, wrongly in the author's view, as synonyms for pressure and volume pre-set.

Both types of apparatus have certain chacteristics which are of importance in relation to their clinical use. In the case of the pressure pre-set apparatus the volume of gas which the machine delivers to the patient falls off rapidly as resistance to inflation increases. As obstruction to output builds up, a progressively larger proportion of the pressure is dissipated in pushing gas past the obstruction, so that virtually no pressure is left over to expand the alveoli and ventilate the lungs. Further, in many such machines when obstruction to output occurs, the duration of inspiration decreases and the short inspirations are not as effective in inflating the chest.[64] On the other hand, a pressure pre-set machine is capable of compensating for a leak in the apparatus or in the junction between the patient and the machine. Under such circumstances the output will be increased until the capacity of the delivery mechanism is reached. The pressure pre-set apparatus will usually give more obvious audible warning in the form of a change in its rhythm and very often in the sound of its valves when it is working against an obstruction. On the obverse, if the pressure pre-set machine is also pressure cycled, a leak which is so large that cycling pressure is never reached may result in total arrest of the machine. A pressure pre-set machine cannot build up dangerous pressure and apply this to the patient.

By contrast the volume pre-set machine is capable of building up greater pressure to overcome an obstruction and thus of maintaining its tidal volume. Most machines however are fitted with a safety valve which lifts at a pressure of some 30 cm of water, so that compensation for obstruction is by no means complete. In addition the increased inspiratory pressure may be capable of pushing the required tidal volume into the lungs but the weaker passive forces of expiration may not be able to expel this tidal volume against the obstruction, with the result that a permanent over-distension of the chest occurs. This will be associated with a positive pressure in the alveoli which will be transmitted to the great veins, there to interfere with venous return and to cause poor cardiac filling and hypotension. The volume pre-set apparatus too, cannot increase its output to cope with a leak.

Though it is convenient to classify respirators as volume pre-set or pressure pre-set, it is in fact possible to use a number of these machines in either way. This is more true of machines used by anæsthetists in the operating theatre than it is of those employed during long-term artificial respiration.[75, 76] Machines which satisfy the requirements of either classification, depending on how they are used, include especially those types of apparatus such as the Clutton-Brock or Mortimer in which a bellows or piston replaces the bag in an anæsthetic machine. Where the expiratory valve is kept closed and only basal oxygen is admitted to a closed circuit, the machine operates essentially as a volume pre-set apparatus. Where however a fairly large flow is used with a spillover it is in fact the pressure in the apparatus which is pre-set by the tension in the spring-loaded expiratory valve.

CYCLING

It is in some respects difficult to delineate the methods by which respirators cycle, that is, trip from the inspiratory into the expiratory phase. There is, however, no problem with pressure cycled machines in which inflation comes automatically to an end when the pressure in the machine is built up to a pre-fixed level. It is, however, important to appreciate that the inflation pressure shown on the gauge of the machine is frequently much lower than that at the point of delivery of the gases.[34] In the vast majority of machines of this type the rate of build-up of the pressure is governed by the magnitude of a gas flow and control of duration of inspiration is obtained by altering this flow. For a given flow the duration of inspiration is set by the resistance of the patient to the output of the machine. If this increases, the inspiration automatically shortens. The actual contrivance which produces cycling varies from machine to machine. In some the increasing pressure breaks the attraction of a magnet for soft iron; in others a diaphragm springs over or a toggle mechanism brings about the change.

The other methods of cycling are difficult to define. These are time cycling and volume cycling. Mushin and his colleagues[30] require that an auxiliary timing mechanism must be present before the former designation can be used. The author, however, regards as time-cycled any machine in which duration of inspiration and expiration are set by the operator. He would limit the term "volume cycled" to machines in which the end of inspiration is brought about by a mechanical contrivance operated by the moving parts of the delivery mechanism; for example, in the Stephenson respirator a bellows opens a trip valve at the top of its travel. By these definitions all machines operated by engines—electric motors, windscreen-wiper motors, sine wave pumps etc.—are regarded as time cycled. Such include the Beaver, the Smith-Clarke, the Clutton-Brock, the Mortimer, the Engström, the Radcliffe respirators, and the Starling pump. In addition this group also includes machines which have an auxiliary timing mechanism like the Barnet. The essential feature of time cycling is that changes in resistance to inflation do not affect the duration of inspiration. Some volume pre-set machines are driven by compressed air delivered at a pressure many times that used for inflation of the lungs. The result is that changes in the resistance to the output of the machine make only a negligible difference to the load[75, 76] and consequently duration of inspiration scarcely varies, i.e. the machine is substantially time cycled. Where entraining devices are employed to reduce consumption of driving gases the effective pressure of the driving gases may, however, be reduced to the point at which an appreciable prolongation of inspiration occurs when load increases, i.e. the characteristics of volume cycling appear.

Finally, the cycling mechanism determines only the probable alteration in duration of inspiration in the presence of increased resistance. The effect on tidal volume depends on whether the machine is pressure or volume pre-set (*vide supra*).

Ventilators also cycle from expiration into inspiration. Except with patient triggered respirators the duration of expiration is only rarely influenced by clinical considerations. The actual type of cycling is therefore of slight importance. In most ventilators it is fixed by a timing mechanism.

PATIENT-TRIGGERED VENTILATORS

As Pask indicated some years ago,[48] it is obviously desirable that a respirator should be able to follow spontaneous respiration when this is present but insufficient. Machines which are capable of doing this are known as patient-triggered respirators. The trigger may be actuated either by the inspiration of a very small amount of air or by the very small pressure change produced by the start of a breath.

It is suggested that a triggered machine should have the following characteristics. It should be sensitive to 0·5 cm of water pressure difference produced by inspiration[54,77] or to a respiratory displacement of 5 to 10 ml.[51, 77] It is possible to make such machines respond to smaller changes of pressure or volume, e.g. to 2·5 ml respiratory displacement. An apparatus with such a sensitivity may however be triggered by the alteration in the chest capacity produced by a cardiac contraction, an obviously undesirable result. The delay in delivery of gas should not exceed 0·2 second.[77] There should be an open passage for inspiration, should triggering not occur, and in all respects the machine should "fail safe". There should be an automatic delivery of air after a selected interval, say 6 seconds, should the patient fail to trigger the machine. There should be provision for adequate humidification.

There is always a delay between the onset of inspiration and the build-up of the inflation stroke of the pump. This delay is greatest where the trigger sets mechanical parts in motion. It is less where the trigger operates a solenoid valve and releases a stream of compressed air. The result of this delay in the mechanically operated respirator is that such machines cannot in fact be used with patient triggering in those whose respiratory rate is extremely rapid, for it is almost impossible for a mechanical contrivance to empty itself against the resistance which the lungs and air passages offer to the entry of air into them within the comparatively short period which inspiration must occupy if the entire respiratory cycle is of the order of $1\frac{1}{2}$ seconds or less. Indeed it is all too common for the patient whose inspiration is already rapid and jerky to begin to breathe out before the machine has completed its inflation stroke. He inevitably tends to strain against this forced inflation with the result that a very high pressure is built up in the mediastinum, the venous return is disturbed and the blood pressure in consequence falls seriously. Patient triggering brings yet another problem to the operation of a respirator; it is impossible to combine patient triggering with a negative phase. In fact, in the Blease apparatus the negative pressure control can be used to increase the sensitivity of the trigger. This it will do to the point at which the extremely small negative pressure produced when the negative phase sucks air toward the machine through an open ended catheter mount is sufficient to operate the trigger mechanism.

It has become apparent, particularly with patient-triggered ventilators, that it is always desirable for a respirator to have a nearly unlimited output. Cylinder-supplied machines, e.g. the Barnet, where the gas flow to the machine must be pre-set, may not be satisfactory in this respect over a long period.[78] The B.O.C. "Cyclator" Type P is said to be free from this disadvantage. So also is the Blease apparatus which draws in outside air to the capacity of the bellows. Campbell and Duggan[79] state that their machine will deliver no more than 12 L/min. It can, however, vary its output to meet the needs of a patient. None the less, this may limit its usefulness in the presence of gross hyperventilation. It might seem difficult to visualize circumstances where such gross hyperventilation could achieve anything useful. It could, however, be needed during the management of some chest injuries and perhaps in the treatment of carbon dioxide narcosis (vide pp. 297 and 301).

The following indications for the use of a patient-triggered respirator are given[59]:

Post-operative respiratory failure where sedation, hyperventilation or curarization is undesirable;

Respiratory failure in the presence of gross hypertrophic pulmonary emphysema accompanied by right heart failure. In such cases a negative phase is of no value and may be dangerous, while sedation and curarization are contraindicated (not all will agree with the last statement).

Atelectasis neonatorum;

After prolonged artificial ventilation where "weaning" from a non-triggered ventilator has proved difficult;

As an alternative method of ventilation during anæsthesia in patients with poor lung function.

DETERMINING THE EXTENT OF MECHANICAL VENTILATION

In a patient in whom mechanical ventilation of the lungs is being used for an hour or two during a surgical operation the ordinary clinical guides to efficacy of ventilation are all that are required, so great is the tolerance of the body to divergences from normal, particularly if these are on the side of over-ventilation. The patient who is undergoing long-term artificial ventilation for therapeutic purposes, however, is attached to a mechanical ventilator by an anæsthetist and thereafter left to the care of a nurse. It is therefore essential that the minute volume of respiration should approximate fairly closely to the patient's requirements as errors which are insignificant over an hour or two can, particularly if they are on the side of under-ventilation, have serious consequences if they are allowed to continue uncorrected for periods of a day or more.

The first consideration to be determined in relation to long-term artificial respiration is the rate. This to some extent depends on the characteristics of the ventilator. If a square-wave ventilator like the Radcliffe apparatus is being employed, a given pressure will produce its maximum tidal volume with a duration of inspiration of approximately 1·25 second.[58] If expiration is to be twice as long as inspiration, the entire respiratory cycle will occupy some 3·75 seconds and the respiratory rate will be 16 per minute. It is however customary to use rather more rapid respiratory rates of the order of 20–24 in children and rates of up to 30 or more in infants.[55, 80] Slower rates may be preferred during mechanical ventilation of the lungs in the presence of bronchial obstruction [51, 55] or with triangular wave machines.

The next absolute consideration is that of the tidal volume. This should be regarded as the amount of alveolar ventilation which will maintain the alveolar Pco_2 at normal levels. This amount will obviously depend on the carbon dioxide output of the body. The balance can be expressed mathematically as the equation:

$$\text{Alveolar } CO_2 \% = \frac{CO_2 \text{ output} \times 100}{\text{alveolar ventilation (ml)}} + \text{inhaled } CO_2 \%^{[81]}$$

Since this last item in the equation is substantially zero in the patient inhaling atmospheric air, it can be disregarded. Since carbon dioxide output varies with metabolic activity, the actual level for an individual patient will be obtainable from a consideration of his body weight, or more accurately from his body surface area. Tables are available to give these figures.[82] The next step therefore is to substitute the figure 5·6 % for alveolar CO_2 in the equation and calculate the alveolar ventilation from the patient's CO_2 production.

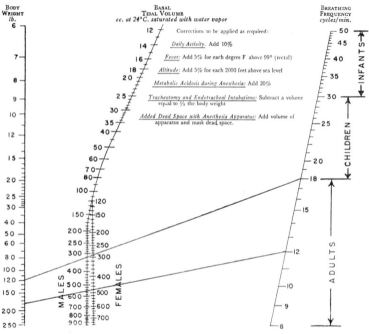

FIG. 43. Radford Nomogram.
(by courtesy of the Editor, the *Brit. J. Anæsth.*)

Thereafter it is necessary to convert alveolar ventilation to actual ventilation by addition of the volume necessary to fill the dead space at each breath. Radford[83] assumed that the dead space in ml was numerically equal to the number of pounds in the body weight. Further, he believed, and his conclusions have since been confirmed, that intubation or tracheostomy halves the anatomical dead space. On these assumptions he constructed his well known nomogram, from which it is possible to derive the basal tidal volume required at any respiratory rate between 8 and 50 by a patient of any weight between 6 and 250 lb if the alveolar CO_2 is to remain at the normal level of $5 \cdot 6 \%$.[84] As far as a spontaneously breathing unanæsthetized patient is concerned his figures have since been found to be a fairly accurate prediction of the ventilation required.

Some considerations of special importance to anæsthetists have however emerged since his work was done. Radford allowed 10 per cent for the reduction in metabolic activity produced by anæsthesia. It would appear that this reduction is insufficient and that 15 per cent would be a more appropriate correction.[82] Secondly, it has become apparent that though the anatomical dead space remains unaltered, the physiological dead space during anæsthesia is some 70 ml greater,[82] and during artificial ventilation the total dead space is more accurately represented by one-third of the tidal volume.[85] The result is that the figures in the Radford nomogram reflect the tidal volume necessary to maintain a normal P_{CO_2} in the alveoli of the anæsthetized patient only if no correction is made for the depression of metabolism produced by anæsthesia nor for the alteration in dead space produced by intubation. Equally it is not surprising that where artificial ventilation of the lungs has been conducted in unanæsthetized subjects whose basal metabolic rates have not been reduced by drugs, the use of the figures in the Radford nomogram as a guide to the appropriate tidal volume leads to substantial under-ventilation.

Another reason for this apparent contradiction may be the defects inherent in apparatus for mechanical ventilation. For example, every machine has valves in it and very few of these are absolutely airtight, though the extent of the leakage is usually small. Secondly, there are a number of jam-fit metal to metal joints between the machine and the patient. When these are carefully machined leakage at such sites is negligible. The presence, however, of a very small amount of dirt or other foreign material can lead to appreciable losses of tidal volume. The most outstanding mechanical source of loss of volume however lies in the elasticity of the rubber unkinkable hose which connects the patient to the respirator. So variable is the nature of these hoses, and so much do they change their character with repeated sterilization, that it is impossible to give an estimate of this loss. It has however been measured roughly by the writer on a Blease P6 apparatus with a new unkinkable hose made of non-conducting rubber. It was found that this machine would produce an apparent tidal volume of some 200 ml with an inflation pressure of $+25$ cm H_2O when the output at the end of the double hose was totally obstructed. The newer models of this machine have been fitted with piano wire in the hoses and the losses have been correspondingly reduced. The old-fashioned red rubber hoses, particularly after repeated sterilization, became very elastic and the loss in one of them can probably amount to the normal tidal volume of the patient or even more.

In addition to these rather obvious mechanical faults there is another reason why the tidal volume given by the Radford nomogram may prove inadequate. The distribution of gases which enter the lungs as a result of intermittent positive pressure respiration is different from that during normal quiet breathing.[87, 88] During spontaneous respiration the maximum expanding force is applied to the alveoli adjacent to the diaphragm and chest wall, while during artificial ventilation by intermittent positive pressure the alveoli most remote from the chest wall and the diaphragm are those which bear the largest proportion of the pressure applied to the lungs. If the blood-gas exchange is to remain unaltered there must be an accompanying alteration in the perfusion of the alveoli so that those which are now best ventilated receive the best blood supply, and those whose ventilation is no longer as effective suffer a corresponding reduction. There is evidence that compensation of this type is in fact incomplete and though carbon dioxide elimination is not impaired oxygen uptake may be. This disturbance is very much more serious in the patient with emphysema than it is in the normal subject.

MONITORING THE VENTILATOR

Clinical Assessment. Whether or not it is possible to set the ventilator to deliver the tidal volume required by the patient it is necessary to check its effectiveness. The most important guide is the clinical picture. If ventilation is adequate the patient is of a good colour, has a stable pulse rate within normal limits and a normal blood pressure for him. The under-ventilated patient who is conscious will be uncomfortable and a little restless if he has sufficient muscle power to show such manifestations. Inadequate ventilation will also lead to rise in pulse rate, rise in blood pressure, though not usually to a greater extent than some 20 points. Sweating and cyanosis may also occur.

Because the absence of cyanosis is so valuable a guide to the efficiency of ventilation it is better not to use oxygen except when a pulmonary shunt is present, for with normal gas mixtures and normal lungs oxygen supply and carbon dioxide elimination fail simultaneously. When an oxygen-rich mixture is used considerable increases in blood carbon dioxide can be masked because cyanosis does not appear at the same time. Apart from these considerations however, oxygen, though extremely valuable in the short term in resuscitation after acute respiratory failure, is an unsatisfactory gas to use over a long period. It is now accepted that when it is so used, e.g. in aviation, it may lead to bronchial irritation and if the findings in small animals are to be transferred to the human subject it may even cause pneumonia. This gas has no other adverse effects in the adult but in the new-born child the inhalation of more than 40 per cent of oxygen may lead to loss of vision as a result of the deposition of fibrous tissue behind the lens of the eye retrolental fibroplasia.

The only clinical sign of over-ventilation which is likely to declare itself is increased muscular irritability which initially will be manifested by twitching and ultimately by tetany, though of course these signs will not be obtainable in totally paralysed muscles. It now seems fairly clear that excessive washing out of carbon dioxide does not of itself lead to hypotension, as was once believed. Fall in blood pressure under such circumstances is the result of the transmission of the excessive inflation pressures to the great veins in the mediastinum rather than a direct manifestation of an abnormally low blood carbon dioxide content.

Measurement of Expired Minute Volume. Clinical guides are not alone sufficient; it is also necessary to measure the amount of air which is actually ventilating the patient. This is most conveniently done by measuring the expired minute volume. The most reliable method of so doing is to place a Wright anemometer periodically between the tracheostomy tube and the hose leading to the patient. This meter, however, cannot be left there indefinitely as it is soon put out of action by the condensation of the water vapour in the humidified air. With the possible exceptions of the Dräger volumeter and its American counterpart the Bennett ventilation meter, the more ordinary meters used in respiratory physiology so greatly increase the dead space that they cannot be used in this situation, though a pneumotachograph could be so employed. This apparatus, however, essentially measures the instantaneous respiratory gas flow. It is therefore necessary to employ also an integrator in order to convert flow into minute volume or alternatively to use a tedious process of counting the squares included in the area under the tracing.

By far the most usual method of measuring the expired air is to use an apparatus with a twin hose. The meter is then placed in the expiratory channel, usually just beyond a trap to prevent the entry of condensed water into it. This method of measuring respiratory displacement is not by any means completely reliable. Some of the mechanical factors which made it impossible to use a nomogram as the sole guide to tidal volume can also interfere with the assessment of the ventilation by measurement of the expired air, though in this connection the only leaks which are of importance are those between the meter and the expiratory valve. Another fallacy can vitiate the assessment of the ventilation by metering the expired air. The diaphragm of a Beaver valve is liable to chatter, if a patient is breathing to some extent for himself while the machine is in use. Under such circumstances air can pass directly from the hose outwards through the expiratory port and if the expired minute volume is being metered here a grossly inflated value will be obtained (p. 263).

BIOCHEMICAL CONTROL OF VENTILATION

Ventilation is sometimes uneven during intermittent positive pressure respiration particularly in the presence of sputum retention. Under such circumstances the over-ventilation of the remaining normal alveoli can cause sufficient local reduction in the carbon dioxide of the blood there to compensate for the lack of ventilation elsewhere in the lung. On the other hand, since over-ventilation is unlikely to increase the partial pressure of oxygen in any alveolus by more than a few per cent, and since the hæmoglobin is nearly completely oxygenated at a partial pressure of oxygen of 95mm of mercury, it is not possible for over-ventilation to compensate for the lack of oxygen uptake in the under-ventilated alveoli. The result is that the carbon dioxide tension of the blood may be normal while the oxygen content is definitely below this level. It is therefore necessary to measure both Pco_2 and Po_2 in assessing the efficiency of a ventilator by biochemical means. The remedy for a low Po_2 is not more ventilation but administration of additional oxygen. This will raise the oxygen tension in the healthy alveoli to a point at which the additional oxygen taken up in solution in the plasma will, when the blood becomes mixed in the left atrium, largely make good the deficiency of oxygen uptake in other parts of the lungs.

Determination of blood Carbon Dioxide. The most certain control of ventilation is obtained by examination of the arterial blood obtained by direct puncture of a vessel. A number of direct methods are available for the determination of the amount of carbon dioxide in the blood obtained. The best known of the earlier methods was that of Riley,[89] in which the gas in a very small quantity of blood was allowed to come out of solution into a bubble of limited size and known composition, approximating to that of alveolar air; thereafter the amount of carbon dioxide and other gases in the bubble was estimated by differential absorption. The whole process took place in a water bath at body temperature. A graduated capillary tube was used for gas measurements. This method could only be used in a patient breathing air. Anæsthetic gases came out of solution into the bubble and were estimated as CO_2. Even if anæsthetic gases were added to the equilibrating mixture they would still cause error as they would be absorbed by the solutions used to take up O_2 and CO_2 from the bubble.

Astrup during the Copenhagen poliomyleitis epidemic obtained the P_{CO_2} of the blood indirectly from the pH and the total CO_2 content.[90] A nomogram is available for this purpose. Blood pH however must be determined within 15 minutes of its withdrawal. If blood stands any longer than this spontaneous glycolysis occurs with the production of acid products which falsify the result. If it is not possible immediately to determine the blood pH, the plasma must be separated and kept on ice. Its pH can then be determined at leisure and a correction applied for the temperature and for the red blood corpuscles which are no longer present as in whole blood.

More recently a method has been described in which the pH of the blood is determined directly. It is thereafter exposed to two or three known tensions of carbon dioxide. The new pH's are measured; these are plotted against the logarithm of the carbon dioxide tension; as there is a linear relationship between pH of the log P_{CO_2} it is possible to obtain the P_{CO_2} of the original specimen by an intrapolation method[91] (*vide* Fig. 47, p. 279).

Rebreathing Methods. It is possible to obtain the P_{CO_2} of the mixed venous blood, which is normally 6 mm higher than that of the arterial, by direct measurement. The principle of the method is as follows. In the normal individual it requires some 20 seconds for a given amount of blood to complete the shortest circulatory circuit, i.e. within this period there is no re-circulation of blood through the lungs. If a patient is given a limited amount of gas to rebreathe for this period its CO_2 content will, providing the difference is not too great, come into equilibrium with the blood entering the lungs, i.e. the mixed venous blood. Two ways are described of obtaining mixtures for rebreathing containing a satisfactory amount of carbon dioxide. The original method was described by Hackney, Sears and Collier.[92] They used various concentrations of CO_2 in oxygen in a bag for this purpose. While the patient was rebreathing them small samples were withdrawn continuously and passed through an infrared analyser with a direct writer. Provided that the carbon dioxide concentration was correct it could be seen in the resulting tracing that as 15 to 20 seconds approached the carbon dioxide content of the expired gases fell to a minimum and remained at this level for some seconds. Thereafter as rebreathing occurred the concentration rose. Further, before this minimum was reached the concentration of carbon dioxide in the inspired air was greater than that in the expired, while after the minimum had been reached the reverse took place and the carbon dioxide content of the expired air was greater than that in the inspired (Fig. 44).

Campbell and Howell modified this method.[93] In their technique the subject rebreathed 1,500 ml of oxygen continuously for 90 seconds. Thereafter he was given two minutes rest; he was then given the contents of the bag to rebreathe once more for 15 seconds or 5

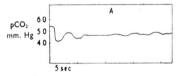

FIG. 44. The changes in CO_2 concentration during rebreathing from a bag. (After Campbell & Howell.) (*Brit. med. J.*, 1960.)

breaths. This method took advantage of the fact that though disease processes might possibly prolong the period required for the minimum total circuit of the circulation or for the intrapulmonary mixing, it was most unlikely that this period would be shortened. The continuously running infra-red analyser was therefore dispensed with and the contents of the bag analysed at leisure by any convenient method. Campbell has described a very simple gas burette and absorption apparatus, a modification of the Haldane, which is quite accurate enough for ordinary working purposes[94] (Fig. 45).

This rebreathing principle has also been utilized by Cooper and Smith of Newcastle.[95] In their technique one litre of 5 per cent carbon dioxide in oxygen is rebreathed on four successive occasions, each lasting 15 seconds. Each period of rebreathing is separated from its predecessor by not less than a minute. Again the contents of the rebreathed bag can be estimated by any convenient method. The writer has used this latter method to a considerable extent in patients on intermittent positive pressure respiration and has encountered the following difficulties. First, if gas taps are not absolutely airtight it is difficult to carry out four 15-second periods of artificial respiration with only one litre of gas. It has been found necessary to completely fill a one gallon bag if a reasonable amount of gas is going to be available at the end of the test for analysis. The use of this larger volume of gas, of course, makes equilibration between the mixed

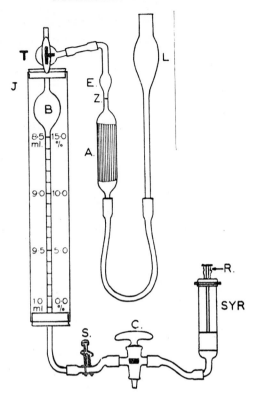

FIG. 45. Modified Haldane Apparatus for estimation of CO_2 in expired air. (For key to diagram see Campbell, *Brit. med. J.*, 1960.)

venous blood and the contents of the bag less complete within the time of rebreathing. In consequence results appreciably lower than those found by the Campbell and Howell method have been obtained when the blood P_{CO_2} was grossly raised. On the other hand, when the mixed venous P_{CO_2} has been at its normal value, or below it, the two methods have given comparable results. Further, the Newcastle method and its modification involve less discomfort for the patient who has only to rebreathe a mixture containing a high proportion of carbon dioxide for 15 seconds at a time. Also, although the absolute figures given for the P_{CO_2} by the modified method are not accurate the trend of the results is still a most useful indication of the patient's progress.

Interpreting the Results

While it is obvious that changes in the Pco_2 must be the main guide to the efficacy of artificial respiration, it is not sufficient to depend solely upon changes in this quantity, nor is it desirable to endeavour so to set the ventilator in every patient that the Pco_2 is retained at the normal value of 40 mm of mercury in the arterial blood and 46 in the mixed venous. The maintenance of the pH of the blood at normal levels is even more important to the body than the maintenance of the Pco_2. These two quantities are of course to some extent interdependent and their relationship one to the other is given by the Henderson-Hasselbach equation, which states that

$$pH = pK' + \log \frac{[B.HCO_3]^*}{[H.HCO_3]}$$

i.e. a third variable, the concentration of the bicarbonate in the blood is also involved in determining pH. Since the amount of dissolved carbonic acid in the blood bears a relation to its Pco_2 this equation can also be written[96]

$$pH = pK' + \log \frac{[B.HCO_3]^*}{\alpha Pco_2}$$

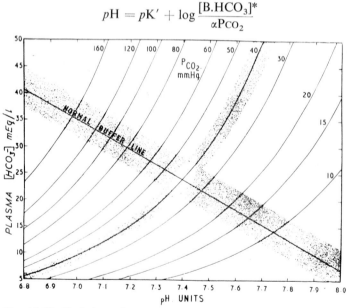

Fig. 46. The Variations of pH, Pco_2 and plasma bicarbonate in the blood. (After Davenport, modified by Campbell. *Post grad. med. J.*)

* The numerical values[91] of PK' and α are given as $5·97 — 6·21$ and $0·0301$ respectively.

The concentration of the bicarbonate in the plasma used to be measured as the alkali reserve but more recently the tendency has been to use the term "standard bicarbonate" to define this quantity. (The standard bicarbonate is the carbon dioxide combining power of the blood measured at a Pco_2 of 40 mm Hg with the hæmoglobin fully oxygenated and at a temperature of 38° C).[98]

Since three variables are involved it is not possible to plot on a

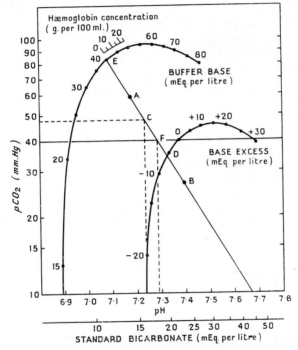

FIG. 47. The Variations of pH, Pco_2 and Plasma Bicarbonate in the blood. Points A & B are the pHC determined for a sample. E, A, C, F, B, D is the line joining them to cut base excess at —3 mEq/L, i.e. the plasma bicarbonate is 21 mEq/L (the normal is 24 mEq/L).

single graph the variation of Pco_2 with pH but it is relatively easy to show how pH will vary as the plasma bicarbonate changes, if the Pco_2 is kept constant. A diagram of this kind will be seen in Fig. 46. This diagram may be used to work out what in fact should be the correct Pco_2 for a patient on artificial respiration if the pH of his blood is to be retained at a normal value of 7·4. For example a patient who fails to breathe adequately at the end of a gastrectomy for a peptic ulcer which has for many years been intensively treated with an alkali, may have a plasma bicarbonate which is elevated to about

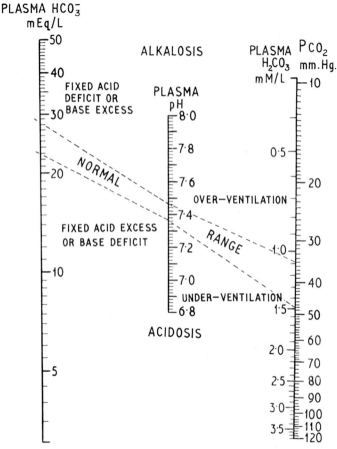

FIG. 48. Nomogram modified from Singer and Hastings. Only the scales for Plasma HCO₃ —pH and Pco₂ have been included. The original nomogram had scales for hæmatocrit and buffer base, i.e. plasma bicarbonate plus all other blood buffers including hæmoglobin and protein.

30 m-equiv/L. It can be seen from the diagram that if the blood pH is to remain at 7·4 the appropriate P_{CO_2} would be nearly 50. If hyperventilation were carried out until the P_{CO_2} was 40 mm Hg,

the blood pH would in fact become something more like 7·5, always providing that the standard bicarbonate did not change during this process—a situation in fact not likely to occur in clinical circumstances. By contrast, if the plasma bicarbonate had been depleted until its value was 15 m-equiv/L the P_{CO_2} which would give rise to a pH of 7·4, is only some 23 mm Hg. If a P_{CO_2} of 40 were produced by reducing the tidal volume of artificial ventilation, the blood pH would, in the absence of compensatory changes in the plasma bicarbonate, fall to the acid value of 7·2.

The diagram shown in Fig. 46 which was designed by Davenport is not the only known graphic method of setting out the interdependence of pH P_{CO_2} and standard bicarbonate. The changes in these variables can also be obtained from Astrup's diagram (Fig. 47)[96] and from the nomogram made by Singer and Hastings (Fig. 48).[99] It is, however, sufficient that those who carry out artificial respiration should familarize themselves with one diagram and appreciate its significance.

While it is most desirable to know the P_{CO_2} and the pH of the blood wherever possible, it is feasible to monitor the performance of a mechanical ventilator simply by following the changes in the plasma bicarbonate. This of course is satisfactory only as long as the body's compensatory mechanisms are able to maintain the arterial blood pH at the normal level of 7·35 to 7·4. It is not even necessary to determine the standard bicarbonate within the strict limits laid down by Astrup.[98] The plasma bicarbonate determined by the classical method of van Slyke and Cullen,[100, 101] which in its volumetric or manometric form is the standard method in most departments of clinical pathology, will serve equally well. If the plasma bicarbonate falls to 20 m-equiv/L or less, the patient is almost certainly being over-ventilated. If it rises seriously beyond 26 m-equiv/L, under-ventilation is likely to be present. Under such circumstances the trend of a daily determination is of much more significance than any single isolated estimation. If the plasma bicarbonate is tending to rise, cumulative under-ventilation is occurring. If the plasma bicarbonate is falling below normal, the patient is being over-ventilated. Lastly, when this type of control is being employed it is essential to be certain that the concentrations of the other electrolytes in the plasma are substantially normal. They must therefore be determined at the beginning of the treatment and subsequently whenever there is any suggestion that they may have been upset, e.g. by the development of paralytic ileus in the course of poliomyelitis. If evidence of an upset is obtained, the trend of the plasma bicarbonate is no longer a useful guide and blood pH or P_{CO_2} must be determined also.

Some Characteristics of the Commoner Ventilators

Name	Classification		End of inflation stroke			Wave form			Driving mechanism	
	Pressure Preset	Volume Preset	Pressure Cycled	Volume Cycled	Time Cycled	Square	Intermediate	Triangular	Electric	Gas or Air Pressure
Radcliffe (Both)	—					—			—	
Smith-Clarke		—			—				—	
Beaver	—	—			—				—	
Barnett	—	—			—	—	—			—
Engström	—		—				—	—		—
Blease	—		—					—		—
Aintree	—		—					—		—
Fazakerley	—		—					—		—
Newcastle	—		—			—				—
Emerson Controller Assister*	—			—			—			—
Jefferson*	—				—	—		—		—
Morch Surgical Respirator*	or	or		—†	—†					—
Stephenson*		—		—						—
Starling Pump	or	or			—		—		—	
Clutton-Brock	or	or			—		—		—	—
Mortimer	—				—	—?				
Donald and Green	—				—		—			—

*From data of Elam et al.

†Has some characteristics of both.

References

1. LASSEN, H. C. A. (1953). *Lancet*, **1**, 37.
2. PEARCE, D. J. (1961). *Anæsthesia*, **16**, 308.
3. WALSH, R. S. (1961). *Proc. Roy. Soc. Med.*, **54**, 799.
4. SPALDING, J. M. K., and YOUNG, S. A., (1955) *Lancet*, **2**, 227.
5. ABLETT, J. J. L. (1961). Awaiting publication.
6. FAIRLEY, H. B., and CHAMBERS, R. A. (1960). *Canad. Anæsth. Soc. J.*, **7**, 447.
7. STRÖM, J. (Ed.) (1956). *Acta med. Scandinav.*, Suppl. 316, 122 154.
8. BJÖRK, V. O., and ENGSTRÖM, C. G. (1955). *J. thorac. Surg.*, **30**, 356.
9. BJÖRK, V. O., and ENGSTRÖM, C. G. (1957). *J. thorac. Surg.*, **34**, 228.
10. WOOLF, C. R. (1961). *Canad. med. Ass. J.*, **84**, 466.
11. HILLARD, E. K., and MUSHIN, W. W. (1960). *Brit. med. J.*, **2**, 729.
12. RUBEN, H., KNUDSEN, E. J., WINKEL, E., and HJORTH, A. A. (1958). *Lancet*, **1**, 460.
13. RUBEN, H. (1955). *Anesthesiology*, **16**, 643.
14. SPENCER, W. A. (1957). *Ann. N.Y. Acad. Sci.*, **66**, 891.
15. SPALDING, J. M. K. (1959). *Proc. Roy. Soc. Med.*, **52**, 664.
16. KELLEHER, W. H. (1961). *Lancet*, **2**, 1113.
17. BRAGG, W. H. (1938). *Brit. med. J.*, **2**, 254.
18. PINKERTON, H. H. (1957). *Brit. J. Anæsth.*, **29**, 421.
19. BRYCE SMITH, R., and DAVIS, H. S. (1954). *Curr. Res. Anesth.* 33, 73.
20. COLLIER, C. R., and AFFELDT, J. E. (1954). *J. appl. Physiol.*, **6**, 531.
21. GREEN, R. A., and COLEMAN, D. J. (1955). *Anæsthesia*, **10**, 369.
22. BAYUK, A. J. (1957). *Anesthesiology*, **18**, 135.
23. NUNN, J. F. (1957). *Brit. J. Anæsth.* **29**, 540.
24. COMROE, J. H., NISELL, O. I., and NIMS, R. G. (1954). *J. appl. Physiol.*, **7**, 225.
25. NEWMAN, H. D., CAMPBELL, E. J. M., and DINNICK, O. P. (1959). *Brit. J. Anæsth.* **31**, 282.
26. DITTMER, D. S., and GREBE, R. S. (1958) in National Academy of Sciences *Handbook of Respiration*. Saunders, Philadelphia.
27. NIMS, R. G., CONNER, E. H., and COMROE, J. H. (1955). *J. Clin. Invest.* **34**, 744.
28. BUTLER, J., and SMITH, B. H. (1957). *Clin. Sci.*, **16**, 125.
29. FERRIS, B. G., MEAD, J., WHITTENBERGER, J. L., and SAXTON, G. A. (1952). *New Engl. J. Med.*, **247**, 390.
30. MUSHIN, W. W., RENDELL-BAKER, L., and THOMPSON, P. W. (1959). *Automatic Ventilation of the Lungs*. Blackwell, Oxford.
31. COMROE, J. H. (Ed.) (1955). *The Lung*, Year Book Publishers, Chicago.
32. COOPER, E. A. (1961). *J. Laryngol.*, **75**, 142.
33. OTIS, A. B., MCKERROW, C. B., BARTLETT, R. A., MEAD, J., MCILROY, M. B., SELVERSTONE, N. J., and RADFORD, E. P. (1956). *J. appl. Physiol.*, **8**, 427.
34. MUSHIN, W. W. (1961). *Proc. Roy. Soc. Med.*, **54**, 798.
35. SPALDING, J. M. K. (1959). *Proc. Roy. Soc. Med.*, **52**, 664.
36. MALONEY, J. V., and WHITTENBERGER, J. L. (1951). *Amer. J. med. Sci.*, **221**, 425.
37. GORDON, A. S., FRYE, C. W., and LANGSTON, H. T. (1956). *J. thorac. Surg.*, **32**, 431.
38. MALONEY, J. V., and WHITTENBERGER, J. L. (1957). *Ann. N.Y. Acad. Sci.*, **66**, 931.
39. HUBAY, C. A., WALTZ, R. C., BRECHER, G. A., PRAGLIN, J. and HINGSON, R. A. (1954). *Anesthesiology*, **15**, 445.
40. MOTLEY, H. L., COURNAND, D. A., WERKO, L., DRESDEL, D. T., HIMMELSTEIN, A., and RICHARDS, D. W. (1948). *J. Amer. med. Ass.*, **137**, 370.

41. MALONEY, J. V., ELAM, J. O., HANDFORD, S. W., BALLA, G. A., EASTWOOD, D. W., BROWN, E. S., and TEN PASS, R. H. (1953). *J. Amer. med. Ass.*, **152,** 212.
42. SPENCER, F. C., BENSON, D. W., LIU, W. C., and BAHNSON, H. T. (1959). *J. thorac. Surg.*, **38,** 758.
43. BRAUNWALD, E., BINION, J. T., MORGAN, W. L., and SARNOFF, S. J. (1957). *Circulation Res.*, **5,** 670.
44. PRICE, H. L., CONNER, E. H., and DRIPPS, R. D. (1954). *J. appl. Physiol.*, **6,** 517.
45. MALONEY, J. V., and HANDFORD, S. W. (1954). *J. appl. Physiol.*, **6,** 453.
46. OPIE, L. H., SPALDING, J. M. K., and CRAMPTON SMITH, A. (1961). *Lancet*, **1,** 911.
47. COURNAND, A., MOTLEY, H. L., WERKO, L., and RICHARDS, D. W. (1948). *Amer. J. Physiol.*, **152,** 162.
48. PASK, E. A. (1955). *Proc. Roy. Soc. Med.*, **48,** 239.
49. HORTON, J. A. G., INKSTER, J. S., and PASK, E. A. (1956). *Brit. J. Anæsth.*, **28,** 169.
50. PASK, E. A. (1957). *Lancet*, **2,** 676.
51. ROBSON, J. G. (1959). *Canad. Anæsth. Soc. J.*, **6,** 215.
52. NORLANDER, O. P., BJÖRK, V. O., CRAFOORD, C., FRIBERG, O., HOLMDAHL, M., SWENSSON, A., and WIDMAN, B. (1961). *Anæsthesia*, **16,** 285.
53. ROCHFORD, J., WELCH, R. F., and WINKS, D. P. (1958). *Brit. J. Anæsth.*, **30,** 23.
54. FAIRLEY, H. B. (1959). *Canad. Anæsth. Soc. J.*, **6,** 219.
55. BEAVER, R. A. (1961). *J. Laryngol.*, **75,** 149.
56. SIEKER, H. O., HICKAM, J. B., and PRYOR, W. W. (1956). *Amer. Rev. Tuberc.*, **74,** 309.
57. Chemical Corps Medical Laboratory. Special Report. No. 38, (1954). U.S. Army Chemical Centre, Mld.
58. OPIE, L. H., SPALDING, J. M. K., and STOTT, F. D. (1959). *Lancet*, **1,** 545.
59. CAMPBELL, D. (1961). *Proc. Roy. Soc. Med.*, **54,** 793.
60. RUSSELL, W. R., and SCHUSTER, E. (1953). *Lancet*, **2,** 707.
61. RUSSELL, W. R., SCHUSTER, E., CRAMPTON SMITH, A., and SPALDING, J. M. K. (1956). *Lancet*, **1,** 539.
62. HICKAM, J. B., SIEKER, H. O., PRYOR, W. W., and FRAYSER, R., (1957). *Ann. N.Y. Acad. Sci.*, **66,** 866.
63. HARMEL, M. H., ELDER, J. D., and NORLANDER, O. (1960). *Acta anæsth. Scandinav.* Supplementum VI, 62.
64. HUNTER, A. R. (1962). *Anæsthesia*, **17,** 3.
65. SMITH-CLARKE, G. T., and GALPINE, J. F. (1955). *Lancet*, **1,** 1299.
66. HUNTER, A. R. (1961). *Anæsthesia*, **16,** 231.
67. NUNN, J. F. (1958). *Brit. J. Anæsth.*, **30,** 134.
68. VAN BERGEN, F. H., BUCKLEY, J. J., WEATHERHEAD, D. S. P., SCHULTZ, E. A., and GORDON, J. R. (1956). *Anesthesiology*, **17,** 708.
69. RUBEN, H., and RUBEN, A. (1957). *Lancet*, **2,** 373.
70. FINK, B. R. (1954). *Anesthesiology*, **15,** 471.
71. HUNTER, A. R. (1962). To be published.
72. BEAVER, R. A. (1954). Unpublished.
73. MUSHIN, W. W., and RENDELL-BAKER, L. (1954). *Brit. J. Anæsth.*, **26,** 131.
74. ELAM, J. O., KERR, J. H., and JANNEY, C. D. (1958). *Anesthesiology*, **19,** 56.
75. MAPLESON, W. W. (1961). *Anæsthesia*, **16,** 572.
76. HUNTER, A. R. (1962). *Anæsthesia*, **17,** 109.
77. BEAVER, R. A. (1961). *Proc. Roy. Soc. Med.*, **54,** 797.
78. WILSON KINNIER, A. B. (1961). *Proc. Roy. Soc. Med.*, **54,** 798.
79. CAMPBELL, D., and DUGGAN, T. C. (1960). *Brit. J. Anæsth.* **32,** 429.
80. ANDERSEN, E. W., and IBSEN, B. (1954). *Brit. Med. J.*, **1,** 786.
81. DRIPPS, R. D., and SEVERINGHAUS, J. W. (1955). *Physiol. Rev.*, **35,** 741.
82. NUNN, J. F. (1960). *Anæsthesia*, **15,** 123.

83. RADFORD, E. P. (1955). *J. appl Physiol.*, **7**, 451.
84. RADFORD, E. P., FERRIS, B. G., and KRIETE, B. C. (1954). *New Engl. J. Med.* **251**, 877.
85. NUNN, J. F. (1962). *Anæsthesia*, **17**, 77.
86. CAMPBELL, E. J. M., NUNN, J. F., and PECKETT, B. W. (1958). *Brit. J. Anæsth.*, **30**, 166.
87. HOWELL, J. B. L., and PECKETT, B. W. (1957). *J. Physiol.*, **136**, 1.
88. BATES, D. V., FOWLER, W. S., FORSTER, R. G., and VAN LINGEM, B. (1959). *J. appl. Physiol.*, **10**, 958.
89. RILEY, R. L., PROEMMEL, D. D., and FRANKE, R. E. (1945). *J. Biol. Chem.*, **161**, 621.
90. ASTRUP, P., GØTZCHE, H., and NEUKIRCH, F. (1954). *Brit. med. J.*, **1**, 780.
91. ROBINSON, J. S., and UTTING, J. E. (1961). *Brit. J. Anæsth.*, **33**, 327.
92. HACKNEY, J. D., SEARS, C. H., and COLLIER, C. R. (1958). *J. appl. Physiol.*, **12**, 425.
93. CAMPBELL, E. J. M., and HOWELL, J. B. L. (1960). *Brit. med. J.*, **1**, 458.
94. CAMPBELL, E. J. M. (1960). *Brit. med. J.*, **1**, 457.
95. COOPER, E. A., and SMITH, H. (1961). *Anæsthesia*, **16**, 445.
96. ASTRUP, P., JORGENSEN, K., ANDERSEN, S. D., and ENGEL, K. (1960). *Lancet*, **1**, 1035.
97. DAVENPORT, H. W. (1958). *A B C of Acid Base Chemistry*. University of Chicago Press.
98. JORGENSEN, K., and ASTRUP, P. (1957). *Scand. J. clin. Lab. Invest.*, **9**, 122.
99. SINGER, R. B., and HASTINGS, A. B. (1948). *Medicine*, **27**, 223.
100. VAN SLYKE, D. D., CULLEN, G. E. (1917). *J. Biol. Chem.*, **30**, 289.
101. VAN SLYKE, D. D., and NEALL, J. M. (1924). *J. Biol. Chem.*, **61**, 523.
102. MAPLESON, W. W. (1962). *Anæsthesia*, **17**, 300.
103. WATSON, W. E. (1961). *Brit. J. Anæsth.*, **33**, 600.
104. WATSON, W. E., SEELYE, E. (1962). *Brit. J. Anæsth.*, **34**, 74.
105. WATSON, W. E., SMITH, A. C., SPALDING, J. M. K. (1962). *Brit. J. Anæsth.*, **34**, 278.
106. SMITH, A. C. (1962). To be published.

CHAPTER 10

THE MANAGEMENT OF PATIENTS DURING ARTIFICIAL VENTILATION

A. R. HUNTER

Artificial Ventilation during Anæsthesia—Resuscitation—Cardiac Resuscitation—Long-term Artificial Ventilation—Crush Injuries of the Chest—Tetanus—Status Epilepticus—Other Indications for Artificial Respiration—Tracheostomy—Chest Physiotherapy— Suction—Fluid Balance—Mobilisation of the Respirator Patient— Glossopharyngeal Breathing.

ARTIFICIAL ventilation of the lungs is employed in three separate sets of circumstances. First it is part and parcel of the management of anæsthesia involving the administration of drugs which interfere with the normal breathing. Secondly, artificial respiration is used as a first-aid procedure in the resuscitation of the apparently dead. Lastly, long term artificial ventilation of the lungs is a valuable therapeutic measure in the management of a number of diseases which produce reversible insufficiency of breathing.

ARTIFICIAL VENTILATION DURING ANÆSTHESIA

The requirements of the patient in terms of tidal volume and rate, and some characteristics of the pumps used have been discussed in the preceding chapter. Some anæsthetists, however, ventilate by intermittent bag compression without much idea of the tidal volume they are producing. Little useful work can be done on the quantitative aspects of such ventilation. The type of circuit used, however, is of importance. For example the Mapleson "D" with a T-piece and the expiratory valve close to the bag at the end of this expiratory hose is the most satisfactory, if carbon dioxide absorption is not to be employed.[1] The standard Magill attachment which gives extremely good carbon dioxide elimination[2] in a spontaneously breathing patient, is the least satisfactory for artificial ventilation.[1, 3]

RESUSCITATION

The resuscitation of the apparently dead presents two separate problems. The first is the restoration of the respiratory exchange and the second the maintenance of the circulation. When sudden respiratory arrest occurs in the operating theatre artificial respiration is very readily carried out by intermittent inflation of the lungs by compression of the bag on the anæsthetic machine. For the patient whose respiration suddenly fails in the wards of a well-equipped hospital an apparatus such as the Oxford Bellows, the Cardiff Inflator, the Ambu Resuscitator, or simply a bag, expiratory valve and face piece ready for connection to an oxygen cylinder, will be available. When, however, respiratory failure occurs remote from hospital, other methods of artificial respiration must be found.

Fifty years ago the Sylvester method was preferred. It had the drawback, however, that the patient lay supine and in this position it required a third person to keep the airway clear. Artificial respiration too was best done by two operators working simultaneously. The Schaefer method, in which the patient lay prone and a single operator astride the small of his back intermittently compressed his lower chest, seemed preferable because in this position the patient's trachea and air passages would drain naturally. For this reason the method was said to be particularly applicable to drowned persons. Some doubt, however, was presently cast on the tidal exchange produced by the Schæfer method[4] and the Holger–Neilson method, which is a compound of the Sylvester and the Schæfer, was employed instead. Gradually, however, it was appreciated that the reason for the all too frequent failure of first-aid artificial respiration lay not in the method employed but in the fact that even in the prone position it was exceedingly difficult to keep the airway clear.[5, 6, 163] Presently Safar, Elam and others showed that it was possible to obtain an adequate tidal exchange, a reasonable blood oxygen level and carbon dioxide output in a curarized artificially ventilated subject by expired air resuscitation.[7, 8]

Expired Air Resuscitation. In this technique the operator applies his mouth to the patient's mouth, pinches the patient's nose and expires forcibly. He then withdraws his mouth from the patient's lips and allows passive expiration to occur. Though the oxygen and carbon dioxide contents of the gases blown in are not ideal, a reasonable respiratory exchange can be maintained. The donor subject of course must hyperventilate but provided that not more than 12 respirations per minute are produced it is most unlikely that any ill effects will result; indeed the carbon dioxide content of the donor's end expiratory air usually settles somewhere between 2·75 and 4% of CO_2.[9, 10] Some workers have, however, reported dizziness and faintness.[9, 11, 163]

Mouth to mouth artificial ventilation with expired air is, of course, not new; indeed the earliest extant account of it is contained in the

Bible.[12] It was for long regarded as the ideal method of resuscitation of the new-born child. In adults, however, it has obvious social disadvantages and it is particularly revolting if the subject's mouth is full of vomitus.[13] No apparatus, however, is required although a handkerchief or piece of rag may be placed between the lips of the subject and the lips of the donor. Gastric distension rather than inflation of the lungs may of course be produced, but in adults this does not seem to matter, and though the pressure of 20 to 25 cm of water which is required to breach the œsophageal sphincter[14] can readily be achieved during this type of lung inflation, the lungs should be safe from rupture. The development of a pneumothorax in new-born infants following mouth to mouth resuscitation has been reported.[91]

Expired air resuscitation is a form of intermittent positive pressure respiration and as such must have an adverse effect on the venous return but it is obviously preferable to have some respiratory exchange with its accompanying adverse effect on the venous return, rather than no ventilation. Expired air resuscitation has the supreme advantage that it can be carried out by a single operator and maintained for a long period. It seems, too, to be successful with the minimum of training. An instance is reported where a man carried out the procedure quite satisfactorily on his wife after having seen it demonstrated once on television.[15] The use of mouth to nose[6] rather than mouth to mouth artificial ventilation has been suggested as an alternative which avoids some at least of the æsthetic drawbacks of the more ordinary method.

The Airway. Expired air resuscitation is performed in the supine position. The question of maintaining the patency of the airway therefore arises. An anæsthetist or a trained nurse will presumably know how to hold the jaw forward and have no difficulty with it. The untrained worker, however, should be taught that if the subject's head is extended by an operator with one hand on top of the head and the other below the back of the neck, a clear airway will be produced. This method is easy to teach to laymen, easy for them to use and does not give rise to any difficulties in endentulous patients.

A number of artificial airways, have been developed for this form of treatment.[7] One was intended primarily for small children[16] and consisted of two airways, one to fit a child and another to fit an adult, cemented together by their flanged ends. It is sometimes said that the tube of the airway to be inserted into the mouths of adults should be quite short so that its end will not press against the back of the throat and cause vomiting.[17] The Brook airway[18] has a large flange which fits over the patient's mouth to give an airtight fit there. It also has a valve in it which permits the patient's exhaled gases to escape to the exterior while directing the gases which the rescuer blows down into the patient's lungs.

It has been quite clearly shown of late that very small amounts of oxygen are sufficient to prolong the lives of experimental animals subjected to acute hypoxia. Artificial ventilation even with as little as 2% oxygen will prevent the deaths of dogs already apnœic from asphyxia.[19] Even the most inefficient artificial ventilation will therefore be of value.

Resuscitation of the Drowned

Death from drowning is not simple asphyxia.[20] When large quantities of sea water find their way into the lungs the high sodium chloride concentration in this rapidly draws body water across the pulmonary endothelium into the lungs. Massive pulmonary œdema soon develops and the hematocrit and plasma sodium levels rise sharply. The simultaneous impact on the heart of hypoxia, increased viscosity of the blood and electrolyte disturbance very quickly lead to its total failure. On the other hand when fresh water is inhaled the osmotic gradient is in the opposite direction and water rapidly enters the circulation, so that the blood may be diluted by 50% within 2 to 3 minutes. This reduction in plasma osmotic pressure leads to rupture of red cells which release their high potassium content into the plasma. The simultaneous occurrence of hypoxia, over-filling of the heart and hyperpotassæmia leads to ventricular fibrillation.[21] Spasm of the glottis and bronchi may, however, protect the patient from these extremely severe osmotic effects for a time and at this stage the state is in fact one of asphyxia with a reasonable chance of recovery following artificial respiration. Because of these facts attempts at drainage of the tracheo-bronchial tree in such cases are largely a waste of time, particularly after immersion in fresh water. A certain amount of fluid can be removed from the trachea and larger bronchi after sea water drowning but the œdema fluid in the smaller sub-divisions of the bronchial tree remains and constitutes the major obstruction.[22]

The treatment of drowning, therefore, consists first and foremost in expired air resuscitation and closed chest cardiac compression. Thereafter the patient must be transferred to hospital where ventricular fibrillation, if it is present, can be converted to sinus rhythm with a defibrillator and the massive electrolyte disturbance corrected under laboratory control. The administration of plasma will apparently improve matters also.[139]

CARDIAC RESUSCITATION

The second part of the resuscitation of the apparently dead patient consists in the restoration of cardiac function. The immediate problem can be dealt with by instituting what was originally known as external cardiac massage,[23] perhaps better referred to as closed chest cardiac compression. This manœuvre consists essentially in forcibly depressing the lower end of the sternum sharply about once every second. The backward displacement of the sternum compresses the heart against the vertebral column. The fibrous pericardium largely prevents compensatory lateral expansion of the heart and the result is that blood is pushed out of the various chambers. Because the valves of the heart are unidirectional, the flow is directed into the arteries where it can be detected as a peripheral pulse with a systolic peak of some 60–100 mm of mercury, though the diastolic pressure may only be some 30 mm.[24] This form of cardiac compression can be maintained for quite considerable periods by one individual.

If closed chest cardiac compression is to be effective, the patient should be lying on a rigid support. In such circumstances a backward displacement of 3–4 cm of the sternum will be sufficient to produce an effective circulation.[25] The ordinary hospital bed, however, is too springy to act as a suitable rigid support. For this reason a fracture board may be pushed through under the spring mattress before external cardiac massage is commenced. If this is not available, very vigorous compression producing a total displacement of some 3–4 in. will compensate for the give in the average spring mattress.[26]

In a certain number of patients the force which must be exerted in order to produce an effective circulation will be such that dislocation at the costal-condral junction or fracture of a rib or costal cartilage may result.[27] Even more serious damage may be produced.[28, 29] Patients who have been subjected to external cardiac massage should therefore be observed very carefully for the next 24 to 48 hours.

Closed circuit cardiac compression is essentially a first-aid procedure, aimed primarily at restoring sufficient cerebral circulation to ensure that the oxygen supply to the brain is restored as quickly as possible. Once this has been done the question of restoration of spontaneous cardiac activity arises.[30]   A diagnosis of the cause of cardiac arrest is essential however at this stage. The patient must therefore be connected to an electrocardiograph. If continuing P-waves and the absence of ventricular complexes indicate a complete heart block, the remedy is isoprenaline[186] or noradrenaline[143] injected intravenously. An artificial pacemaker may be required if the cause of the arrest is total asystole. It is quite possible that the restoration of the circulation by external cardiac massage will have restarted spontaneous cardiac rhythm. (Even a blow on the chest[31] or the sudden refilling of the venous side of the heart[32] by elevating the lower limbs will often cure such cases.) If the electrocardiograph shows the presence of ventricular fibrillation, electric defibrillation will be needed.[33] This can be done satisfactorily by external electrodes, but the voltage is of the order of 400 to 700 volts and the amperage about $\frac{1}{2}$ amp. Such currents are extremely dangerous and only an apparatus in which the operator is securely insulated from the source should be employed. The effect of this current is analogous to that of an electric shock and may produce an asystolic heart. This will, however, very often respond to the mechanical stimulation of further massage; if it does not, an artificial external pace-maker may be tried but it too may fail.

Closed chest cardiac compression is unlikely to be of value in the treatment of cardiac arrest due to massive hæmorrhage, cardiac tamponade, or air embolism,[26] but it may occasionally be of service even in these cases and, provided the appropriate remedy to the condition is promptly applied, it may buy the time necessary to avert a fatality. Some mechanical devices for closed chest cardiac compression have been described but it is much too early to do more than draw attention to their existence.

LONG-TERM ARTIFICIAL VENTILATION
Indications

Poliomyelitis. The development of treatment by artificial ventilation came from the need for effective therapy for poliomyelitis.[34] This disease has an initial period of spreading paralysis which lasts for a week or so. The condition then stabilizes itself, and gradual recession of the paralysis occurs. Recovery is sometimes incomplete. There is, however, no way of forecasting the extent of regression. For this reason all cases must be fully treated.

Respiratory insufficiency may arise in poliomyelitis in three ways.[35] First there may be paralysis of the intercostal muscles and the diaphragm in a patient whose swallowing mechanism remains unimpaired. This is known as spinal poliomyelitis[36] and such cases, because secretions do not accumulate in the airway, are often referred to as "dry" cases. The second cause of respiratory insufficiency is bulbar poliomyelitis.[37] In this the muscles of respiration remain unaffected but because the virus invades the medulla oblongata, the respiratory centre itself, or more often the reflexes of swallowing and those which protect the respiratory tract from inhalation of foreign material, are put out of action. The characteristic sign is bulbar breathing, i.e. breathing in which the saliva and other secretions are gargled in the airway (death rattle).[35] Lung collapse is an extremely frequent complication. A third cause of respiratory failure in cases of poliomyelitis is anoxia of the respiratory centre arising as a secondary phenomenon from the combination of airway obstruction and pulmonary atelectasis.

Assessment of Disability. The indication for respirator treatment is any detectable weakness of respiration or significant fall in vital capacity, for it is felt that if the patient is put in the respirator early, the neurones responsible for the maintenance of breathing may be allowed to rest and thus be less liable to succumb to the virus. It is quite wrong to wait for the appearance of restlessness and laboured shallow respiration, increasing cyanosis and distress[38] (see also p. 307).

Bulbar poliomyelitis can in some instances be treated satisfactorily simply by posture, i.e. by laying the patient in the semi-prone position in a bed inclined steeply head down.[36] This position, however, though it ensures the clearance of the lower lobes of the lungs and of the upper air passages, can lead to sputum retention in the bronchi of the upper lobes.

Complications. Certain complications[34] may develop in patients with poliomyelitis. In bulbar cases the virus may spread upwards in the brain stem. If this occurs hyperpyrexia develops.[39] It is not uncommon to have an associated severe fall in blood pressure.[40] Hyperpyrexia is managed by cooling the patient with wet sheets, on to which a stream of air can be blown with a fan. In addition chlorpromazine may be given to aid the reduction in the temperature, although some regard this drug with suspicion because it may further lower a blood pressure which has already reached nearly critical levels. Hypotension also causes problems where intermittent positive pressure is being applied to the lungs. For it adds to the severity of the upset caused by interference with the venous return to the heart. The use of a noradrenaline drip has been suggested to correct hypotension.

Pulmonary œdema may develop. It has an extremely bad prognosis and treatment has very little effect on it. Paralytic ileus and acute dilatation of the stomach can also complicate poliomyelitis. The appearance of these complications is an absolute indication for tracheostomy and the insertion of a cuffed tube to protect the patient against inhalation of vomitus. This risk is especially serious in the patient in a tank respirator who cannot hope to "hold his breath" against the negative pressure applied to his chest in inspiration, for long enough to clear his throat after a vomit.[41]

In addition to playing a part in treating poliomyelitis the anæsthetist can render a valuable service in ensuring the safe transport of patients to hospital, especially those with bulbar palsy.[42, 45]

Myasthenia Gravis. The etiology and pathogenesis of myasthenia gravis is extremely complicated.[46, 47] The muscle weakness which characterizes the condition, however, not infrequently extends to the respiratory muscles and the muscles of swallowing. The problems which appear during the management of respiratory failure are therefore similar to those with poliomyelitis, save only that the graver complications of this latter disease, such as hyperpyrexia and paralytic ileus, do not normally appear.[48] The outstanding and as yet totally unexplained feature of myasthenia gravis is the variation of its severity from time to time in the same patient.[49] Indeed spontaneous cure is by no means unknown in quite severe cases. For this reason artificial respiration is always well worth while. Indeed there need be no hesitation in embarking on this form of treatment repeatedly in the same patient.

In myasthenia gravis artificial respiration is simply a means to the end of stabilizing the patient on appropriate doses of anticholinesterase drugs in such a way that he can recover sufficient muscle power to breathe for himself.[50] A neostigmine drip may be employed at first; in this 5 mg of the drug are put in 500 ml of normal saline and run in at a rate of 1 mg per hour. Thereafter neostigmine can be given orally or by a Ryle's tube. The simultaneous administration of neostigmine and the performance of artificial respiration adds greatly to the patient's comfort and in the writer's experience is an effective method of treatment. Providing the neostigmine dosage is not excessive the abolition of spontaneous respiratory movements by mild hyperventilation rests the endplates of the respiratory muscles sufficiently to allow their recovery.

The disease itself, however, is not the only possible cause of respiratory difficulty. If unduly large doses of anticholinesterase are given to a patient with myasthenia gravis, respiratory paralysis may ensue. This arises because the large amounts of acetylcholine which persist at the endplate produce a permanent depolarization analogous to that caused by decamethonium. The essential distinction between this type of respiratory insufficiency and that due to the disease is that edrophonium intensifies respiratory difficulties when they are due to excessive dosage of anticholinesterase,[50] while it produces some improvement in those in whom the condition is due to the myasthenia itself. Respiratory insufficiency due to excessive anticholinesterase dosage is treated by artificial respiration and temporary interruption of the supply of neostigmine.

There is a type of myasthenia gravis in which the muscle endplates become fatigued. Blocking these end plates with d-tubocurarine and thus preventing the access of acetylcholine to them is said to rest them, and cases have been described where recovery has followed a period of curarization and artificial respiration.[51, 52] The writer, however, has seen perfectly satisfactory recovery in myasthenics following a period of artificial respiration without curarization, and in a disease in which the clinical picture varies so much from time to time, it is impossible to be certain that any recovery which occurs is not of the nature of a spontaneous remission.

There is one practical point in the management of the myasthenic. The use of aperients at times at which muscle power is not satisfactory is very liable to produce a sharp aggravation of the condition and may make artificial respiration once more necessary in a patient who had recovered sufficiently to breathe for himself.

Polyneuritis. Acute toxic polyneuritis in the spinal nerves produces respiratory failure of some 3 to 4 weeks' duration.[53-55] The condition may spread to the cranial nerves to produce also the manifestations of bulbar palsy. In addition to artificial ventilation of the lungs, steroids may be employed in its treatment in order to diminish the possibility of residual damage to nerves by fibrous tissue produced by inflammatory reaction.[56] It has, however, been suggested that steroids may aggravate tendencies to tracheal ulceration. Acute toxic polyneuritis is a most rewarding condition to treat and almost complete recovery can be confidently forecast, providing the patient can be tided over the period of respiratory insufficiency.

Poisoning. Tracheostomy and artificial respiration have become routine treatment in cases of barbiturate poisoning where respiratory insufficiency threatens to supervene or where the coma carries with it the risk of inhalation of secretions from the pharynx. It is, however, possible to manage such cases with the aid of cuffed endotracheal tube if the period of respiratory depression is not likely to exceed 48 hours. A case has been reported where intermittent positive pressure respiration was combined with blood dialysis through an artificial kidney in order to accelerate the elimination of the barbiturate.[57] Intermittent positive pressure respiration could also be applied satisfactorily to the treatment of morphine poisoning.

Elimination of the Work of Breathing. Artificial ventilation of the lungs has been employed to eliminate the work of breathing in critically ill patients. This form of treatment has been combined with the use of an artificial kidney in the treatment of uræmia.[58] Since the work of breathing increases if the lung becomes consolidated, it may be that some of the good results obtained by artificial ventilation in patients with bronchopneumonia superimposed on chronic bronchitis and emphysema may be partly due to this cause also. This factor may also account for the salvage of patients with combined head and chest injuries by intermittent positive pressure respiration. Two cases have been reported where imminent circulatory failure was reversed immediately following the institution of this measure in patients with a normal blood carbon dioxide content.[59]

Artificial Ventilation in Infancy and Childhood. It has been reported that the combination of artificial ventilation with tracheostomy and suction through the tracheostomy has improved respiratory insufficiency presenting in the new-born child, and particularly that due to hyaline membrane.[60] It is also of value in acute tracheobronchitis occurring in infants.[61]

Prolonged Action of Relaxant Drugs. Artificial respiration also finds an application in the treatment of "neostigmine resistant curarization".[62] This, however, is essentially a syndrome and not a diagnosis.[63] It includes such diverse conditions as dystrophia myotonica, latent myasthenia gravis, carbon dioxide narcosis and genuine idiopathic prolongation of the action of relaxant drugs. It has recently been suggested[64] that extreme metabolic acidosis may play a part in the etiology of this condition. The intravenous injection of $2 \cdot 74\%$ sodium bicarbonate in doses of 300 to 400 ml has been recommended. This solution not only improves breathing in appropriate cases; it also corrects the profound circulatory upset which is so often present. The problem is fully dealt with elsewhere in this volume. Carbon dioxide narcosis in this connection is discussed on page 297 *et seq.* Suxamethonium apnœa, unless unwisely treated with neostigmine, should rarely require more than about an hour's artificial respiration.

Neuromuscular Block by Antibiotics. Respiratory paralysis has been noted at the end of operations in which relatively large quantities of antibiotics have been instilled into a serous cavity. A considerable number have followed the use of neomycin[178] but polymyxin and streptomycin[179, 180] are also occasionally responsible. The condition is basically one of myoneural block of a nondepolarizing type and therefore more severe in the patient under ether anæsthesia. It is, however, often so intense as not to be reversible by neostigmine. It will, however, pass off spontaneously over a few hours if the patient is ventilated artificially.

Hypokalæmia. Hypokalæmia is a well known cause of muscle paralysis. It has in fact been suggested as a cause of neostigmine resistant curarization.[62] So far, however, no cases of familial periodic paralysis, the idiopathic type of hypokalæmia, seem to have required treatment by artificial ventilation. This measure has, however, been necessary in two patients[181, 182] who developed hypokalæmia as part of the electrolyte disturbance[183] which follows uretero-sigmoid-ostomy. All cases of hypokalæmia may, however, be expected to respond to potassium and it is unlikely that artificial respiration will be required for more than a short interval.

Other Neurological Conditions. Artificial ventilation is not of value in patients in whom acute cerebral compression has caused respiratory arrest, except where it is possible immediately to lower the intracranial pressure and thus to restart breathing within a comparatively short time. Artificial respiration will keep alive for many weeks those with cervical spinal cord transaction caused by injury or disease. The late results in such cases are, however, depressing.

Dystrophia Myotonica. Patients with this disease sometimes show profound respiratory depression after a general anæsthetic (p. 60). They will usually recover spontaneously after some hours' artificial respiration.

Polymyositis. This rare disease causes subcutaneous œdema, anthralgia and widespread muscle weakness. The muscles of the pharynx are often involved and tracheostomy and the insertion of a cuffed tube are required to prevent soiling of the lungs. A case has been recorded in which artificial ventilation was also necessary because the muscles of respiration became inefficient.[184] The disease runs a remitting course and the use of this method of treatment in a respiratory crisis is fully justified. Steroid therapy is also necessary.

Status Asthmaticus. Tracheal intubation and the instillation of trypsin into the bronchial tree followed by removal of mucus by suction may be of value in status asthmaticus, especially in combination with artificial respiration.[185] The inflation pressures required in asthmatics are, however, considerable and there is always a risk of over-distending localized areas of lung and making the situation worse.

CARBON DIOXIDE NARCOSIS

Carbon dioxide narcosis as an indication for artificial ventilation may appear in two distinct forms. Classically it develops as a complication of an acute respiratory infection in a patient with long-standing chronic bronchitis and emphysema. It may, however, be the result of simple hypoventilation of a patient with substantially normal lung alveoli.[65, 66] In this latter form it is one of the causes of post-anæsthetic respiratory insufficiency. Under such circumstances a cause for it will usually be apparent. Thus the writer has seen it where an anæsthetist failed to appreciate that an 8-month pregnancy constituted a load on artificial respiration during curarization and did not ventilate the patient appropriately vigorously. He has also seen it as a complication of anæsthesia for the evacuation of a very large post-pneumonectomy hæmothorax, conducted with curarization and artificial ventilation, again where the need for additional inflation pressure was not appreciated and the enormous amount of blood in the upper hemithorax compressed the under lung as the patient lay in the lateral position. The remedy is hyperventilation with a non-return valve or through soda lime. Usually an hour or so will suffice.

Where anæsthesia is induced in a patient with pre-existing chronic bronchitis and carbon dioxide accumulates during the operation, a much more persistent and intractable form of the condition is liable to develop. Many precipitating factors may be involved, e.g. curarization with inadequate artificial ventilation, the load imposed on respiration by the Trendelenburg position, sputum retention and bronchospasm. Opiate premedication may add to the problem and pre-operative transfusion of blood, if too generously performed, may add an element of pulmonary œdema. The diagnosis depends on the absence of the stigmata and dystrophia myotonica, the normal response of muscle to stimulation of its nerve and the demonstration of a gross elevation of the mixed venous blood P_{CO_2}[67] and plasma bicarbonate or pH fall.

Treatment is by hyperventilation to a point just short of that at which the positive inflation pressure causes blood pressure fall. Because much of the alveolar membrane is abnormal, treatment may need to be prolonged for many hours. Humidification of the inspired gases is therefore essential. Because of the pre-existing tracheo-bronchial infection the endotracheal tube should be replaced by a tracheostomy within 24 hours. It will be necessary to interrupt the artificial respiration every hour at first to assess progress. Even where there is gross carbon dioxide retention the first result of hyper-ventilation will be to reduce the sensitivity of the respiratory centre. There will, therefore, be no spontaneous respiratory effort on stop-ping artificial ventilation. Such improvement in exchange as is produced will not be apparent until respiration has re-established itself. It is obviously undesirable in such cases to use either endo-genous or additional carbon dioxide to restart breathing on stopping ventilation. Nikethamide in a dose of 4 ml can, however, be injected intravenously for this purpose. This avoids anoxia and the additional build-up of carbon dioxide during the test period.

Sooner or later the maintenance of circulatory stability will become a problem. A noradrenaline drip is then extremely valuable. The patient's progress should be followed by 12-hourly determina-tions of blood pH and Pco_2. If a rebreathing method is employed the Campbell and Howell technique is to be preferred[67] (p. 276). Further, because there is always a serious defect in mixing and diffusion the second period of rebreathing should be prolonged to 40 seconds and a correction factor of 2 mm Hg deducted from the Pco_2 of the gases in the bag to correct for the accumulation of endogenous CO_2 during the longer rebreathing period.[68]

Carbon dioxide narcosis arising as a result of acute infection in chronic bronchitis and emphysema is a difficult and complex problem.[69-71] The basic lesion is a pulmonary insufficiency caused by the development of broncho-pneumonia in an already diseased lung. The clinical picture[71, 72] is of a patient with severe dyspnœa, cyanosis, confusion, drowsiness or coma and a variable amount of secretion. There may be irregular muscle twitching. The signs of congestive heart failure may be present. Blood pressure is often high but falls later.

Effective treatment must obviate several disabilities.[73] Failure of air entry into the lung results from the bronchospasm which is part of the basic disease. This is aggravated by sputum retention. In time this leads to an inadequate blood gas exchange, a process which is also hindered by pnemonic exudate in the alveoli and by the pre-existing alveolar damage produced by the emphysema. In addition the respiratory centre is often depressed by the accumulated carbon dioxide. Indeed it may have totally ceased to respond to this gas and the continuation of breathing may depend on an anoxic stimulus from the chemoreceptors of the carotid sinus. All too frequently the position has been made worse by the misguided administration of an opiate analgesic.[69] Even a simple sedative like chloral can depress the respiratory centre[74] sufficiently to precipitate acute symptoms which necessitate the patient's admission to hospital.

Treatment. No single therapeutic procedure gives uniform results. Oxygen has been given in limited quantities, 24 to 35%[75] by mask or 2 to 4 L/min well humidified and blown into a tracheostomy.[74] (It has been calculated that for every mm Hg the tension of the oxygen in the inhaled air is increased there is in theory a nearly equal rise in the arterial blood CO_2 tension. In practice the rise is always rather less.)[75] This form of therapy is safer than intermittent oxygen in higher concentrations as these carry the risk of producing quite prolonged apnœa with serious anoxia.[75] Analeptics like nike-thamide[76] and aminophylline[77] are of value in restarting breathing should it be arrested by giving too much oxygen. A nikethamide drip has also been used as a therapeutic measure but can cause restlessness and anxiety.[76]

Tracheostomy has been employed to provide a path for the ready removal of secretions.[74] It also reduces the dead space and may thus convert an inadequate tidal volume into effective ventilation. In those who seem to be respiratory cripples the tracheostomy may be so designed that it can be kept permanently open (Tracheal fenestration).[78] Tracheostomy too is a necessary preliminary to intermittent positive pressure respiration.

Artificial ventilation has been attempted by many workers in the treatment of carbon dioxide narcosis. Tank respirators are quite useless.[79] It is also suggested by some that square wave respirators are unsatisfactory; in the presence of bronchial obstruction a machine which slowly builds up inflation pressure[80] (a triangular or sine wave respirator or flow generator[81]) is more satisfactory. A negative phase may not be of much value as it can exaggerate trapping. It can be exceedingly difficult to persuade such dyspnœic patients to accommodate themselves to a respirator. For this reason patient-triggered machines are preferred by some, e.g. the Bird assistor. The administration of relaxants has in the author's limited experience of this type of work, been unsatisfactory. The element of bronchospasm in such cases has been so great that after a relaxant has been given it has proved impossible adequately to oxygenate the patient even with oxygen rich mixtures. With suxamethonium it has been possible to tide the patient over the period of respiratory repression with considerable difficulty. A longer acting relaxant might well have produced an immediate fatality. The administration of pethidine is a safer way of helping the patient to accommodate himself to the respirator.

Such patients may also be treated by the administration of the organic carbon dioxide buffers such as THAM[82] (tris-(hydroxymethyl)amino-methane). This substance, said to act partly by promoting renal excretion of CO_2, has proved to be a valuable agent for taking up carbon dioxide in experimental animals. Its use in the human subject has not been uniformly satisfactory.[83] Indeed it has provoked tetany. Another drug which aids carbon dioxide elimination is dichlorphenamide.[84, 187] This is basically a carbonic anhydrase inhibitor, 30 times as potent as the more familiar compound acetazolamide (Diamox) which is used as a diuretic. Dichlorphenamide does not depend however for its action on diuresis but is said to improve the alveolar ventilation. The full mechanism of its action has yet to be worked out. It may simply be an analeptic.

It has been suggested that the intravenous injection of M/6 sodium lactate solution may be of value in cases which may have been of carbon dioxide narcosis.[85] This solution is in fact a source of ionizable base; for the lactate portion of the molecule is readily· metabolized in the liver to carbon dioxide and water to leave the sodium free to combine with any acidic ions in the blood, in other words to add to the alkali reserve. It is a little difficult to see how the comparatively small amount of base supplied in 1 L of M/6 lactate, viz. 7 m-equiv., which represents only a minute fraction of an adult's total base, would contribute much to the improvement of a case of carbon dioxide narcosis unless it is believed that the pH change is responsible for the coma rather than the accumulated CO_2. Such an opinion is contrary to current beliefs. Indeed improvement in a patient with carbon dioxide narcosis is sometimes obtained by deliberate reduction of the body's bicarbonate by the administration of ammonium chloride. Dichlorphenamide also decreases the alkali reserve.[84] It may be, however, that the cases which have responded well to M/6 lactate may not have been due to carbon dioxide narcosis but to other causes such as metabolic acidosis[64] (vide p. 295).

CRUSH INJURIES OF THE CHEST

(Stove-in Chest)

The management of the patient with a stove-in chest presents several problems to the anæsthetist.[86] Immediately on the patient's admission the airway must be cleared by passing an endotracheal tube, if necessary under general anæsthesia. Paradoxical chest movement is then prevented by controlling the respiration. Any blood, secretion or foreign material in the air passages is next sucked out. Urgent surgical procedures like pleural drainage to allow escape of blood or air, arrest of hæmorrhage, repair of ruptured diaphragm, relief of cardiac tamponade are then performed. At the conclusion of those the endotracheal tube is replaced by a tracheostomy if the injuries are severe. These measures alone may be sufficient to set the patient on the way to recovery.

Where, however, there is mobilization of a large area of chest wall—flail chest[87]—with severe paradoxical movement or progressive rise of pulse rate it will be necessary to have recourse to artificial ventilation of the lungs. The problem here, however, is not solely one of preventing the respiratory insufficiency associated with paradoxical movement; for it is possible for some patients to progress almost to the point of respiratory death without any increase in the mixed venous blood CO_2 tension.[59] It seems that there is a reflex shutdown in the pulmonary circulation in the lung underlying the fractured ribs.[88] Further, where patients die after chest injuries the lungs may show areas of collapse, consolidation and œdema which manifest themselves in life as a progressive increase in resistance to inflation, and death may be due to the development of acute cor pulmonale.[86]

Once it has been decided that artificial ventilation of the lungs is necessary some means must be found of facilitating the replacement of spontaneous by artificial respiration. Curarizing drugs are best avoided. Analgesics and sedatives are preferable.[89] The administration of the former with controlled respiration indeed affords the best method of pain relief in such cases, but on their own analgesics can cause fatal respiratory depression. Where the patient is dyspnœic and in extremis when he is first seen the use of a relaxant drug may, however, be the only way of obtaining control of the respiration[59] without the employment of inflation pressures so high as to produce blood pressure fall. Where obstruction to inflation is a feature the degree of passive hyerventilation possible may at first fall far short of that required to avoid hypercarbia and maintain apnœa. In these circumstances too a relaxant drug may be needed. The use of a relaxant drug is, however, never to be embarked on light-heartedly and only in circumstances where suitable medical help can be available within a minute or so. Because bronchial obstruction is frequent, a respirator with a triangular or sine wave form and a moderately slow build-up of positive pressure, e.g. the Engström, Blease or Newcastle apparatus, is more likely to be tolerated in these cases too than the square wave type of apparatus such as the Radcliffe and the Barnet. Whatever method of treatment is employed there is a risk of tracheobronchial flooding by sputum released by change of posture. This will cause sudden asphyxial death, unless the condition is promptly recognised and suitable skilled help is available at once to clear the airway (p. 311).

The results of treatment of stove-in chest are not good. The largest recent published series records 9 survivors out of 38 cases,[86] though better results have been obtained with the freer use of intermittent positive pressure respiration.[90]

TETANUS

Tetanus is an extremely serious life-threatening disease but to which there are no serious sequelæ in those who survive. Furthermore the condition is self-limiting.

The severity of a particular attack has a bearing on the method of treatment.[92, 93] The most severe cases are those in which the incubation period is of the order of 7 days or less, and in which the interval between the onset of the first symptom and the appearance of the first tetanic spasm is under 24 hours. Severe cases can also be recognised by the fact that the spasms occur with increasing severity and frequency after heavy sedation. The presence of a temperature higher than 103° F is also an indication of a severe attack of the disease.

The dangers of tetanus are these:

First, the generalized muscular rigidity leads to hypoventilation by fixing the respiratory muscles. Secondly, when a patient develops a tetanic spasm the intense tonic contraction of all the muscles of the body prevents breathing. This disturbance may be sufficiently prolonged to result in death from acute asphyxia.[94] The airway is threatened because the tonic rigidity of the muscles of mastication leads to tight closure of the lower jaw—trismus, the feature which gives the disease its popular title of lock-jaw. In addition the tongue may be bitten during a spasm and become swollen as a result of bruising or infection. The toxin of tetanus may invade the medulla oblongata and give rise to disturbances of the function of the cranial nerves.[92, 93, 95, 96] Disorganization of swallowing results. Saliva may therefore accumulate in the back of the throat and because the larynx is also insensitive this saliva is readily inhaled into the trachea and lungs. For these reasons too there is a very serious danger of inhalation of gastric content should the patient vomit. The bulbar disturbance also depresses the cough reflex. Laryngeal stridor may occur.[92] Secretion may accumulate in the lungs and bronchi. In addition the sedative drugs which are often used for the treatment are depressors of the cough reflex and tend to lead to sputum retention.[97]

Disturbances of medullary function[95, 98, 99] may also upset the vasomotor centre causing episodes of hypertension, motor instability and frank hypotension. Hyperpyrexia[93] occurs in some patients and as in bulbar poliomyelitis this too is almost certainly a direct effect of the disease on the brain stem. Tetanus may also affect the myocardium.[95, 104]

Principles of Management

The first basic principle in the management of the patient with tetanus is the maintenance of the patency of the airway. In addition, the spasms are controlled to minimize the disturbance of respiration. Specific measures to deal with the infection are required; 100,000 to 200,000 units of antitoxin should be given intramuscularly when the patient is first seen.[100] If there is an obvious wound with anaerobic infection in it, it should be excised at once. Wherever there is any difficulty with breathing either because spasms are interfering with it momentarily or because secretions are accumulating in the back of the throat or in the lungs, a tracheostomy should be performed.[92] If the spasms are recurring frequently in spite of adequate doses of sedative drugs or if the patient is becoming cyanotic during the spasms, curarization and intermittent positive pressure respiration should be instituted.

The patient's position must be regularly changed and physiotherapy applied to loosen sputum retained in the smaller bronchi (p. 315). Physiotherapy directed to the maintenance of the limb muscles must also be carried out regularly. The patient, however, must be fully relaxed before any attempt is made to do anything such as physiotherapy, or even tracheal suction, lest a spasm be precipitated. The normal rules governing the degree of ventilation apply. A loss of compliance, however, may be due either to the return of the tetanic rigidity or to the accumulation of sputum in one of the large bronchi.

When this method of treatment was first introduced the patients were kept anæsthetized during intermittent positive pressure respiration with nitrous oxide. Presently it became apparent that this anæsthetic gas was capable of producing severe bone marrow depression[101-103] and more recently chlorpromazine and amylobarbitone have been used for sedation,[105, 106] Many patients, however have no memory for the period of this acute illness.[95] Sedation may not therefore be necessary.[107] On the other hand Ablett has indicated that the performance of prolonged tracheal suction on the curarized patient who does remember gives rise to a most unpleasant sensation of choking and impending death. In the unsedated, paralysed patient tracheal suction should therefore be carried out as expeditiously as is consistent with effective removal of secretion.

Relaxants

The initial curarization of a patient with tetanus[108] will normally be carried out under the anæsthetic administered for the tracheostomy and the dose of drug will be similar to that required to produce abdominal relaxation, i.e. some 20 to 40 mg of d-tubocurarine in an adult. Thereafter intramuscular doses of this drug of the order of 40 mg 2–4 hourly will be sufficient to maintain paralysis. It is, however, essential that the nurse who is looking after the patient should be free to inject 20 mg of the drug into the drip if at any time a serious spasm occurs. There is an extreme variation in the sensitivity of patients and some workers quote figures varying from 4 to 30 mg intramuscularly every 1 to 2 hours, while yet others have given as much as 7,640 mg of the drug to a child aged 7 in the course of 26 days.[99] Such enormous doses of relaxant drugs are cumulative and the myoneural block produced by them may well persist for many hours or even a day or two after they are discontinued. Under such circumstances the use of a triggered respirator is a help if it is certain that the patient will not develop further serious spasms; otherwise the period of weaning can be one of considerable anxiety.

Twitching of the trachea on gentle manipulation of the tube is the earliest sign that more relaxant is required.[95] Occasionally there may be a diaphragmatic flicker at the end of inspiration. Twitching of the fingers is a more obvious indication[98] but by this time there will usually also be some visible fall in the compliance of the patient, indicating a return of muscular rigidity.

The stimulator designed by Churchill-Davidson[109] is useful in testing the degree of relaxation which is present. The application of this stimulus is however liable to precipitate a disturbance whose severity will be inversely proportional to the intensity of the myoneural block.

Laudexium which has much less ganglion blocking action, has been preferred by some.[93] The dose varied in one case[110] from 12 mg per hour in the early stages of the disease to 2 mg per hour later. The alkaloid toxiferine[111] may have some claim to be employed as it has an extremely long period of action but virtually no effect on the blood pressure. Suxamethonium,[112] which was given in some of the early cases, is now no longer used.

The use of neostigmine as an antidote to reverse curarization in these patients is undesirable as the effect of this drug rarely lasts for more than a matter of an hour or so, with the result that patients may become recurarized and paralysed after its effects have worn off.

Fluid Balance

Though the ordinary patient on artificial respiration is normally fed by a stomach tube there is something to be said for intravenous feeding of the patient with tetanus. An intravenous drip for fluid administration allows a better control of the electrolytes[93, 97, 113] which are liable to be upset as in poliomyelitis.[189] It also provides a route for immediate intravenous injection should a spasm occur when the effect of the relaxant drug is wearing thin. It is also helpful in that gastric hypersecretion[98] sometimes occurs during the first day or two of the treatment.

Neonatal Tetanus

This condition, in which the portal of entry of the organism is the umbilicus of the newborn child, occurs mainly in tropical countries and is a major problem in Africa where the mortality has been very serious indeed,[114, 115] being of the order of 70 to 90 per cent[116] in some areas. There has, however, been a glimmer of hope for infants with severe tetanus as a result of the substitution of curarization and intermittent positive pressure for older methods of treatment.[117, 119] Other cases have been treated with chlorpromazine without intermittent positive pressure and yet others with chlorpromazine and paraldehyde.[115].

Other Drugs in the Treatment of Tetanus

Curarization and intermittent positive pressure is by no means the only method of treating tetanus. As far back as the 1870's Oré used intravenous chloral for this purpose.[120] Extremely good results (15 successive cases thus without a single death[121]) have been reported from the control of tetanic spasms with a slow intravenous drip of thiopentone.[122, 123] Tribromethanol has also been successfully employed.[124, 125] Since excessive activity of the spinal reflexes is a basic feature of tetanus, it is logical to treat it with mephenesin.[126-128] Though a few successes have been reported from this drug, the overall picture has been far from encouraging.[115, 129, 130] The drug which has the most outstanding claim to be used in the treatment of tetanus, however, is chlorpromazine.[100, 131-133, 138, 139] Not only does this relieve the tremendous anxiety of the patient who suffers from this disease, it has also been shown to possess the power of reversing the local action of the toxin in the limb muscles on an experimental animal.[134] This experimental work is transferable to the human subject, for in patients with localized tetanus the administration of chlorpromazine gives rise to a tremendous improvement in the muscular rigidity.[135-137]

The results of the administration of chlorpromazine in the treatment of tetanus, however, have not been encouraging in all centres.[90] In addition chlorpromazine has caused toxic effects[105, 116] including jaundice.[192] There is an additional problem too in that there appears to be an optimum dosage of the drug[133] and if this is exceeded the result may be to increase the number of spasms. Epilepsy from the sudden withdrawal of chlorpromazine has also been noted.[97] Where, however, chlorpromazine has been employed in combination with other sedatives such as amylobarbitone or paraldehyde,the results have been more encouraging. It may be that much of the variation in the results of the treatment of tetanus is traceable to the variable nature of the disease.

STATUS EPILEPTICUS

The vast majority of patients in status epilepticus are satisfactorily treated with the new intramuscular preparation of Diphenyl hydantoin (Epanutin). In a few, however, and especially in those in whom there is an obvious cause of cortical irritation, such as subdural pus, convulsions persist in spite of appropriate doses of anticonvulsants. When the convulsion is actually occurring respiration is arrested during the tonic stage and may be grossly disturbed during the clonic stage. In the post-epileptic coma the laryngeal reflexes are extremely profoundly depressed and inhalation of secretion and saliva from the back of the throat occur extremely readily. The situation is thus one of acute episodes of respiratory failure superimposed on respiratory insufficiency due to inhaled foreign material. In such cases curarization and artificial respiration,[140] exactly as in tetanus, will often tide the patient over the acute phase of his illness which will usually only last for 3 or 4 days. Some of these patients, however, are extremely toxic and may tolerate the hypotensive effects of d-tubocurarine badly. Perhaps laudexium would be more suitable.

CLINICAL ARTIFICIAL RESPIRATION

Indications

The clinical signs of the need for commencing artificial ventilation[142] of the lungs vary from disease to disease. Restlessness and sleeplessness are important. The fact that a patient has to take a breath in the middle of a sentence may indicate a diminished vital capacity; so also may be an inability to count up to a reasonable number before taking a second breath. This test is very easy in that the physician can readily compare the patient's performance with his own. In more scientific terms, artificial respiration is likely to be required when the vital capacity has fallen[38] to some 25 to 30 per cent of the normal value and will be imperative when tidal volume and vital capacity approximate to one another. Tachycardia and a slight rise in the blood pressure may indicate failure of carbon dioxide elimination. The use of the accessory muscles of respiration is another indication for commencing artificial respiration, while cyanosis and panting respiration indicate that respiratory failure has already occurred. If mental haziness is developing into coma the need is urgent. Diminished minute volume of respiration may also be demonstrated but by the time this has occurred, again the need for artificial respiration is clamant. In some cases of seeming respiratory insufficiency, however, secretions have already been inhaled into the lungs[35, 39] or atelectasis has already occurred because of deficient movement of a portion of the chest wall. In such circumstances there is thus always the possibility that tracheostomy and removal of retained sputum by suction may be sufficient to improve respiratory function dramatically and perhaps even avert, at least for the time being, the need for artificial respiration.

The Airway

Whatever the cause of the respiratory insufficiency, it is vital that a clear airway should be established as a first step in treatment. The supra-laryngeal portion of the airway is threatened in these cases for two reasons. First if the patient is comatose, muscular relaxation occurs in the throat, tongue and jaw muscles, just as during anæsthesia. Second, patients with bulbar involvement are unable to swallow. Saliva and other secretions accumulate in the back of the throat and produce a variable degree of respiratory obstruction.

The main threat to the lower airway in the patient with respiratory insufficiency lies in the accumulation of secretions in the trachea and bronchi. These may be inhaled from above in those who are comatose or are suffering from laryngeal paralysis as a result of bulbar palsy. They are retained because the patient often has no cough reflex. In those in whom the cause of the respiratory insufficiency is an acute episode superimposed on chronic bronchitis and emphysema the source of the secretions will be the inflammatory process in the lungs and bronchi. Secretions which have accumulated in the lower respiratory tract may be removed by bronchoscopy and suction. The effects of this procedure are, however, short-lived[39] and if the patency of the airway is to be maintained, provision must be made for suction at frequent intervals. Where the respiratory insufficiency is likely to be transient, e.g. as in barbiturate or morphine poisoning, the provision may be the passage of an endotracheal tube. If the tube has a cuff on it this can be inflated to prevent the access of further secretion. Intubation, if repeated, however, tends to lead to some degree of laceration of the larynx[188] and in very young children œdema glottidis may result.[143] Endotracheal tubes have been left *in situ* for a week without ill effect in unconscious patients without bronchial infection. In the presence of infection, however, an endotracheal tube left for 48 hours will give rise to considerable inflammation of the tracheal wall. This may in some instances, however, be a reaction to rubber since such a tube in the trachea can by its mere presence provoke increased secretion.[144] Endotracheal tubes are notoriously difficult to fix[143] and it is all too easy for them to become disconnected, kinked, or to slip down into the right main bronchus, with disastrous results to the patient.

Tracheostomy

The vast majority of patients with respiratory insufficiency will be subjected to tracheostomy.[145] This assures the patency of the airway. Secondly, an immediate and easy portal of entry for a suction catheter is provided and no special skill is needed in passing it. Thirdly, the respiratory dead space is reduced by 1·1 ml per kg (0·5 ml per lb) body weight.[146] Lastly, a tracheostomy tube with inflatable cuff isolates the lower respiratory passages from the pharynx in which secretion may tend to accumulate. It affords absolute protection against death from inhalation of vomitus, either immediately by asphyxia or subsequently as a result of the ensuing pulmonary infection.[147] A cuffed tube in the trachea also provides a means of ensuring an airtight fit between the patient and any intermittent positive pressure respirator to which he may need to be connected.

The Operation. In patients with respiratory insufficiency tracheostomy should be conducted under general anæsthesia.[34] The agent used is not of great importance. During the Danish poliomyelitis epidemic, cyclopropane and oxygen seems to have been employed; more recently nitrous oxide and oxygen with or without halothane have proved satisfactory. A preliminary bronchoscopy[39] after the induction dose of thiopentone and suxamethonium is often desirable in those in whom there is much soiling of the tracheo-bronchial tree by inhaled secretions. Thereafter an endotracheal tube is passed, preferably a cuffed tube, and respiration is controlled from the beginning of the procedure. When the surgeon is ready to make his window in the trachea the endotracheal tube is withdrawn part way until the end of it is just above the proposed site of the opening in the tracheal wall and spontaneous respiration is re-established. If a standard pattern silver tube is to be introduced it may not even be necessary to withdraw the endotracheal tube so far, as the diameter of the trachea may well be such that it will accommodate both the endotracheal tube and the tracheostomy tube.

The following points are important in relation to the treatment of patients with respiratory insufficiency. First, where the first tracheal ring was breached as it was in many cases in Denmark,[34] tracheal stenosis not infrequently resulted. Secondly, it has been found necessary to cut out a portion of the tracheal wall if cuffed tracheostomy tubes are repeatedly to be introduced into the trachea through the tracheostome. The classical linear incision in the trachea is not satisfactory. A window, large enough to accommodate the tube to be passed, should be cut out as tracheal stenosis has resulted from the infolding of a portion of the tracheal wall by a tube introduced through too small a hole.[145] On the other hand not more than one-third of the entire circumference of the trachea should be sacrificed in order to make the opening.[34] If larger holes are made, tracheal stenosis may occur subsequently.

Though it is important to avoid the first ring,[148] and according to some authors the second ring also,[145] tracheostomy should not be performed at too low a level.[148] Cuffed tracheostomy tubes are not easy to introduce and the longer path through the tissues of the neck at lower levels makes low tracheostomy unsatisfactory. Secondly, low tracheostomy brings the lower end of the tracheostomy tube within the trachea uncomfortably close to the bifurcation.[148] Under such circumstances the tube may find its way into the right main bronchus and the left lung may be shut off completely. A high tracheostomy offers a positive advantage. It makes it possible to use tubes with fairly long cuffs. This increases the area of tracheal mucosa over which the pressure of the inflated cuff may be spread and thus reduces the risk of necrosis. When a tube is changed it is also possible with a high tracheostomy to replace it by another with its cuff in a slightly different place, and thus again to avoid continuous pressure on the same area of tracheal mucous membrane.[149]

Post-operative Care. The performance of the operation of tracheostomy short-circuits the inspired air past the normal humidifying mechanisms of the upper respiratory tract. Provision must therefore be made for artificial humidification of the inspired gases. If this is not done a certain proportion of patients will develop fibrinous tracheo-bronchitis. Fibrinous crusts will then appear in the trachea and bronchi and in extreme instances an entire cast of the trachea and larger bronchi may be formed. This last result almost invariably gives rise to a fatality from asphyxia.

Humidification. Some respirators such as the Smith-Clarke have a humidifier built into them to prevent fibrinous tracheitis; in others a separate humidifier[150] must be employed. A humidifier consists essentially of a large airtight can of water kept at a temperature of 110° F by an electric heater and thermostat. The humidifier is interposed in the inspiratory hose and the air going to the patient is blown through it.

Where a tracheostomy has recently been performed and artificial respiration is not necessary the Oxford blower may be employed.[151] This consists of a vacuum cleaner type fan motor which drives a stream of air over the surface of warm water in an air-tight can. The output is delivered to a little plastic mask which is applied loosely to the patient's neck over the tracheostomy.

Attempts have been made to utilise the water vapour which condenses from the expired air for purposes of humidification.[152] Basically such contrivances consist of layers of wire gauze interposed between the open end of the tracheostomy tube and the exterior. These devices will often prevent fibrinous tracheitis, though they are not effective in its treatment once it has developed. There is also available a nebulizer for humidification of inspired air during artificial respiration. This apparatus, however, requires compressed gas to make it work and it can only be employed with an apparatus like the Bird assistor, in which the motive force for artificial respiration comes from the intermittent release of a supply of air or oxygen from a cylinder.

The treatment of fibrinous tracheo-bronchitis when it appears after tracheostomy is not very satisfactory. It is essential in such cases to have a bronchoscope by the patient's bed and to be prepared to remove the tracheostomy tube and carry out bronchoscopy through the tracheal stoma should the signs of respiratory obstruction appear. In an emergency an ordinary metal pharyngeal sucker thrust into the trachea and bronchi may be more rapidly effective than formal bronchoscopy. Protein digesting substances such as Trypsin[153] and detergent aerosols[154] like Alevaire may be instilled into the trachea but the results of such treatment are by no means universally satisfactory. Fortunately the condition is self-limiting and if the patient can be tided over the first week after his tracheostomy no further trouble from this cause need be anticipated.

Cuff Deflation. The rubber cuff of a tracheostomy tube is inflated until it presses outwards sufficiently to prevent the escape past it of air blown into the patient by a respirator. It will then also be impossible for secretions to run down from the upper airway into the lower trachea. Most workers fear that if this pressure is allowed to continue without intermission the necrosis of tracheal mucous membrane will occur. With this in mind they recommend that the cuff of the tracheostomy tube or, where it is present, the cuff of an endotracheal tube, should be deflated for some 5 minutes every 4 hours.[147] It is vitally important that the patient's trachea should be sucked out immediately after the cuff has been deflated because secretions which had been dammed back in the upper portion of the trachea will almost certainly find their way past the tracheostomy tube at this stage.

Some workers believe that it is unnecessary to release tracheostomy cuffs[145] at all except when the tube requires to be changed. This should be done every 5 to 7 days. If the cuff must be deflated the output of the respirator must be increased so that sufficient will be available to inflate the chest and to allow a considerable escape of gas past the cuff to the exterior through the upper respiratory passages. If the cuff is to be deflated only every 4 hours, patients will greatly appreciate it if the 2 a.m. deflation can be avoided; this makes an uninterrupted night's sleep possible.

Tracheal Suction. The removal of secretions from the trachea is an integral part of the management of patients with respiratory insufficiency, whether they are being treated on a respirator or not. Tiemann's catheters were originally used for this purpose because it was possible to direct their stiff points alternately into the right or left main bronchus. These catheters are, however, relatively rigid and their sharp points are liable to excoriate the tracheal mucous membrane.[39] A popular catheter at the moment is of plastic with a number of side holes in its end.[148] This, however, has the drawback that it will not remove secretion which does not cover all the holes in the catheter. The author's preference is still for the standard Jacques rubber urethral catheter (Size 6 or 8, English catheter gauge) with a single lateral hole in the end.

It is frequently necessary to lubricate suction catheters, particularly in order to persuade them through the right-angled Radcliffe tracheostomy tube. Glycerine is the most satisfactory substance for this purpose. Liquid paraffin should certainly not be used, as this may produce lung tumours. Any water-soluble jelly type lubricant will also serve. The plastic catheters used by anæsthetists for passage through endotracheal tubes for suction purposes are much too rigid and too sharp at the end to be safe.

It is currently believed by many that tracheal suction should be carried out as nearly as possible as an aseptic operation[92] and that the portion of the catheter which is to be introduced into the tracheostomy should be held with forceps only. A side tube is attached to the connection at the proximal end of the catheter.[155] This side tube is left open during the passage of the catheter as it descends, to prevent the suction end from adhering to the tracheal wall; when it is desired to suck the side tube is covered with the tip of a finger and secretion is then removed from the trachea. There is no doubt that there is much to be said for the aseptic tracheal suction. It is, however, rarely effective in its aim of preventing infection. It is also the author's experience that where secretion is difficult to reach, or where it is viscid, a much more effective clearance of the tracheo-bronchial tree can be obtained when an ordinary soft rubber urethral catheter is passed through the tracheostomy tube, grasped between the finger and thumb of the operator, and made to rotate to and fro as it descends in the trachea. It is of course vital that the nurse who performs suction should wash her hands immediately before performing the operation. Catheters too should be boiled before use, used once and then rejected for re-sterilization.

Some degree of tracheo-bronchial infection inevitably results from the performance of tracheostomy. Indeed so seriously do some regard this complication[152] that they feel that tank respirators should be employed whenever possible in the management of respiratory paralysis.[157, 158] Most workers, however, simply give such patients anti-infective agents. Penicillin is unlikely to be satisfactory because the infection picked up will almost certainly be by organisms resident in the hospital which are very likely to be penicillin resistant. The tetracyclines are unsatisfactory in those who are receiving large quantities of milk as they are thereby deprived of the protection from enteric infection normally afforded by the gastric hydrochloric acid. Chloramphenicol is of course too toxic for constant use. Mixtures of penicillin and streptomycin, and perhaps the more modern wide-spectrum penicillins, may be satisfactory. It is, however, the author's view that sulphamezathine in a dose of 1 G 6-hourly given over the whole period during which the tracheostomy is open will prevent any serious respiratory infection. Should an acute exacerbation occur the sensitivities of the predominant organisms in the sputum should be determined and the appropriate antibiotic administered.

Complications of Tracheostomy

The more serious complications of tracheostomy appear to have been comparatively rare during intermittent positive pressure respiration. A tube has, however, ulcerated into a major artery and caused a fatal hæmorrhage.[97] Steroid administration may aggravate this risk. Tracheo-œsophageal fistula has also been produced by tracheostomy tube.[72]

Though pneumothorax and surgical emphysema have been reported as complications of tracheostomy it seems more likely that the cases in which these have arisen during intermittent positive pressure respiration[159] have been due to the application of excessive pressures to the patient rather than the direct result of the tracheostomy. Pneumothorax after tracheostomy is almost always the result of vigorous inspiratory efforts made in an attempt to overcome obstruction of the tube in the spontaneously breathing and fully active patient.

Tubes for Tracheostomy

A large number of different types of tube have been described for insertion into a tracheostomy performed to facilitate artificial respiration. The mere fact that there are so many indicates that none is completely satisfactory. In Copenhagen[34] a cut down cuffed endo-tracheal tube was used. Others prefer a cut down endobronchial tube with the idea that the shorter cuff may be placed at different levels in the trachea on different inflations and thus the area subjected to pressure changed from time to time.[92] The length of the trachea from the bifurcation to the vocal cords is only about 4 in. (10 cm). The distance from the lower margin of tracheostomy to the bifurcation of the trachea may be as little as 2 in. in a small adult. It is, therefore, not surprising that when tubes of this type were used it was quite common for them to find their way accidentally into the right main bronchus, with disastrous consequences to the ventilation. They are also exceedingly difficult to secure.

The tracheostomy tube which has found widest application is the Radcliffe tube.[160] This is right-angled and has a square-cut end. It is probably the most difficult of all to insert but the flange on the external end of it completely prevents the tube from slipping too far down; on the other hand if the track from the trachea to the exterior is unduly long it is very easy for the tube to be only partly inserted into the tracheostomy. In this position it is very unstable and the risk of its coming out is not inconsiderable. It is also possible for the white metal end, into which the connection fits, to slip out of the rubber. Further, fixation of the whole tube into the neck is not easy. Wings, like those on the classical silver tracheostomy tube, are sometimes supplied with Radcliffe tubes. It is, however, almost impossible, unless the track from the skin to the trachea is exceedingly short, to use these wings to fix the tube in the manner in which an ordinary silver tube is fixed. Magnetic connections to prevent the accidental separation of the connector from the tracheostomy tube have been proposed for the Radcliffe tracheostomy tube. In an endeavour to eliminate the irritation produced by red rubber tubes, a Radcliffe tracheostomy tube has been manufactured from latex rubber and reinforced with a nylon thread.[161]

Bullough[162] has described a tube made from a No. 12 endotracheal tube, for intermittent positive pressure respiration. The end in the trachea is cut square, while that which protrudes from the patient's neck is secured by a rubber collar. There is a special connection with a side-arm and plug which can be removed for purposes of suction. This side-arm is so designed that its internal diameter is exactly equal to that of a suction catheter, in the hope that during suction artificial ventilation might be continued. The advantages of this, however are somewhat dubious (p. 316). Another type of tracheostomy tube is made by placing the cuffed portion of a Magill endotracheal tube over a silver tracheostomy tube. The suggestion has also been made that cuffed tubes should be dispensed with entirely and the output of the respirator increased to make good the inevitable leak. This allows the patient to talk but such an arrangement would not afford protection against the inhalation of vomitus. Further, the extent of the leak must vary tremendously from time to time and the degree of ventilation of the patient's lungs will be correspondingly erratic.

CONTROL OF VENTILATION

In addition to observing the clinical signs of the adequacy of ventilation (p. 272) it is necessary to perform biochemical estimations.

These may be performed on arterial blood, or arterialized venous blood.[164] Indirect determinations of the P_{CO_2} of the mixed venous blood may be made by rebreathing methods (see pp. 274 *et seq.*). The frequency with which such determinations are required will vary from patient to patient. They will, however, normally be necessary twice daily in the very early stages of the treatment. The need for them will progressively diminish as treatment goes on but even in long-term cases an occasional check is desirable.

CHEST PHYSIOTHERAPY

The simplest form of physiotherapy applied during artificial respiration is the removal of sputum by means of a suction catheter passed into the trachea. It is necessary in addition to take special measures to mobilize sputum which is beyond the immediate reach of the suction catheter and to these procedures the term " physiotherapy" is more often applied. Two distinct steps are involved. The first consists in placing the patient so that the part of the lung to be drained is elevated and its bronchus drains as nearly vertically downwards as can be arranged. (It is not usually desirable to place patients on a respirator face down, though this has obvious advantages from the point of view of promoting drainage, in view of the anterior inclination of the trachea.) Once the patient has been placed in the appropriate position the sputum in the bronchi is released by vibratory massage or tapôtement. This consists essentially of a series of slaps applied to the chest wall; their vigour will be determined by the tenderness of the patient's skin. After this process has gone on for a few minutes the physiotherapist vigorously squeezes the part of the chest she has been treating, immediately at the end of an inspiratory stroke of the pump. The effect of this type of treatment can be further improved if manual compression of a rubber bag is substituted for machine artificial ventilation at this point and a maximal inflation immediately precedes the application of external pressure. A second operator should be available to pass the suction catheter into the trachea and remove secretion as soon as it is displaced into the larger bronchi by physiotherapy.

SUCTION

The suction apparatus is an essential part of the equipment for managing a patient on long-term artificial respiration. Their characteristics have recently been studied in detail.[166, 167] First, the apparatus should be capable of developing a negative pressure of the order of 25 in. of mercury (64 cm). Smaller pressures will fail to take up viscous sputum. Secondly, it is important that this negative pressure should be attained fairly quickly. To this end the air intake into the freely open suction bottle should be at a rate of 30 L/min.

The introduction of a thick suction catheter through a comparatively narrow bore tracheal tube can create a very considerable negative pressure in the lungs. This negative pressure will give rise to a sudden increase in venous return and this may in fact cause sudden death where the resulting enormous load is suddenly imposed on an already anoxic heart. The outside diameter of a suction catheter should therefore never exceed more than half the inside diameter of the tube through which it is to be introduced. In a practical test of a number of catheters it was found that those with external diameters of from 0·1 to 0·16 in. were satisfactory; finer catheters were unable effectively to remove viscous material from a model.

FLUID BALANCE AND ELECTROLYTE DISTURBANCES

Nutrition. Where the patient can swallow there is no difficulty; an ordinary hospital diet can be taken. Where, however, a Ryle's tube must be passed for feeding a fluid diet of milk and eggs, to it is added an appropriate amount of minerals (5 G of sodium chloride) and vitamins. The proprietary food Complan is best avoided as it is liable to cause diarrhœa. In general the same principles govern the feeding of these patients as do the treatment of those with head injuries. The daily protein intake should not exceed 80 G while the blood urea is elevated over 80 mg per 100 ml. Once it has fallen larger amounts of protein may be given. Special tube feed diets, again designed initially for patients with head injuries, have been developed for this purpose.[168] The daily intake of fluid should be 5 to 6 pints.

Control of Fluid Intake. During the first week, or until it is apparent that they have settled to a normal level, the concentrations of the electrolytes in the patient's blood should be determined daily. The serum sodium level provides the best guide to the degree of hydration. Determinations based on the hæmatocrit and hæmoglobin level are unsatisfactory because hæmolysis and other factors can upset these in patients with acute illnesses.

SEDATIVES

A period of treatment on a respirator is a most anxious time for the patient. The administration of 50 mg of chlorpromazine 8-hourly to produce tranquillity is always well worthwhile unless this drug proves to have an adverse effect on circulatory stability. Alternatively, paraldehyde may be injected intramuscularly or down the Ryle's rube. Soluble phenobarbitone has also been used as a sedative. Paraldehyde and chloral are satisfactory drugs for night sedation. Opiates, particularly pethidine given intravenously, are most valuable in those who have a tendency to "fight the pump".

MOBILIZATION OF THE RESPIRATOR PATIENT

The need to mobilize a patient on a respirator arises mainly in connection with cases of poliomyelitis where the recession of paralysis does not result in the spontaneous recovery of the respiratory muscles.[169] This situation arose in 25 of the 345 cases who required artificial respiration during the Copenhagen epidemic. If the patient's respiratory mechanism remains totally paralysed it is necessary, unless he has become a frog breather, to mobilize him with his respirator. Adaptations of the Radcliffe[110] and of the Barnet ventilators have been described for the purpose. In these the machine is secured to the back of an invalid chair in which the patient is transported. Arrangements can also be made to place the respirator in the back of a motor car in which the patient is travelling. A special harness round the neck ensures that the tracheostomy tube cannot be pulled out accidentally. An apparatus using a battery-operated version of the ordinary domestic "dustette" may also be employed[171]; with this simple apparatus the output of gas from the machine is delivered to a mouthpiece held between the patient's teeth. Closing the mouth and naso-pharynx permits the gases to be blown down the trachea, while in expiration the mouthpiece is still held between the teeth but the gases are allowed to escape from the lungs around it.

If some slight recovery of respiratory activity occurs it may be possible to mobilize the patient with the aid of a cuirass respirator. The negative pressure varieties which operate with the aid of a thoraco-abdominal shell—such as the Monaghan or the Rota-ventilator—permit the patient to remain in the sitting position while being respired. The Bragg-Paul, though less efficient in itself and requiring that the patient possesses even more spontaneous respiratory movement of his own, gives a greater degree of freedom than any of the other cuirass machines.

All respirators, however, should be regarded only as aids to recovery. The real aim of the treatment is to allow the patient ultimately to breathe normally. To this end he must be encouraged to breathe for himself for short periods which are within his compass on several occasions each day as soon as this is possible. It is, however, essential to strike a balance between the risk of fatiguing weak muscles by overworking them for too long periods and failing to exercise them sufficiently to ensure that they recover as quickly as possible. No rules however can be laid down in this matter; each case must be decided on its merits.

Even after the restoration of apparently adequate spontaneous breathing the patient's troubles are not over. It is all too common for those in whom part of the respiratory mechanism still remains paralysed to develop sputum retention with every attack of common cold.[172] The partly paralysed muscles of respiration cannot compensate for the reduction in effective ventilation and the patient is again precipitated into respiratory failure. Further, patients on the margin of insufficiency are often acclimatized to a high alkali reserve and the hyperventilation employed to wash out this accumulated carbon dioxide may tend to produce tetany[173] if treatment is too vigorous.

GLOSSOPHARYNGEAL BREATHING (FROG BREATHING)

A failure of the muscles of normal respiration to recover following an attack of poliomyelitis does not necessarily doom a patient permanently and totally to life with a respirator. In 1951 Dail noticed that some paralysed poliomyelitis patients were breathing in an odd way which involved something not unlike swallowing movements.[174] He found that they had worked out a method of using the muscles of the throat and floor of the mouth to pump air into their lungs. The technique was as follows: the mouth and throat were filled with air as fully as possible by depressing the floor of the mouth and pulling down the larynx; the lips were closed and the soft palate elevated to trap the air which had been taken in. With the larynx open the floor of the mouth and the larynx were raised and this, together with the motion of the tongue, forced the air in the mouth down the trachea; the larynx was then closed to trap this air and the cycle began again. After some 4 to 8 such cycles the cords relaxed and the air pushed into the trachea and lungs escaped passively as in normal respiration. This form of breathing was of course possible only when the tracheostomy had been occluded; each stroke took 0·3 to 0·6 of a second and displaced just under 60 ml.[175] More than 90 per cent of the patients were ultimately taught the method. This form of breathing is known as glossopharyngeal breathing, or frog breathing.

Glossopharyngeal breathing is not easy for all to learn. Some may find it very difficult when a tracheostomy tube is *in situ*,[176] either because it is not possible to occlude the stoma properly or because the irritation of the tube itself makes laryngeal movement painful. Many such patients, however, will master the technique after closure of the tracheostomy while in a cabinet or cuirass respirator.[177] Occasionally patients complain of dryness or irritation of the throat during frog breathing. This, however, usually disappears after a few weeks and it is always less troublesome if the patient can be trained to take in the air through his nose. Glossopharyngeal breathing is a conscious activity and patients who depend on it must receive artificial respiration when they are asleep. Similarly, when they are eating it is desirable that artificial respiration should be provided. Indeed the patient who is depending on this form of breathing should not be left alone, as if he chokes he may asphyxiate. He is in like straits if the plug in the tracheostomy tube comes out and he himself is unable to replace it. Glossopharyngeal breathing offers especial advantages to patients with nearly total respiratory paralysis. It is possible with its aid to push quite a considerable volume of air down into the lungs; this air can be released with a rush not unlike a natural cough; this manoeuvre can be of value in getting up secretions when the normal cough mechanism is unsatis-factory and will go far to prevent the development of pulmonary complications when the patient contracts an upper respiratory infection.

Apart from the inability of the patient to learn the technique, there seems to be no contra-indication to this method of breathing. Occasionally, however, patients complain of a fullness in the head and a feeling of faintness during a full glossopharyngeal breath; this is probably to be related to the fact that the procedure is in effect a Valsalva manoeuvre. However, breaths of up to a quarter of the normal vital capacity have no effect on the circulation and in quiet glossopharyngeal breathing a normal circulatory system is just as well able to cope with this form of intermittent positive pressure respiration as with any other.

References

1. WATERS, D. J., and MAPLESON, W. W. (1961). *Brit. J. Anæsth.*, **33**, 374.
2. MAPLESON, W. W. (1954). *Brit. J. Anæsth.*, **26**, 323.
3. SYKES, M. K. (1959). *Brit. J. Anæsth.*, **31**, 247.
4. MACINTOSH, R. R., and MUSHIN, W. W. (1946). *Brit. med. J.*, **1**, 908.
5. SAFAR, P. (1958). *Lancet*, **2**, 266.
6. RUBEN, A., ELAM, J. O., and RUBEN, H. (1959). *Lancet*, **2**, 69.
7. SAFAR, P., LOURDES, A. E., ESCARRAGA, L. A., and ELAM, J. O. (1958). *New Engl. J. Med.*, **258**, 671.
8. SAFAR, P. (1958). *J. Amer. med. Ass.*, **167**, 335.
9. COX, J., WOOLMER, R., and THOMAS, V. (1960). *Lancet*, **1**, 727.

10. ELAM, J. O., GREENE, D. G., BROWN, E. S., and CLEMENTS, J. A. (1958). *J. Amer. med. Ass.*, **167**, 328.
11. ELAM, J. O., BROWN, E. S., and ELDON, J. D. (1954). *New Engl. J. Med.*, **250**, 749.
12. Holy Bible, Kings II, **4**, 34.
13. MATTHEWS, G. (1960). *Lancet*, **2**, 601.
14. MUSHIN, W. W., and MORTON, H. J. V. (1958). *Brit. med. J.*, **1**, 215.
15. SKOGH, M. (1960). *Lancet*, **1**, 1415.
16. WULFSOHN, N. L. (1961). *Lancet*, **1**, 1410.
17. DOBKIN, A. B. (1960). *Lancet*, **1**, 982.
18. BROOK, M. H., and BROOK, J. (1960). *Canad. med. Ass. J.*, **82**, 245.
19. BRUCER, M., and SWANN, H. G. (1950). *J. appl. Physiol.*, **3**, 479.
20. EDITORIAL. (1962). *Lancet*, **1**, 468.
21. LONG, W. R. (1962). *Brit. med. J.*, **1**, 578.
22. RUBEN, A., and RUBEN, H. (1962). *Lancet*, **1**, 780.
23. KOUWENHOVEN, W. B., JUDE, J. R., and KNICKERBOCKER, G. G. (1960). *J. Amer. med. Ass.*, **173**, 1064.
24. NIXON, P. G. F. (1961). *Lancet*, **2**, 844.
25. EDITORIAL. (1960). *Brit. med. J.*, **2**, 1582.
26. BENTALL, H. H. (1962). *Proc. roy. Soc. Med.*, **55**, 653.
27. MILSTEIN, B. B. (1961). *Brit. J. Anæsth.*, **33**, 498.
28. BARINGER, J. R., SALZMAN, E. W., JONES, W. A., and FRIEDLICH, A. L. (1961). *New Engl. J. Med.*, **265**, 62.
29. MORGAN, R. R. (1961). *New Engl. J. Med.*, **265**, 82.
30. EDITORIAL. (1960). *Lancet*, **2**, 1333.
31. SCHEOF, D. and, BORNEMANN, C. (1960). *Amer. J. Cardiol.*, **5**, 30.
32. RAINER, E. H., and BULLOUGH, J. (1957). *Brit. med. J.*, **2**, 1024.
33. JULIAN, D. G. (1961). *Lancet*, **2**, 840.
34. LASSEN, H. C. A. (1956). *Management of Life-Threatening Poliomyelitis.* Livingstone, Edinburgh.
35. RUSSELL, W. R. (1955). *Brit. med. J.*, **1**, 98.
36. RUSSELL, W. R. (1959). *Brit. med. J.*, **1**, 613.
37. SMITH, A. CRAMPTON (1956). *Brit. med. J.*, **2**, 163.
38. BREEN, G. E. (1956). *Brit. med. J.*, **2**, 175.
39. HARRIES, J. R., and LAWES, W. E. (1955). *Brit. med. J.*, **1**, 448.
40. JAMES, E. (1955). *Brit. med. J.*, **1**, 726.
41. ANNOTATION. (1957). *Lancet*, **1**, 416.
42. SCOTT, A. F. C., and KNOX, B. R. (1956). *Lancet*, **1**, 515.
43. SPALDING, J. M. K., and CRAMPTON SMITH, A. (1956). *Lancet*, **1**, 639.
44. TRUETA, J., and AGERHOLM, M. (1956). *Lancet*, **1**, 859.
45. SANDIFORD, H. B. C. (1957). *Lancet*, **2**, 823.
46. EDITORIAL. (1956). *Lancet*, **1**, 495.
47. PATERSON, J. H. (1956). *Proc. roy. Soc. Med.*, **49**, 789.
48. GRIFFIN, S. G., NATTRASS, F. J., and PASK, E. A. (1956). *Lancet*, **2**, 704.
49. GARLAND, H., and CLARK, A. N. G. (1956). *Brit. med. J.*, **1**, 1259.
50. TURNER, J. W. A. (1959). *Brit. med. J.*, **1**, 778.
51. CHURCHILL-DAVIDSON, H. C., and RICHARDSON, A. T. (1957). *Lancet*, **1**, 1221.
52. VAN SPIJK, D. v. d. M., and LAMMERS, W. (1957). *Lancet*, **2**, 94.
53. SMITH, A. C., SPALDING, J. M. K., and RUSSELL, W. R. (1954). *Lancet*, **1**, 939.
54. KELLEHER, W. H., MEDLOCK, J. M., and POWELL, D. G. B. (1956). *Lancet*, **2**, 68.
55. WISLICKI, L. (1955). *Brit. J. Anæsth.*, **27**, 303.
56. GRAVESON, G. S. (1957). *Lancet*, **1**, 340.
57. HONEY, G. E., and JACKSON, R. C. (1959). *Brit. med. J.*, **2**, 1134.
58. NORLANDER, O. P., BJORK, V. O., CRAFOORD, C., FRIBERG, O., HOLMDAHL, M., SWENSSON, A., and WIDMAN, B. (1961). *Anæsthesia*, **16**, 285.

59. HUNTER, A. R. (1962). (To be published.)
60. DONALD, I. (1957). *Brit. J. Anæsth.*, **29**, 553.
61. NISBET, H. I. A., and WILSON, F. (1958). *Brit. J. Anæsth.*, **30**, 419.
62. HUNTER, A. R. (1956). *Brit. med. J.*, **2**, 919.
63. EDITORIAL. (1961). *Lancet*, **1**, 34.
64. BROOKS, D. K., and FELDMAN, S. A. (1962). *Anæsthesia*, **17**, 161.
65. SCURR, C. F. (1954). *Brit. med. J.*, **1**, 565.
66. GRAY, T. C., and FENTON, E. S. N. (1954). *Brit. med. J.*, **1**, 820.
67. CAMPBELL, E. J. M., and HOWELL, J. B. L. (1960). *Brit. med. J.*, **1**, 458.
68. HOWELL, J. B. L. (1961). Personal communication.
69. EDITORIAL. (1953). *Lancet*, **1**, 381.
70. WESTLAKE, E. K. (1954). *Brit. med. J.*, **2**, 1012.
71. SIMPSON, T. (1954). *Brit. med. J.*, **1**, 297.
72. MUNCK, O., KRISTENSEN, H. S., and LASSEN, H. C. A. (1961). *Lancet*, **1**, 66.
73. EDITORIAL. (1959). *Brit. med. J.*, **1**, 289.
74. DAVIDSON, L. A. G. (1959). *Lancet*, **1**, 597.
75. CAMPBELL, E. J. M. (1960). *Lancet*, **2**, 10 and 12.
76. WESTLAKE, E. K., and CAMPBELL, E. J. M. (1959). *Brit. med. J.*, **1**, 274.
77. GALDSTON, M., and GELLER, J. (1957). *Amer. J. Med.*, **23**, 183.
78. EDITORIAL. (1959). *Lancet*, **1**, 84.
79. STONE, D. J., SCHWARTZ, A., NEWMAN, W., FELTMAN, J. A., and LOVELOCK,
    F. J. (1953). *Amer. J. Med.*, **14**, 14.
80. HICKMAN, J. B., SICKER, H. O., PRYOR, W. W., and FRAYSER, R. (1956).
    Ann. N.Y. Acad. Sci., **66**, 866.
81. MUSHIN, W. W., RENDELL-BAKER, L., and THOMPSON, P. W. (1959).
    Automatic Ventilation of the Lungs. Blackwell, Oxford.
82. EDITORIAL. (1960). *Brit. med. J.*, **2**, 1943.
83. CAMPBELL, E. J. M. (1961). *Brit. med. J.*, **1**, 286.
84. EDITORIAL. (1960). *Lancet*, **1**, 1120.
85. KENNY, S. (1956). *Brit. med. J.*, **2**, 1113.
86. GRIFFITHS, H. W. C. (1960). *J. roy. Coll. Surg., Edin.*, **6**, 13.
87. SELLORS, T. HOLMES (1961). *Thorax*, **16**, 1.
88. Quoted by BARRETT, N. R. (1960). *Lancet*, **1**, 293.
89. AVERY, E. E., MORCH, E. T., and BENSON, D. W. (1956). *J. thorac. Surg.*,
    32, 291.
90. WINDSOR, H. M., and DWYER, N. (1961). *Thorax*, **16**, 3.
91. EMMERT, F. (1930). *Amer. J. Dis. Child*, **39**, 1268.
92. ABLETT, J. J. L. (1956). *Brit. J. Anæsth.*, **28**, 258.
93. GLOSSOP, M. W., and LOW, M. D. W. (1957). *Brit. J. Anæsth.*, **29**, 326.
94. BODMAN, R. I., MORTON, H. J. V., and THOMAS, E. T. (1955). *Lancet*, **2**, 230.
95. ALHADY, S. M. A., BOWLER, D. P., REID, H. A., and SCOTT, L. T. (1960).
    Brit. med. J., **1**, 540.
96. ADAMS, E. B. (1958). *Proc. roy. Soc. Med.*, **51**, 1002.
97. GARLAND, H. (1959). *Proc. roy. Soc. Med.*, **52**, 877.
98. POWELL, K. J., BRIMBLECOMBE, F. S. W., and STONEHAM, M. E. R. (1958).
    Lancet, **1**, 713.
99. SMITH, A. C., HILL, E. E., and HOPSON, J. A. (1956). *Lancet*, **2**, 550.
100. SHANKER, A., and MEHROTRA, L. S. (1959). *Brit. med. J.*, **2**, 1150.
101. SANDO, M. J. W., and LAWRENCE, J. R. (1958). *Lancet*, **1**, 588.
102. LASSEN, H. C. A., HENRIKSEN, E., NEUKIRCH, F., and KRISTENSEN, H. S.
     (1956). *Lancet*, **1**, 527.
103. WILSON, P., MARTIN, F. I. R., and LAST, P. M. (1956). *Lancet*, **2**, 422.
104. MATTS, S. G. F. (1960). *Brit. med. J.*, **1**, 1057.
105. PACKARD, R. S., CARTMILL, T. B., and HENRY, J. G. (1958). *Brit. med. J.*,
     1, 16.
106. LAURENCE, D. R., BERMAN, E., SCRAGG, J. N., and ADAMS, E. B. (1958).
     Lancet, **1**, 987.
107. HELSINGER, N. (1956). *Lancet*, **2**, 1163.

108. ABLETT, J. J. L. Awaiting Publication.
109. CHRISTIE, T. H., and CHURCHILL DAVIDSON, H. C. (1958). *Lancet*, **1**, 776.
110. WALTON, W. J. (1961). *Brit. J. Anæsth.*, **33**, 589.
111. FOLDES, F. F., WOLFSON, B., and SOKOLL, M. (1961). *Anesthesiology*, **22**, 93.
112. ANDREWS, J. D. B., MARCUS, A., and MUIRHEAD, K. M. (1956). *Lancet*, **2**, 652.
113. WILSON, G., and CARE, A. D. (1955). *Lancet*, **1**, 1303.
114. GALLOWAY, W. H., and WILSON, H. B. (1955). *Anæsthesia*, **10**, 303.
115. WILKINSON, J. L. (1961). *Brit. med. J.*, **1**, 1721.
116. LAURENCE, D. R., BERMAN, E., SCRAGG, J. N., and ADAMS, E. B. (1958). *Lancet*, **1**, 987.
117. WRIGHT, R., and ADAMS, E. B. (1960). *Brit. med. J.*, **1**, 345.
118. SYKES, M. K. (1960). *Anæsthesia*, **15**, 401.
119. WRIGHT, R., SYKES, M. K., JACKSON, B. G., and MANN, N. M. (1961). *Lancet*, **2**, 678.
120. ORGANE, G. (1962). *Ann. Roy. Coll. Surg.* (To be published.)
121. FORBES, G. B., and AULD, M. (1955). *Amer. J. Med.*, **18**, 947.
122. BATTEN, R. (1956). *Lancet*, **1**, 231.
123. LAWSON, E. A., and BANKOLE, M. A. (1959). *Lancet*, **2**, 917.
124. COOKE, J. V. (1953). *J. Pædiat.*, **43**, 220.
125. MAYON-WHITE, R. M. (1956). *Lancet*, **2**, 841.
126. BELFRAGE, D. H. (1947). *Lancet*, **2**, 889.
127. DAVISON, M. H. A., WARD, A. B., and PASK, E. A. (1949). *Brit. med. J.*, **1**, 616.
128. PLEWES, L. W., and WILSON, D. (1951). *Anæsthesia*, **6**, 15.
129. JOHNSTONE, D. D., (1958). *Brit. med. J.*, **1**, 12.
130. SHACKLETON, P. (1954). *Lancet*, **2**, 155.
131. HUTCHINSON, J., and HURRELL, G. D. (1958). *Brit. med. J.*, **2**, 429.
132. LAURENCE, D. R. (1958). *Lancet*, **1**, 1106.
133. ADAMS, E. B., WRIGHT, R., BERMAN, E., and LAURENCE, D. R. (1959). *Lancet*, **1**, 755.
134. LAURENCE, D. R., and WEBSTER, R. A. (1958). *Brit. J. Pharmacol.*, **13**, 330.
135. BARR, M. N. (1958). *Lancet*, **1**, 991.
136. KELLY, R. E., and LAURENCE, D. R. (1956). *Lancet*, **1**, 118.
137. LAURENCE, D. R. (1958). *Proc. roy. Soc. Med.*, **51**, 1000.
138. VAKIL, B. J. (1960). *Brit. med. J.*, **1**, 56.
139. REDDING, J. S., VOIGT, G. C., SAFAR, P. (1960). *J. appl. Physiol.*, **15**, 1113.
140. EVANSON, J. M. (1959). *Lancet*, **2**, 72.
142. EDITORIAL. (1959). *Brit. med. J.*, **1**, 1098.
143. CHURCHER, M. D. (1962). *Brit. med. J.*, **1**, 1320.
144. SMITH, A. C. (1955). *Proc. roy. Soc. Med.*, **48**, 952.
145. HEWLETT, A. B., and RANGER, D. (1961). *Postgrad. med. J.*, **37**, 18.
146. PITMAN, R. G., and WILSON, F. (1955). *Lancet*, **2**, 523.
147. SMITH, A. C., SPALDING, J. M. K., and RUSSELL, W. R. (1954). *Lancet*, **1**, 939.
148. ANDREW, J. (1956). *Brit. med. J.*, **2**, 328.
149. ABLETT, J. J. (Personal communication.)
150. MARSHALL, J., and SPALDING, J. M. K. (1953). *Lancet*, **2**, 1022.
151. SPALDING, J. M. K. (1956). *Lancet*, **2**, 1140.
152. WALLEY, R. V. (1956). *Lancet*, **1**, 781.
153. STEIGMAN, A. J., and SCOTT, C. H. (1952). *J. Amer. med. Ass.*, **150**, 1403.
154. RAVENEL, S. F. (1953). *J. Amer. med. Ass.*, **151**, 707.
155. PLUM, F., and DUNNING, M. F. (1956). *New Engl. J. Med.*, **254**, 193.
156. SANDIFORD, H. B. C. (1957). *Lancet*, **2**, 823.
157. JAMES, E. (1957). *Lancet*, **2**, 948.
158. TRUETA, J., and AGERHOLM, M. (1956). *Lancet*, **1**, 859.
159. HAY, P. (1954). *Lancet*, **2**, 1156.

160. Spalding, J. M. K., and Crampton Smith, A. (1956). *Lancet*, **2**, 1247.
161. Salt, R. H., Parkhouse, J., and Simpson, B. R. (1960). *Lancet*, **2**, 407.
162. Bullough, J. (1957). *Lancet*, **2**, 373.
163. Poulsen, H., Skall-Johnson, J., Staffeldt, I., and Lange, M. (1959). *Acta. anæsth. Scand.*, **3**, 129.
164. Brooks, D., and Wynn, V. (1959). *Lancet*, **1**, 227.
165. Opie, L. H., and Spalding, J. M. K. (1958). *Lancet*, **2**, 671.
166. Rosen, M., and Hilliard, E. K. (1960). *Brit. J. Anæsth.*, **32**, 486.
167. Rosen, M., and Hilliard, E. K. (1962). *Curr. Res. Anesth.*, **41**, 50.
168. Higgins, G., Lewin, W., O'Brien, J. R. P., and Taylor, W. H. (1954). *Lancet*, **1**, 61.
169. Annotation. (1958). *Lancet*, **2**, 405.
170. Sutcliffe, R. L. G., and Spalding, J. M. K. (1959). *Lancet*, **1**, 706.
171. Macrae, T., Walley, R. V., and Lucas, H. K. (1959). *Lancet*, **1**, 452.
172. Wilson, A. B. Kinnier, and Stevenson, F. H. (1957). *Lancet*, **2**, 820.
173. Joels, N., Hurwitz, L. J., and Dreifuss, F. E. (1957). *Lancet*, **1**, 194.
174. Dail, C. W. (1951). *Calif. Med.*, **75**, 217.
175. Dail, C. W., Affeldt, J. E., and Collier, C. R. (1955). *J. Amer. med. Ass.*, **158**, 445.
176. Annotation. (1959). *Brit. med. J.*, **2**, 749.
177. Agerholm, M. (1959). *Brit. med. J.*, **2**, 1021.
178. Pittinger, C. B., and Long, J. P. (1958). *Surgery*, **43**, 445.
179. Bush, C. H. (1961). *Brit. med. J.*, **1**, 557.
180. Fisk, G. C. (1961). *Brit. med. J.*, **1**, 556.
181. Steinbeck, A. W., and Tyrer, J. H. (1959). *Brit. J. Urol.*, **31**, 280.
182. Straffon, R. A., and Coppridge, A. J. (1959). *J. Amer. med. Ass.*, **171**, 139.
183. Lowe, K. G., Stowers, J. M., and Walker, W. F. (1959). *Scot. Med. J.*, **4**, 473.
184. James, J. L., and Park, H. W. T. (1961). *Lancet*, **2**, 1281.
185. Broom, B. (1960). *Lancet*, **1**, 899.
186. Chandler, D., and Rosenbaum, J. (1955). *Amer. Heart J.*, **49**, 295.
187. Christensen, P. J. (1962). *Lancet*, **1**, 881.
188. Gusterson, F. R. (1955). *Anæsthesia*, **10**, 300.
189. Astrup, P., Gøtzche, H., and Neukirch, F. (1954). *Brit. med. J.*, **1**, 780.

CHAPTER 11

ANÆSTHESIA ASSOCIATED WITH IATROGENIC CONDITIONS

JOHN W. DUNDEE

Hypotensive—Drugs Antibiotics—Phenothiazines—Other Tranquillizers—Analgesics and Sedatives—Drugs used in Parkinsonism—Oral Fluids—Radiation Therapy—Pitocin and Oxytocin—Colchinine — Diortho-Cresol — Oestrogens — Citrate Intoxication—Surgical Conditions—Steroid Therapy—Iatrogenic Disease causing Respiratory Insufficiency—General Comment.

IT is essential to define precisely the meaning attached to "iatrogenic conditions" in this chapter. A number of commonly used therapeutic agents produce effects which only come into prominence when other drugs such as anæsthetics are administered. These effects are termed iatrogenic (or iatrogenetic) because they are "induced by the physician".

The anæsthetist is very concerned with iatrogenic conditions, because they have an adverse effect on the course of anæsthesia. Their danger lies in the fact that many of the drugs have no obvious toxic effects in the conscious patient, or else the complications which they cause during anæsthesia are quite different from those normally associated with their use. Furthermore, the iatrogenic effects of some agents may last for a considerable time after their administration has been stopped.

Iatrogenic disease, as a condition affecting the course of anæsthesia, first came into prominence with the introduction of the hypotensive drugs and the corticosteroids.[1] The effects of the latter drugs result from the body's inability to respond to the stress of anæsthesia and surgery but they can have similar effects in the presence of other stimuli such as acute infections or parturition. A large number of drugs have since been added to this list, but they all cause problems which are of specific interest to the anæsthetist. Most of the drugs which cause iatrogenic disease are given before the induction of anæsthesia, but recently there have been examples of drugs given routinely by surgeons and obstetricians affecting the course of anæsthesia. Some operative procedures also affect the patient's response to a subsequent anæsthetic.

It will be seen throughout this chapter that awareness of the possible effects of some drugs is the main factor in preventing catastrophies during anæsthesia. When trouble does arise it can be more easily managed if the toxicology of all non-anæsthetic drugs given to the patient is known. The incidence of iatrogenic disturbances during anæsthesia is likely to increase as new drugs are introduced, for it is the preparations which have not undergone long-term clinical trial which are likely to cause most trouble. Anæsthetists, physicians and surgeons now know that certain drugs are best avoided before operation, but no one can tell what may happen with some of the newer ones. Thus we are likely to get a changing pattern of emphasis on different drugs as time goes on, and in a few years a chapter similar to this may deal with quite a different group than those to be discussed.

Since this chapter is a new addition to a book of this nature it includes as many drugs as can be implicated, even on purely theoretical grounds, as causing iatrogenic disease which will affect anæsthesia. No apology is made for referring on occasions to purely experimental data, for with one of the groups to be discussed proper knowledge of the basic pharmacology would have incriminated certain compounds as potential agents in the production of iatrogenic disease.

Brief mention is also made of surgical iatrogenic conditions of interest to the anæsthetist and the chapter ends with a discussion of some non-anæsthetic problems due to drug therapy or surgery in which the advice or help of the anæsthetist may be requested. All sequelæ of anæsthesia, especially those with long-term effects (e.g. neurological sequelæ of spinal anæsthesia) are iatrogenic conditions, but these are not discussed in this chapter.

HYPOTENSIVE DRUGS

Irrespective of their exact mode of action, hypotensive drugs produce their therapeutic effect by a reduction in peripheral vascular tone. It is not surprising to find that their hypotensive action can be augmented by general anæsthetics, all of which produce some degree of vasodilatation. Changes in posture during operation will accentuate the fall in blood pressure and patients will be unusually sensitive to hæmorrhage.

Methonium Compounds. When pentamethonium and hexamethonium were being widely used as therapy for peptic ulceration, Davison warned anæsthetists that should the ulcer perforate the patient would be in a very grave pre-operative condition.[2] Dundee showed that this was more than a theoretical consideration by reporting a fatality which occurred under these circumstances.[1] In one further patient, who was receiving pentolinium for essential hypertension, the severe bout of hypotension which accompanied the induction of anæsthesia was followed by several days of mental clouding and the possibility of cerebral thrombosis was considered.

In these, and other reported cases, the anæsthetist was not aware that the patients were on methonium therapy. Once the dangers of the pre-operative use of these drugs was appreciated, no further fatalities were reported. This may be partly due to the eclipse of the methonium drugs by newer hypotensive agents, but the same danger exists with the more recently introduced drugs.

Rauwolfia Compounds. Reserpine reduces blood pressure by a peripheral block of the sympathetic nervous system due to a depletion of its adrenergic mediator, noradrenaline.[3, 4] Although the drug itself rapidly disappears from the body, the depletion of noradrenaline lasts about a fortnight. The degree of depletion of the catechol amine has not been studied with different doses of reserpine, but it must be assumed to have occurred to a significant degree if a clinical dose of the hypotensive agent has been given for some time.[5]

Patients on reserpine should be treated as potentially "poor risks" when their cardiovascular systems have to cope with an increased load as during anæsthesia or labour. Probably only rarely will the load be so severe, the depletion so great or the circulatory reserve so low that cardiovascular collapse will occur.[5] Nevertheless, the risk does exist as evidenced by a report of 24 cases of hypotension during anæsthesia in patients on rauwolfia therapy.[6] The drug could definitely be incriminated in one patient whose blood pressure fell alarmingly during the induction of anæsthesia; the operation was postponed for two weeks during which time the rauwolfia therapy was stopped, at the end of which no untoward effects were found after the administration of the same drugs as had been given on the previous occasion. Theoretically, the greatest danger should exist when thiopentone or halothane are given because of their lack of stimulating effect on the sympathoadrenal system.[7]

As with the methonium compounds, the hypotension which occurs in patients on reserpine may not respond readily to ephedrine, methamphetamine or mephentermine and the continuous infusion of potent amines such as phenylephrine, noradrenaline or methoxamine may be required.[8] Coakley and his colleagues[6] have noted that the hypotension is frequently associated with bradycardia and that marked improvement followed the intravenous injection of atropine or oxyphenonium (Antrenyl). A fall in blood pressure combined with bradycardia is a feature of the action of the veratrum alkaloids, which are frequently combined with rauwolfia in the treatment of hypertension. In one patient who was receiving the combined therapy, the tachycardia associated with the introduction of ether into the anæsthetic circuit and that which followed the intravenous injection of oxyphenonium was on both occasions accompanied by a rise in blood pressure.[1]

It seems almost unnecessary to mention that the rauwolfia compounds potentiate the ganglion-blocking drugs and great care should be exercised if a patient on reserpine is scheduled for controlled hypotension with trimetaphan or one of the methonium compounds. The same care should also be shown to the use of spinal or epidural anæsthesia in these cases. It is also worth noting that fatal hypotension has been reported following the administration of large doses of reserpine in late pregnancy.[9]

In addition to the above, rauwolfia produces nasal congestion and excess salivation. This may lead to difficulties in maintaining a clear airway during anæsthesia and increases the risk of excessive bleeding after nasal intubation.

Methoserpidine is a synthetic isomer of reserpine, which retains the hypotensive action of the parent compound, but has fewer undesirable side effects.[10] Early reports suggest that it is as promising in clinical practice as was hoped from the pharmacological data.[11] By virtue of its mode of action, the same precautions should be taken as for reserpine, if patients under treatment require anæsthesia.

Other Hypotensive Drugs. Data is much less complete as regards the effect of other hypotensive agents on the course of anæsthesia. Apart from experiments which showed that hexamethonium and trimetaphan produced neuromuscular block after the administration of mecamylamine in cats,[12] there is nothing to suggest that it produces any deleterious effects during anæsthesia other than would be expected from a ganglion-blocking drug.

Guanethidine acts in a manner similar to reserpine by releasing the stores of noradrenaline from the walls of the arteries, the heart and other organs possessing a sympathetic innervation.[4] This suggests that patients receiving this drug present the same difficulties as already described for those on rauwolfia therapy. Since the hypotensive action of guanethidine lasts for at least seven days after cessation of treatment[13] an adequate period of time should elapse between stopping the drug and the administration of anæsthesia. It has recently been pointed out that both bretylium and guanethidine potentiate tubocurarine,[88] and this may well be of importance to the anæsthetist.

In relation to the effects of all the hypotensive agents on the course of anæsthesia, it is worth noting that their action is reputed to be enhanced during a heat wave.[14] This could of course be explained on the higher incidence of dehydration, but on the other hand may be due to the vasodilation caused by the high environmental temperature. While there is no evidence to suggest that the operating theatre temperature can influence their action, it should be borne in mind and those who do not work in air conditioned theatres may have to take extra precautions so that a patient who is undergoing therapy for essential hypertension is not subjected to the added risk of induction of anæsthesia, except as an emergency life saving procedure.

ANTIBIOTICS

The suggestion that the use of sulphonamides precluded the use of sulphur containing barbiturates, such as thiopentone, in case sulphaemoglobinæmia might occur[15] was probably the first reported incidence of iatrogenic disease affecting the course of anæsthesia. Clinical experience has since shown that thiopentone can safely be given to patients on sulphonamide therapy and until recently the lack of sedative and hypotensive effects of the newer antibiotics suggested that they could be given with safety before and after anæsthesia. However, in 1956, Prigden[16] reported that respiratory arrest occurred in four patients to whom intraperitoneal neomycin had been given under anæsthesia. The outcome of the apnœa was fatal in two of the cases who were children while two adults recovered after three and forty-eight hours' apnœa. Further cases of a similar nature were reported in the following year[17-20] and these led to an extensive investigation of the neuromuscular blocking action of neomycin and other antibiotics. It is interesting to note that the more recent studies only confirmed the initial pharmacological reports on these drugs, but their full significance was not appreciated until the effects during anæsthesia were reported.

Experimental Data. For the sake of simplicity all the antibiotics with relaxant properties will be discussed together. Polymyxin B[21] and streptomycin [22, 23] have been known for some time to be capable of producing neuromuscular block in animals. Streptomycin potentiates the effects of tubocurarine in rabbits,[24] but the block resembles that produced by magnesium and is more easily reversed by calcium than by neostigmine.[22] In a series of studies from the University of Iowa[25-28] it was found that neomycin sulphate, streptomycin sulphate, dihydrostreptomycin sulphate, polymyxin B and kanamycin all produced neuromuscular blockade in animals at various dosage levels. With the exception of polymyxin B, the blocking action of the antibiotics was enhanced by tubocurarine chloride and all were antagonized by neostigmine except polymyxin B and kanamycin. Penicillin G, tetracycline hydrochloride, erythromycin lactobromate, ristocetin and bacitacin have no effect on the myoneural junction.

The studies of Sabawala and Dillon[29] on the effects of antibiotics on human intercostal muscles confirmed the neuromuscular blocking effect of neomycin, streptomycin and polymyxin B and demonstrated their synergism with ether. They observed that the dose of an antibiotic necessary to produce an appreciable neuromuscular block is far above the therapeutic range and considered that cyclopropane is the anæsthetic which is least likely to cause severe respiratory depression in combination with them.

Clinical Reports. The clinical reports of the adverse effects of neomycin on the course of anæsthesia are all very similar. A large dose of the drug was given during anæsthesia into the peritoneal[16-20, 30-32] or pleural[33] cavity. This was followed by apnœa which lasted up to forty-eight hours after administration of the antibiotic. Ether was the commonly used agent in these cases, and the cause appears to be a synergism between the effects of the anæsthetic and neomycin on the myoneural junction.

Reports on the adverse effects of streptomycin are much fewer than those following neomycin. However, in 1948, Loder and Walker[34] described three cases of muscle weakness and visual difficulty after standard intramuscular doses of the drug. The syndrome resembled myasthenia gravis and the symptoms were relieved by neostigmine and stopping the streptomycin. Bush[35] ascribed prolonged neuromuscular block following 8 mg tubocurarine in a six months' old baby to the 1 g dose of streptomycin which was given intraperitoneally during surgery. Doses of 5 g were given into both the peritoneal and pleural cavities in the case described by Fisk.[36] Again tubocurarine was given during anæsthesia and its effect was adequately reversed by neostigmine. Thirty to forty minutes later the patient developed severe respiratory depression in the ward and despite a transient improvement after neostigmine, artificial ventilation was required for forty minutes before return of spontaneous respiration.

One single report[37] implicates the intraperitoneal administration of kanamycin as the cause of apnœa in a child anæsthetized with ether. It was considered to be less potent in this respect than neomycin on a mg for mg basis and in the reported cases the apnœa was not reversed by edrophonium, but there was a dramatic recovery after a single small dose of calcium gluconate.

Comment. There is convincing evidence that large doses of both neomycin and streptomycin can cause a neuromuscular block, but this is unlikely to occur with the therapeutic doses employed in man. This block is potentiated by both ether and non-depolarizing relaxants. If a large dose of either antibiotic is given into either the peritoneal or pleural cavity of a patient who is under the influence of ether, tubocurarine or gallamine prolonged curarisation may occur. If the drug is given immediately before the end of the operation this effect may not be manifested until the patient has returned to the ward. This must be remembered in view of the large doses of neomycin which are recommended for the treatment of acute bacterial peritonitis.[38]

This form of iatrogenic disease is of particular significance to those who are studying the effects of new drugs. In the early pharmacological studies of one of the antibiotics there was ample evidence to suggest that, under appropriate circumstances, the drug could augment the action of certain muscle relaxants. One must not imagine that the use of the depolarizing relaxants eliminates this hazard for the prolonged use of suxamethonium produces a neuromuscular block which will be intensified and prolonged by either neomycin or streptomycin.

The thoroughness with which the effects of these antibiotics and their effect on anæsthetics and muscle relaxants has been investigated is admirable and it testifies to the importance which is being attached to iatrogenic disease. It is important also to note that the experimental findings and clinical reports have appeared in journals devoted to surgery,[16, 18, 19, 25, 30, 32] anæsthesia[26, 29] and antibiotics[27] as well as general medical journals.[20, 31, 33-36] Thus the significance of this side effect of antibiotics is likely to have been brought to the attention of all who are most concerned. One can hope that the neuromuscular effects of any new antibiotics will be fully investigated before they are released for clinical use, and that the relevant findings are brought to the attention of all who use them.

PHENOTHIAZINES

A very large number of these drugs are now in clinical use,[39] and while the definite indications for their administration have decreased over the past few years, the anæsthetist is likely to come across cases who have been receiving them for varying lengths of time, particularly when dealing with psychiatric cases. In view of their widespread effects on the body, one might expect the phenothiazines to be the group of drugs most commonly involved in iatrogenic disease. This has not been the case and it is instructive to consider one possible explanation for this.

Chlorpromazine was one of the first phenothiazines to gain widespread popularity and it is also one of the most toxic members of this series. It was widely used as an adjuvant to anæsthesia either in the technique of artificial hibernation or in the production of hypothermia by surface cooling. Anæsthetists also used it in the management of chronic pain and as an anti-emetic. Thus, within a short time of its introduction both the capabilities and side effects of this drug were known, and the latter were described in some detail in the anæsthetic literature. In fact, anæsthetists placed more emphasis on the toxic effects of chlorpromazine than their medical, surgical or psychiatric colleagues, probably because they commonly gave it by the intravenous or intramuscular route and so detected hypotension, etc. more readily. It is easy to imagine the care that would be taken in the anæsthetic management of a patient who was known to be on chlorpromazine therapy, and this probably prevented many fatalities.

The more recent members of the phenothiazine group of drugs are reputed to be less toxic than their predecessors and (while there may be some doubt about the validity of this statement in respect to some of them) they are thus less likely to upset the course of anæsthesia. Some side-effects (e.g. hypotension) occur with all the phenothiazines, others (e.g. pseudo-Parkinsonism) occur more frequently in compounds with a particular side chain.[39] The long-term effects of the newer compounds have not yet been fully evaluated, and they may well be capable of producing the same severity of liver dysfunction which is known to be associated with chlorpromazine. Thus it is much too early to say that iatrogenic disease is only a feature of the older phenothiazines and can be ignored as far as the newer compounds are concerned.

It would be impossible to survey all the phenothiazines in detail and discuss the effects which they might have on the course of anæsthesia, particularly in the light of the enormous amount of published literature pertaining to their use. As a compromise, individual side effects which can influence anæsthesia will be described with pertinent references to their reported effects on anæsthesia. Their deleterious effects will vary with the duration of their administration and the dose employed and will also depend on the physical condition of the patients.

Central Nervous System. Reports vary as to the potentiating effects of the phenothiazines on anæsthetic drugs. Chlorpromazine definitely prolongs the action of the barbiturates in animals,[40-42] and man,[43] but this will not unduly affect the course of anæsthesia if the barbiturates are only used for induction agents. While Scanlon[44] has reported one case of prolonged apnœa and delayed return of consciousness following the use of thiopentone-gallamine-nitrous oxide-oxygen-ether in a patient who was on chlorpromazine therapy, a reduction in the induction dose of thiopentone should prevent similar occurrences.

In spite of the wide use of chlorpromazine in psychiatry, there are no reports of prolonged narcosis when thiopentone was subsequently given prior to electro-convulsive therapy. In fact, the reverse might be expected, since there is experimental evidence to show that the prolonged use of chlorpromazine causes resistance to the narcotic effects of thiopentone.[45]

The position of the other phenothiazines is much less clear. Animal experiments demonstrate potentiation of thiopentone by promethazine,[42, 46] promazine[47] and triflupromazine.[42] There is no reliable information on this effect in man, but it was found that recovery from a standard operation performed under methohexitone-nitrous oxide-oxygen was prolonged in patients premedicated with 100 mg promazine (Sparine), and 12·5 mg prochlorperazine (Stemetil).[48] It is rather surprising to note that Dundee and Moore[48] found that premedication with those phenothiazines which increased sensitivity to somatic pain (promethazine and pecazine) increased the requirements of methohexitone for the operation of dilatation and curettage, as compared with patients who received atropine alone. While this data is not strictly relevant to phenothiazine-induced iatrogenic disease, it is all that is available to give an indication of what might happen if the anæsthetist encounters a patient who has recently received one of the newer phenothiazines.

Cardiovascular System. All phenothiazines cause peripheral vasodilatation with a fall in blood pressure in susceptible subjects, [43, 49, 50] and it is this effect to which anæsthetists should pay most attention. Chlorpromazine, promazine, triflupromazine, prochloperazine, promethazine and pecazine have all been shown to increase the degree and duration of hypotension which follows a fixed dose of methohexitone[48] and there is good reason to believe that this also applies when thiopentone is given. By virtue of its adrenolytic action, the preoperative use of chlorpromazine may lead to ether and cyclopropane causing severe hypotension,[1] since their sparing effects in blood pressure are largely due to their stimulant action on the sympathoadrenal system.[7] They may also alter the response to vasopressors in the manner already described for reserpine.

It has been estimated that about 1 per cent of patients on long-term chlorpromazine therapy developed liver dysfunction of the obstructive type.[51] This may decrease detoxication of analgesic drugs and increase their duration of action during anæsthesia. If the biliary obstruction leads to any parenchymatous liver damage, the serum cholinesterase level may fall to the extent that the action of suxamethonium will be prolonged and such cases may also show resistance to tubocurarine chloride and gallamine triethiodide. While information on the hepatotoxic effects of other phenothiazines is not available this possibility must always be kept in mind.

A recent German paper incriminates the use of chlorpromazine as a factor in the production of metabolic acidosis.[52] The authors suggest that patients in respiratory difficulties may not be able to hyperventilate to compensate for this and their lives are thus endangered by the sequelæ of acidosis. There is no clinical evidence to support or refute this statement, but it is worth bearing in mind.

Reference has already been made to the increased requirements of barbiturates in patients premedicated with antanalgesic phenothiazines.[48] The same paper also showed that the same drug caused an increased incidence and severity of tremor and spontaneous involuntary muscle movement after methohexitone. It is not known whether their long term use will have a similar effect, but this may happen.

It is worth mentioning briefly another sequel of phenothiazine therapy for which the advice of the anæsthetists might be sought. Compounds with a piperazine side chain[39] cause a high incidence of pseudo-Parkinsonism and oculogyric crisis. This side effect responds quickly to the intramuscular injection of promethazine 25–50 mg but this may have to be repeated at intervals of four to six hours for two days. In the author's experience, this is a very frequent complication of fluphenazine therapy and is also found after the use of the non-phenothiazine antiemetic and tranquillizer, haloperidol.

OTHER TRANQUILLIZERS

Most of these belong to the monoamine oxidase inhibitor series of drugs and their actions are very imperfectly understood. Recent data suggests that their long term use can result in liver dysfunction and Shee[53] has described the overaction of pethidine in patients on iproniazid therapy. The symptoms were coma, muscle twitching, nausea and Cheyne Stokes respiration, which have been previously described for the effect of pethidine in patients with liver damage. [54, 55] There was an immediate abatement of side effects after the administration of 25 mg prednisolone hemisuccinate, which suggests that liver dysfunction may not be the full explanation for the symptoms and the possibility that pethidine and iproniazid degradation products may form a loose chemical complex which causes cerebral irritation or depression has been suggested.[53] These effects are not likely to occur when pethidine is injected during anæsthesia, but may result from its premedicant use.

Mason[87] reports that monoamine oxidase inhibitors make patients unduly susceptible to the effects of methamphetamine, and in those who have had long treatment with these preparations, normal doses of vasopressors may cause excessive hypertension. Drugs with which this has been reported include tranylcypromine ("Parnate"), phenelzine ("Nardil") and isocarboxazid ("Marplan"), and on theoretical grounds this could also occur after the use of nialamide ("Niamid").

ANALGESICS AND SEDATIVES

The effect of these drugs on the course of anæsthesia will depend on the length of time for which they have been given before anæsthesia. The long term use of potent analgesics and sedatives leads to a tolerance to their desired therapeutic effects, and this causes a cross tolerance to the thiopentone and similar drugs.[45] There may be an effect on tolerance to the inhalation agents, but this cannot be measured with the same precision as the dosage of barbiturates. There is also some evidence to suggest that patients who have acquired a tolerance to the analgesics and sedatives will require greater amounts of the antidepolarizing muscle relaxants.

Unfortunately resistance to anæsthetics, resulting from acquired tolerance to other drugs, often occurs in the type of patient who is not able to tolerate the large doses required. This can be counteracted to some extent by increasing the preoperative dose of analgesic and keeping it in proportion to the patient's demand for these drugs and by increasing the dose of relaxants in the cases where these are being used.

It is well known that morphine and similar drugs can cause postural hypotension,[56] but this is not a frequent complication of their use, even after intravenous injection,[57] The large doses which some ambulant patients can take suggest that tolerance to their sedative action is accompanied by a similar tolerance to the cardiovascular effects. Despite belittling the hypotensive effects of these drugs in normal subjects it should be remembered that they are apt to produce a high incidence of blood pressure falls in patients with a decreased blood volume. It is under circumstances like these that they may influence the course of anæsthesia.

There is some experimental evidence to show that analgesics can alter the cardiovascular effects of anæsthetics. The increase in cardiac output normally produced by cyclopropane is prevented by the pre-anæsthetic administration of morphine and this analgesic also increases the depressant effect of some of the volatile agents.[56]

One would expect the phenothiazines to potentiate the cardio-vascular effects of analgesics and the experience of Eckenhoff and Oech[56] shows that the simultaneous administration of both drugs may lead to appreciable hypotension when the patients are moved from the bed to the operating table.

There are no reports in the literature of the long-term preoperative use of analgesics adversely affecting the cardiovascular responses to general anæsthetics, but the above considerations show that this should be borne in mind when one is asked to deal with such cases.

While therapeutic doses of analgesics and sedatives produce no appreciable depression of respiration in the conscious subject, they can augment the depressant effect of thiopentone.[58] Morphine can also prolong the period of apnœa induced by suxamethonium.[59] Apnœa resulting from the potentiation of a large preoperative dose of morphine by neostigmine has been recorded,[60] but this must be a very rare event.

It is possible that the administration of either nalorphine or leval-lorphan to counteract the depressant effects of large doses of analgesia may cause acute withdrawal symptoms, if the patient has developed a physical dependence on potent analgesics. Theoretically, this could be produced by the commercially available mixture of pethidine and levallorphan (pethilorfan).[61]

One very rare complication of phenacetin therapy has been reported recently.[62] The patient developed cyanosis during the anæsthesia and no satisfactory explanation could be offered for this other than methæmoglobinæmia resulting from the analgesic.

OTHER DRUGS

There are some other instances where the relationship between the patient's preoperative therapy and the effect of anæsthesia is less well proven than in the above instances. These are summarized, and both clinical and experimental data is included. It may well be that reporting experimental findings in a chapter of this nature will prevent some catastrophe should the appropriate circumstances arise.

Drugs used in Parkinsonism. Dundee[1] has described three abnormal responses to anæsthesia in two patients receiving benzhexol (Artane; Pipanol). One of these resembled an acute oculogyric crisis, accompanied by apnœa and the other patient had prolonged unconsciousness and respiratory depression. No explanation was offered for these events, and no further cases have been reported in the literature. On the contrary Hurter[63] has described his experiences in anæsthetizing fifty-four patients for thermocoagulation of the globus pallidus and, although all had been treated preoperatively with benzherol 30 mg daily, only one showed any delay in recovery from anæsthesia.

Oral Fluids. Widespread attention has been paid to the hazard of the "full stomach" during the induction of anæsthesia and the frequency of regurgitation and vomiting as a cause of death.[64, 65] It is sufficient to note that, apart from obstetric practice, inadequately prepared routine cases, and those patients with traumatic injuries or intestinal obstruction, a full stomach can unexpectedly be encountered in diabetics who have been given hypertonic glucose solution as part of their routine preoperative preparation.

Radiation Therapy. Animals exposed to X-ray therapy show particularly poor tolerance to cyclopropane, but not to ether, ethylene, nitrous oxide or thiopentone.[66] Foster[67] suggests that these findings may be applicable to man and he described a case to support his thesis. In this patient, who had received X-ray therapy to a carcinoma of the mouth five weeks before anæsthesia, it was not possible to administer cyclopropane satisfactorily because of the unusual degree of respiratory depression which followed even subnarcotic concentrations of the drug. From a review of the literature he postulates the occurrence of increased permeability of the blood-brain barrier resulting from the radiation and points out that the resulting excessive vagal tone may increase the hazards of endotracheal intubation with cyclopropane.

As well as focussing attention on the potential hazards of deep X-ray therapy, this case report shows some of the problems that may have to be met following an atomic explosion.

Pitocin and Oxytocin. A death has been reported from the use of pitocin during emergence from light cyclopropane anæsthesia,[68] and it was attributed to the administration of vasopressin (although in a very dilute form) to a patient with impaired coronary circulation who was in a state of heightened vagal reflex activity (due to the anæsthesia). This theory was supported by evidence showing that deep cyclopropane anæsthesia protects against the coronary constriction caused by vasopressin.[69]

Since the above case was reported this subject has been studied in some detail by Ichiyanagi and Morris[70] and an oxytocic drug free from the vasopressor principle has been included in the investigation (Syntocinon). Both drugs were given with cyclopropane without the sequelæ of serious cardiac irregularities. However, they pointed out that since pitocin is a biological preparation separated from pituitary extract, it may contain some vasopressin which is the cause of its cardiovascular effects.

In addition to the cardiovascular effects of pitocin, there is good clinical evidence to show that its intravenous infusion modifies the action of suxamethonium.[71] Fasciculations are minimal or absent and normal doses of relaxant are ineffectual in producing apnœa. Neuromuscular block of a nondepolarizing type does occur, but its onset is slower than that of the normal suxamethonium-depolarizing block. The total duration of respiratory depression following suxamethonium is prolonged and it can be reversed by neostigmine.

Colchicine. This drug, which once enjoyed some popularity in the treatment of attacks of gout, has been shown to potentiate some hypnotic and anæsthetic agents in animals.[72] Magnesium sulphate, thiopentone, pentobarbitone and hexobarbitone were affected, but the drug has no influence on anæsthesia with chloral hydrate, cyclopropane or nitrous oxide. Potentiation was observed when the colchicine was given one to three hours before the hypnotic and this effect persisted for four to eight hours after its administration. The potentiation was explained on the basis of the mitotic-arresting ability of both the colchinine and the hypnotic.

Diortho-Cresol. This is a constituent of many widely used herbicides and animal experiments have shown that it significantly potentiated the rapidity of onset, depth and duration of the narcotic effect of some barbiturates.[73] The effect was only noted with high doses of the diortho-cresol and it is recommended that thiopentone should not be used for induction of anæsthesia in patients suffering from poisoning with this agent.

Oestrogens. In view of the influence of the sex glands on barbiturate anæsthesia, as demonstrated in animals[74] one might expect stilbœsterol therapy to prolong thiopentone narcosis, but there is no clinical evidence to suggest that this does occur.

Citrate Intoxication. As a result of a rapid massive transfusion in a normal subject or a large transfusion in a patient with hepatic dysfunction is a form of iatrogenic disease which is included for the sake of completeness. It should be suspected in the presence of an unexplained increase in venous pressure with gradual onset of cardiac failure. The treatment of this is well documented in the medical literature[75, 76] and is outside the scope of this chapter.

SURGICAL CONDITIONS

Certain surgical procedures can alter the patient's response to anæsthesia and thus can be classed as iatrogenic disease. However, in clinical practice they do not cause the same problem as alterations in response due to drugs, because the anæsthetist is more likely to be told the nature of previous surgical operations or can quickly elicit the information for himself during the preoperative visit. The presence of obvious scars will invariably lead to an inquiry about the nature of the operations and, if the patient does not know their nature, it may be advisable to postpone the proposed procedure until complete details are available.

The problems of surgical iatrogenic disease mostly fall under the headings of *mechanical* or *hormonal*. These will be discussed very briefly since, strictly speaking, they would require a further full chapter devoted to the choice of anæsthesia in certain pathological conditions.

Among the mechanical problems are those group of patients who have undergone operations which will reduce the ventilating capacity of the lungs. These include pneumonectomy, lobectomy, thoracoplasty, phrenic crush and the induction of an artificial pneumothorax or pneumoperitoneum. It is not possible to generalize about their effects other than stressing the importance of adequate ventilation during anæsthesia and meticulous care to ensure complete decurarization at the end if a muscle relaxant has been given. Caution should also be exercised in the use of pre- and postoperative analgesics as well as in their use during anæsthesia. In some cases there may be dangers of over-inflation of the lungs causing a shift of the mediastinum, while in others secretions before and during anæsthesia may cause particular difficulties. One would expect any of the above-mentioned surgical procedures to predispose to an increased likelihood of postoperative atelectasis following any subsequent operation and emphasis should be placed on good physiotherapy both before and after operation.

A broncho-pleural fistula is another iatrogenic condition which causes difficulty during anæsthesia. For a full description of the problems it presents and suggestions for its management the reader is referred to the very comprehensive review by Parkhouse.[77]

Scarring following thyroidectomy could conceivably lead to difficulties at endotracheal intubation, should this be necessary for a subsequent anæsthetic. However, the absence of case reports indicates that this is not a common occurrence. A more real problem is the patient who has had a granuloma of the vocal cords and who requires a further operation for a pathological condition not associated with the larynx. It would seem reasonable advice to suggest that, if possible, anæsthesia should be carried out without endotracheal intubation. Where this is not feasible attention should be paid to the preoperative nutrition of the patient and the sterility of the tube, particularly emphasizing the avoidance of any antiseptic or lubricant material to which they could conceivably be sensitive. Intubation should be as atraumatic as possible and be carried out under the influence of a muscle relaxant to avoid coughing on the tube. An adequate depth of anæsthesia throughout the procedure will also minimize this latter factor, which may play a part in traumatizing the larynx. If a cuffed tube cannot be avoided, it should be inflated to the minimal pressure necessary for an airtight fit, and, if circumstances permit, the pressure should be released from time to time.

With the increasing use of tracheotomy in the management of imminent or actual respiratory insufficiency, it can be expected that some of the patients who recover will eventually come to operation for a completely different reason. The anæsthetist should be aware of the possibility of tracheal stenosis in such cases and an adequate preoperative examination should detect its presence. The subsequent management will depend on the nature of the proposed operation and the severity of the stenosis. It should be possible to pass a latex flexometallic tube in most cases if necessary. Endotracheal intubation may cause either an inflammatory reaction or œdema at the site of the stenosis and apparatus should be available to carry out an emergency tracheotomy during the postoperative period. Since œdema may subside rapidly, it might be worth treating the first symptoms of dyspnœa with a helium-oxygen mixture and seeing the response to this before embarking on the more major task of tracheotomy.

Patients who have had operations on their spinal cord or vertebra may be more prone to fractures than normal subjects and care should be exercised in their handling while under the influence of anæsthesia.

Bilateral adrenalectomy and hypophysectomy are the two operations which are particularly likely to influence the course of a subsequent anæsthetic. By removal of either the source of the stimulus to the adrenal cortex or the glands themselves one produces a patient who, without exogenous hormone support, will develop acute adrenal insufficiency. The steps to be taken in the prevention of severe hypotension during anæsthesia and its management in established cases are the same, whether the insufficiency has been caused by steroid therapy or surgery, and will be dealt with later in some detail. It must not be forgotten that one adrenal gland may be removed in patients who have, in the past, suffered from a phæochromocytoma. These should present no difficulties, provided the remaining gland is functioning normally. Thyroidectomy can lead to an undetected degree of myœdema and such patients will be unduly sensitive to the depressant effects of all anæsthetics and analgesics. On theoretical grounds patients who have had an orchidectomy may not recover as quickly as expected from the intravenous barbiturates, but there is no data to suggest that this is a real problem in clinical practice.

For the sake of completeness it must be mentioned that re-exploration of an upper abdominal incision can lead to excessive blood loss, particularly if there are large masses of intraperitoneal adhesions. The anæsthetist should budget for this possibility when ordering supplies of blood for the second operation.

STEROID THERAPY

This is discussed separately from the drugs which specifically alter the response to anæsthesia, since steroid therapy may affect the patient's ability to respond to any severe stress, of which anæsthesia is only one form. However, it was the severe falls in blood pressure during and after anæsthesia, sometimes accompanied by respiratory depression and delay in return of consciousness, which first drew attention to steroid therapy as a cause of iatrogenic disease.

The published literature on adrenocortical insufficiency caused by cortisone, its analogues or corticotropine is very great and for the sake of clarity, references are omitted entirely from this section, except to refer the reader to a few comprehensive reviews on the subject.[78-81] From these it will be seen that individual case reports were all in fairly close agreement as to the causation and sequelæ of the impaired response to stress.

Because of their poor tolerance to any severe stress, patients with Addison's disease were once considered too poor risks for any form of surgery. This applies to adrenal insufficiency from any cause, and it is now established that the administration of any of the corticosteroids can result in adrenal hypofunction, which may persist for up to two years after cessation of the therapy. The dosage does not always seem to be an important factor, as some degree of impairment has been detected after a single intra-articular injection of cortisone. Impairment of adrenocortical function is due to inhibition of the pituitary by the exogenous steroid, thus reducing the level of circulating corticotropin (the normal stimulus to the adrenal cortex) once the steroid therapy is stopped. Corticotropin (ACTH) therapy will have a similar effect since it stimulates the adrenal cortex to produce an excessive amount of cortisol, which in turn causes pituitary inhibition.

In adrenocortical insufficiency, patients react to the stress of anæsthesia and surgery by hypotension (out of proportion to the blood loss), respiratory depression and delay in return of consciousness. Different degrees of response are seen depending on the extent of the adrenal hypofunction and the severity of the stress. There are published cases of peripheral circulatory failure developing during or after anæsthesia in patients who had steroid therapy which was stopped for more than one year before operation, and in others in whom the treatment continued right up to the day before surgery, but in whom the all important preoperative dose was missed. It has also occurred in patients who, because of delayed recovery from anæsthesia, missed the dose they were due at the end of the operation. It is worth noting that in many instances the operative procedure was a very minor one and the period of anæsthesia was very brief.

Catastrophies from drug-induced adrenocortical failure are easily preventable. In patients who are already receiving steroid therapy or corticotropine, an increased dose should be given before operation. Where treatment has been stopped for some time cortisone therapy should be started on the day before operation and a double dose given on the morning of the operation. In the preoperative visit, all patients should be questioned routinely regarding steroid therapy. Fortunately, they are now more frequently being told that their tablets are cortisone or a similar drug and asked to pass this information on to those concerned, should an operation be required. Many medical clinics issue cards stating that patients are receiving or have received steroids and this is a very valuable step in preventing collapse from undetected adrenocortical insufficiency.

The problem is greatest in emergency cases, where a history of steroid therapy may not be looked for in the rush to prepare the patient for operation. It is also present in patients admitted in a comatose condition. Even in the absence of direct information on the administration of cortisone and its analogues, a history of any of the many conditions for which the drugs are prescribed may be of help in the event of unexplained hypotension occurring during operation. In addition to the collagen diseases these include various skin conditions, asthma, pulmonary disease, allergies, spondylitis, ulcerative colitis and arthritis. It is also worthwhile knowing the various commercial preparations of cortisone derivatives which are available as some of the proprietory names of these may be most misleading (e.g. Betnesol βmethasone).

Unexplained cardiovascular collapse during operation, where the effect to vasopressors and transfusion is negligible, suggests the occurrence of acute adrenocortical insufficiency. If this diagnosis is correct, the response to the intravenous injection of 100–200 mg cortisol will often be dramatic. Patients who were unresponsive to vasopressors before its use should show a fairly normal response after cortisol.

It is important to remember that steroid therapy should be continued for several days after operation and the dosage gradually reduced depending on the patient's response. An acute respiratory or other infection may act as a stress of sufficient severity to cause post-operative hypotension, and steroid therapy should again be increased temporarily to cope with this. Finally, it is the duty of the anæsthetist to indicate clearly on the case notes of any patient with whom he has had difficulties attributable to acute adrenocortical insufficiency, the nature of these difficulties and the treatment employed.

IATROGENIC DISEASE CAUSING RESPIRATORY INSUFFICIENCY

With the increasing part played by the anæsthetists in some centres in the management of respiratory insufficiency, attention is drawn to two iatrogenic conditions for which their advice might be sought.

Cholinergic crisis in Myasthenics. The pharmacology of myasthenia gravis has been reviewed extensively by Schwab[82] and its diagnosis and management by Wylie and Churchill Davidson.[76] Myasthenic patients sometimes become increasingly unresponsive to anticholinesterase therapy. The exact cause of this is not known, but it usually follows heavy overdosage in a patient with generalized weakness. This can lead to a profound myoneural block due to excessive quantities of acetylcholine and depolarizing drugs at the end plate. The symptoms are widespread muscle fasciculations, sweating, excess secretions, abdominal cramps and muscle weakness. Respiratory inadequacy will occur quickly unless the appropriate treatment is instituted at once.

The first step is to distinguish between myasthenic crisis and cholinergic crisis. A small dose of edrophonium will improve the former but exacerbate the latter.

When the airway is obstructed with secretions, tracheal suction must be carried out and 1–2 mg atropine given intravenously to dry up secretions and antagonize the excessive cholinergic stimulation of the intestinal tract. If this is not sufficient, tracheotomy and positive pressure respiration may be required. Anticholinesterases should be withheld when the patient is on the respirator and if a prolonged period of artificial respiration can be carried out it will usually benefit the patient and when spontaneous respiration returns the patient's response to neostigmine or pyridostigmine may have greatly improved.

It has been suggested that tubocurarine be used to "rest" the end-plate for a time when artificial ventilation is being carried out,[83] but it would seem more logical to restore the cholinesterase to its normal level by giving 1–2 g 2 PAM.[82] One must be careful that the restoration of the cholinesterase by this oxime does not, by removing all anticholinesterase drug effects, shift the patient from the cholinergic crisis to a myasthenic crisis. This is no problem if the patient is already on a respirator, but if this is not the case, means of ventilating the lungs must be readily available.

Postoperative Respiratory Inadequacy. This is most common after thoracic surgery, particularly in tuberculous patients[84, 85] or those with neoplasms.[86] Aetiologically they can be divided into those who developed infection in the one remaining lung and those who already had a compensated respiratory insufficiency before operation. In many patients paradoxical respiration is prevented by IPPR during operation, but can occur postoperatively when spontaneous respiration is resumed. Tracheotomy and controlled respiration is life saving in these cases and can tide them over the acute infection or the period of mobility of the chest wall.

GENERAL COMMENT

The more one hears of the multitude of drugs which can affect the course of anæsthesia in an adverse manner, the greater one becomes aware of the importance of clearly reporting such incidents. There is probably no field in which the saying "forewarned is forearmed" applies with greater truth, and it is important that we be supplied not only with adequate data on the clinical uses of all drugs which our patients receive, but with the side effects of these preparations. Iatrogenic disease will always be a hazard which the anæsthetist has to contend with and a combination of experimental and clinical data will make him aware of its extent and implications.

References

1. DUNDEE, J. W. (1958). *Brit. med. J.*, **1**, 1433.
2. DAVISON, M. H. A. (1951). *Brit. med. J.*, **1**, 584.
3. BURN, J. H., and RAND, M. J. (1958). *Brit. med. J.*, **1**, 903.
4. BURN, J. H. (1961). *Brit. med. J.*, **1**, 1623.
5. Annotation (1961). *Brit. med. J.*, **1**, 1022.
6. COAKLEY, C. S., ALPERT, S., and BOLING, J. S. (1956). *J. Amer. med. Ass.*, **161**, 1143.
7. PRICE, H. I., LINDE, H. W., JONES, R. E., BLACK, G. W., and PRICE, M. L. (1959). *Anesthesiol.*, **20**, 563.
8. EGER, E. I., and HAMILTON, W. K. (1959). *Anesthesiol.*, **20**, 641.
9. NARDONE, A. A., STROUP. P. E., and GILL, R. J. (1960). *Amer. J. Obstet. Gynec.*, **80**, 258.
10. MIR, B. J., and LEWIS, J. J. (1960). *J. Pharm. Pharmacol.*, **12**, 667.
11. JONES, D. L. B., MICHAEL, A. M., and OMMER, J. P. (1961). *Brit. med. J.*, **2**, 1738.
12. PAYNE, J. P. (1957). *Brit. J. Anæsth.*, **29**, 358.
13. BAUER, G. E., CROLL, F. J. T., GOLDRICK, R. B., JEREMY, D., RAFTOS, J., WHYTE, H. M., and YOUNG, A. A. (1961). *Brit. med. J.*, **2**, 410.
14. MONTUSCHI, E., and PICKENS, P. (1961). *Brit. med. J.*, **2**, 174.
15. MALLINSON, F. B. (1941). *Brit. J. Anæsth.*, **17**, 98.
16. PRIGDEN, J. E. (1956). *Surgery*, **40**, 571.
17. Case Report: *Amer. Soc. Anesthesiologists Newsletter* (1957), **21**, 38.
18. POTH, E. (1957). *Amer. J. Surg.*, **88**, 803.
19. WEBBER, B. M. (1957). *A.M.A. Arch. Surg.*, **73**, 174.
20. POTH, E. J. (1957). *J. Amer. med. Ass.*, **163**, 1317.
21. BROWNLEE, G., and BUSHBY, S. R. (1948). *Lancet*, **1**, 131.
22. MOLITOR, H., GRAESSLE, O. E., KINA, S., MUSHETT, C. W., and SILBER, R. H. (1946). *J. Pharmacol. exper. Therap.*, **86**, 151.
23. BRAZIL, O. V., and CORRADO, A. P. (1957). *J. Pharmacol. exper. Therap.*, **120**, 452.
24. BEZZI, G., and GESSA, G. L. (1960). *Nature, London*, **184**, 905.
25. PITTINGER, C. B., and LONG, J. P. (1958). *Surgery*, **43**, 445.
26. PITTINGER, C. B., LONG, J. P., and MILLER, J. R. (1958). *Anesth. and Analg.*, **37**, 276.
27. PITTINGER, C. B., and LONG, J. P. (1958). *Antibiotics and Chemotherap.*, **8**, 198.

28. TIMMERMAN, J. C., LONG, J. P., and PITTINGER, C. B. (1959). *Toxicol. and app. Pharmacol.*, **1**, 299.
29. SABAWALA, P. D., and DILLON, J. B. (1959). *Anesthesiol.*, **20**, 659.
30. FERVARA, B. E., and PHILLIPS, R. D. (1957). *Amer. Surg.*, **23**, 710.
31. MIDDLETON, W. H., MORGAN, D. D., and MOYERS, J. (1957). *J. Amer. med. Ass.*, **165**, 2186.
32. ENGEL, L., and DENSON, J. S. (1957). *Surgery*, **42**, 862.
33. STERCHISHIM, O., VOLOSHIN, P. C., and ALLARD, G. A. (1959). *Canad. med. Ass. J.*, **81**, 32.
34. LODER, R. E., and WALKER, G. F. (1959). *Lancet*, **1**, 812.
35. BUSH, G. H. (1961). *Brit. med. J.*, **1**, 558.
36. FISK, G. C. (1961). *Brit. med. J.*, **1**, 556.
37. MULLETT, R. D., and KEATS, A. S. (1961). *Surgery*, **49**, 530.
38. SCHATTEN, W. E. (1956). *Surg., Gynec. and Obstet.*, **102**, 339.
39. DUNDEE, J. W., and MOORE, J. (1962). *Brit. J. Anæsth.*, 247, **34**.
40. SADOVE, M. S., BALAGOT, R. G., and REYES, R. M. (1956). *Curr. res. Anesth.*, **35**, 165.
41. DUNDEE, J. W., and SCOTT, W. E. B. (1958). *Anæsth. and Analg.*, **37**, 12.
42. DOBKIN, A. B. (1960). *Brit. J. Anæsth.*, **32**, 424.
43. DRIPPS, R. D., VANDAM, L. D., PIERCE, E. C., and OECH, S. R., and LURIES, A. A. (1955). *Ann. Surg.*, **142**, 774.
44. SCANLON, J. W. (1955). *Brit. med. J.*, **1**, 1459.
45. DUNDEE, J. W. (1955). *Brit. J. Anæsth.*, **27**, 165.
46. BLUNDELL, A. E., PILLION, S. W., BODELL, B., and ANSLOO, G. P. (1959). *Curr. res. Anæsth.*, **38**, 328.
47. DOBKIN, A. B. (1960). *Anesthesiol.*, **21**, 292.
48. DUNDEE, J. W., and MOORE, J. (1961). *Brit. J. Anæsth.*, **33**, 382.
49. MILLAR, R. A. (1957). *Canad. Anæsth., Soc. J.* **4**, 346.
50. DOBKIN, A. B., KAIL, A. McL., and WONG, C. (1961). *Anæsthesia*, **16**, 160.
51. DUNDEE, J. W. (1957). *Anæsthesia*, **12**, 215.
52. MAURATH, J., FRANKE, D., and SCHLOSSER, V. (1960). *Anæsthetist*, **9**, 14.
53. SHEE, J. C. (1960). *Brit. med. J.*, **2**, 507.
54. VON BRUCKE, S. (1940). *Wien klin. Wschr.*, **53**, 854.
55. DUNDEE, J. W., and TINCKLER, L. F. (1952). *Brit. med. J.*, **2**, 703.
56. ECKENHOFF, J. E., and OECH, S. R. (1960). *Clin. Pharmacol and Therap.*, **1**, 483.
57. DOBKIN, A. B., and CRISWICK, V. G. (1961). *Anesthesiol.*, **22**, 398.
58. HELRICH, M., ECKENHOFF, J. E., JONES, R. E., and ROLPH, W. C. (1959). *Anesthesiol.*, **17**, 459.
59. DEKORNFELD, T. J. (1957). *Surveys of Anesthesiol.*, **1**, 318.
60. GRAY, T. C., DUNDEE, J. W., and RIDING, J. E. (1958). *Proc. 11th Italian Congress of Anæsthesia*, 520.
61. TELFORD, J., and KEATS, A. S. (1961). *Anesthesiol.*, **22**, 465.
62. SNIPER, W. (1961). *Brit. med. J.*, **2**, 96.
63. HURTER, D. C. (1960). *Brit. J. Anæsth.*, **32**, 160.
64. MORTON, H. J. V., and WYLIE, W. D. (1951). *Anæsthesia*, **6**, 190.
65. EDWARDS, G., MORTON, H. J. V., PASK, E. A., and WYLIE, W. D. (1956). *Anæsthesia*, **11**, 194.
66. WILSON, J. E. (1955). *Anesthesiol.*, **16**, 503.
67. FOSTER, P. A. (1956). *Anesthesiol.*, **17**, 735.
68. LESSER, M., and EASON, G. A. (1954). *Brit. med. J.*, **2**, 79.
69. PARSLOE, C. P., MORRIS. L. E., and ORTH, O. S. (1950). *Anesthesiol.*, **11**, 76.
70. ICHIYANAGI, K., and MORRIS, L. E. (1959). *Anesthesiol.*, **20**, 669.
71. HODGES, R. J. H., BENNETT, J. R., TUNSTALL, M. E., and SHANKS, R. O. F. (1959). *Brit. med. J.*, **1**, 413.
72. BALEK, R. W., KOESIS, J. J., and GEILING, E. M. K. (1957). *Arch. Internat. Pharmacodyn*, **111**, 182.
73. EDSON, E. F., and CAREY, F. M. (1955). *Brit. med. J.*, **2**, 104.

74. BUCHEL, L. (1954). *Anesth. et Analg. (Paris)*, **11**, 229, 268.
75. FIRT, P., and HEJHAL, L. (1957). *Lancet*, **2**, 1132.
76. WYLIE, W. D., and CHURCHILL-DAVIDSON, H. C. (1960). *A Practice of Anæsthesia.* Lloyd-Luke, London.
77. PARKHOUSE, J. (1957). *Brit. J. Anæsth.*, **29**, 217.
78. DUNDEE, J. W. (1957). *Brit. J. Anæsth.*, **29**, 166.
79. MUSHIN, W. W. (1957). *Anæsthesia*, **12**, 15.
80. TANDAN, E. C., ISAAC, M., and KHATARIAN, S. C. (1961). *Indian J. Anæsth.*, **9**, 195.
81. BAYLISS, R. I. S. (1960). *Brit. J. Anæsth.*, **32**, 529.
82. SCHWAB, R. S. (1960). *Clin. Pharmacol. and Therap.*, **1**, 319.
83. CHURCHILL-DAVIDSON, H. C., and RICHARDSON, A. T. (1957). *Lancet*, **1**, 1221.
84. MASSON, A. H. B., and ROBERTSON, J. D. (1958). *Brit. med. J.*, **1**, 1516.
85. GARDINER, A. S. (1960). *Anæsthesia.*, **15**, 246.
86. BJORK, V. O., and ENGSTROM, C. G. (1955). *J. thorac. Surg.*, **30**, 356.
87. MASON, A. (1962). *Lancet*, **i**, 1073.
88. DIXIT, M. B., GULATE, O. D. and GOKHALE, S. D. (1961). *Brit. J. Pharmacol.*, **17**, 31.

INDEX

AM 109, 33–34
Acetazolamide, 300
Abdominal decompression, in obstetrics, 232
Abdominal surgery, reflex disturbances during, 7
Acetylcholine, release of, 84, 91
Acid-base balance, in anæsthesia, 2
in hypothermia, 117, 125
Addison's disease, anæsthesia in, 341
Adrenalectomy, effect on anæsthesia, 340
Adrenaline, effect with halothane, 132
Aintree respirator, 260, 282
Airway, in resuscitation, 288–289
Airway resistance, 253–255
Ambu ventilator, 11, 13, 245, 246, 261, 287
Amethocaine, in bronchoscopy, 193, 194
in obstetric anæsthesia, 216
5-Amino-1:2:3:4:-tetrahydroacridine, 72
Amnesia, 38, 41
Anæsthesia, associated with iatrogenic conditions, 324–344
carbon dioxide narcosis in, 297
dental. *See* Dental anæsthesia
effect on analgesics and sedatives, 334–335
effect of some surgical conditions, 338–340
effect of steroid therapy, 340–342
epidural. *See* Epidural anæsthesia
for hypothermia, 122–123
in elderly patient, 23–24
inhalation. *See* Inhalation anæsthesia
in neurosurgery, 127–156
in obstetrics. *See* Obstetric anæsthesia
intravenous. *See* Intravenous anæsthesia
local. *See* Local anæsthesia
measurement of compliance, 251–253, 254
mechanical ventilation during, 286
mental changes due to, 23, 24
pædiatric, 13, 15
requirements of, 128
spinal. *See* Spinal anæsthesia
with patient co-operation, 153–154

Analeptics, 68–73
Analgesics, effect on anæsthesia, 334–335
toxic effects, 65
Angiocardiography, anæsthesia for, 184–186
Angiography, anæsthesia for, 188
"Anoci-association" theory, 7
Anti-analgesia, 37, 38, 53–54
Antibiotics, causing neuromuscular block, 295–296, 328
effect on anæsthetics, 328–331
Aortography, anæsthesia for, 186–188
Apnœa, prolonged, 107
Arfonad. *See* Trimetaphan
Artane, effect on anæsthesia, 336
Arterial pressure, measurement during cardiac surgery, 169
Artery, injection of thiopentone into, 66–68
Artificial respiration, 286–291
Artificial ventilation. *See* Mechanical ventilation
Asphyxia, inhalational, treatment of, 212–213
prevention of in newborn, 233–234
Aspiration, of stomach content, 21
Aspiration pneumonitis, 212–213
Ataralgesia, in obstetrics, 227–228
Atropine, in premedication, 134, 219
use with halothane, 132
Ayre's T-piece, 133
Azeotec vaporizer, 11

B.82, 35
B.133, 35
B.137, 34–35
Barbiturates, 30–38. *See also under individual names, e.g.* Thiopentone
anti-analgesic effect, 53–54
causing local irritation, 37
causing respiratory depression, 37
detoxication of, 52
distribution in tissue, 49–52
in cerebral angiography, 54–55
plasma binding, 53
poisoning by, 294
reversal of effects of, 68–73
side effects of, 31, 35, 36–37
Barnet respirator, 261, 266, 282, 317
Baytenal, 31–32, 33
Beaver respirator, 259, 260, 266, 282